Congenital and perinatal infections

Perinatal and congenital infections remain a stubborn and major cause of morbidity and mortality in infants throughout the world. This concise, accessible account provides an essential guide to the diagnosis, management and prevention of these infections. The first three chapters underline how and why infections during this critical period can be so devastating. The main section of the book focuses on individual infections, with an emphasis on applying the very latest knowledge and techniques for effective intervention. Another unique feature of this account is its recognition that the severity and types of these infections vary considerably from country to country, and from the developing world to the developed world: the international team of experts involved in this compilation have striven to make this an account that will transcend these boundaries and be suitable for all doctors and allied health professionals around the world charged with the care of the mother and newborn.

Dr Marie-Louise Newell is Reader in Epidemiology in the Department of Epidemiology and Public Health at the Institute of Child Health in London. She is coordinator of the European Collaborative Study on HIV Infections and is well known nationally and internationally for her work on infections in pregnancy and the consequences for the infant.

Professor James McIntyre is Associate Professor in Obstetrics and Gynaecology at the University of Witwatersrand in South Africa. He is co-director of two research units (Perinatal HIV Research Unit and the Reproductive Health Research Unit) and is well known as an international authority on HIV and pregnancy.

D1605302

Congenital
and **perinatal infections**

Prevention, diagnosis and treatment

Edited by

Marie-Louise Newell
Institute of Child Health, UCL, London, UK

and

James McIntyre
University of Witwatersrand, South Africa

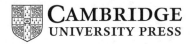
CAMBRIDGE
UNIVERSITY PRESS

PUBLISHED BY THE PRESS SYNDICATE OF THE UNIVERSITY OF CAMBRIDGE
The Pitt Building, Trumpington Street, Cambridge, United Kingdom

CAMBRIDGE UNIVERSITY PRESS
The Edinburgh Building, Cambridge CB2 2RU, UK   http://www.cup.cam.ac.uk
40 West 20th Street, New York, NY 10011–4211, USA   http://www.cup.org
10 Stamford Road, Oakleigh, Melbourne 3166, Australia
Ruiz de Alarcón 13, 28014 Madrid, Spain

First published 2000

Printed in the United Kingdom at the University Press, Cambridge

Typeset in Minion 10.5/14pt [V N]

A catalogue record for this book is available from the British Library

ISBN 0 521 78979 6 paperback

Every effort has been made in preparing this book to provide accurate and up-to-date information which is in accord with accepted standards and practice at the time of publication. Nevertheless, the authors, editors and publisher can make no warranties that the information contained herein is totally free from error, not least because clinical standards are constantly changing through research and regulation. The authors, editors and publisher therefore disclaim all liability for direct or consequential damages resulting from the use of material contained in this book. Readers are strongly advised to pay careful attention to information provided by the manufacturer of any drugs or equipment that they plan to use.

The editors would also like to remind readers of the dosage of µg for micrograms and that particular care should always be taken when reading and writing dosage figures.

Contents

Contributors

Edgardo J. Abalos
Centro Rosarino de Estudios Perinatales
Pueyrredón 985, (2000) Rosario, Argentina

Daynia E. Ballot
Department of Paediatrics
University of the Witwatersrand
Johannesburg Hospital
York Road, Parktown
South Africa, 2193

Guillermo Carroli
Centro Rosarino de Estudios Perinatales
Pueyrredón, (2000) Rosario, Argentina

Gina Dallabetta
HIV/AIDS Department
Family Health International
2101 Wilson Boulevard, Suite 7000
Arlington, Virginia, USA 22201

Suzanne D. Delport
Department of Paediatrics
Kalafong Hospital
P/Bag X396
Pretoria
South Africa, 0001

Marianne Forsgren
Movagen 7
S-18245 Enebyberg
Sweden

Ruth Gilbert
Centre for Evidence Based Child Health
Institute of Child Health
30 Guilford Street
London WC1N 1EH, UK

Robert L. Goldenberg
University of Alabama at Birmingham
560 Old Hilman Building
618 South 20th Street
Birmingham, Al 395294-7333
USA

Glenda Gray
Perinatal HIV Research Unit
University of the Witwatersrand
Chris Hani Baragwanath Hospital
PO Bertsham
Johannesburg
South Africa, 2013

A. Metin Gülmezoglu
Reproductive Health Unit,
WHO, Avenue Appia
1211-Geneva-27
Switzerland

G. Justus Hofmeyr
Department of Obstetrics and Gynaecology
Coronation Hospital and
University of the Witwatersrand
7 York Road, Parktown
Johannesburg, South Africa, 2193

Gunilla Malm
Department of Neuropaediatrics
Huddinge University Hospital
Karolinska Institute Medical School, Sweden

Laurent Mandelbrot
Gynecologie–Obstetrique
Consultation Puzos
Hôpital Cochin Bandelocque – Port Royal
123 Boulevard de Port Royal
75014 Paris
France

Desmond Martin
National Institute for Virology
P/Bag X4, Sandringham
South Africa, 2131

James McIntyre
Perinatal HIV Research Unit
University of the Witwatersrand
Department of Obstetrics and Gynaecology
Chris Hani Baragwanath Hospital
PO Bertsham
South Africa, 2013

Paolo Miotti
National Institutes of Health
Division of AIDS, Room 4109
6700-B Rockledge Drive MSC 7626
Bethesda, MD 20892-7626, USA

Marie-Louise Newell
Department of Epidemiology and Public
Health
Institute of Child Health
30 Guilford Street
London WC1 1EH, UK

Arne Ohlsson
Department of Paediatrics
Mount Sinai Hospital
600 University Avenue, Toronto
Ontario M5G 1X5, Canada

Robert C. Pattinson
MRC Maternal and Infant Health Care
Strategies Unit
Kalafong Hospital
P/Bag X396
Pretoria
South Africa, 0001

Catherine S. Peckham
Department of Epidemiology and
Public Health
Institute of Child Health
30 Guilford Street
London WC1 1EH
UK

Mirja Puranen
Department of Oral Pathology and
Radiology
Insitute of Dentistry
Lemminkäisenkatu 2
Fin-20520 Turku
Finland

Patrick S. Ramsay
University of Alabama at Birmingham
560 Old Hilman Building
618 South 20th Street
Birmingham, AL 35294-7333
USA

Barry Schoub
National Institute for Virology
P/Bag X4
Sandringham
South Africa, 2131

Vibhuti Shah
Department of Paediatrics
Mount Sinai Hospital
600 University Avenue, Toronto
Ontario M5G 1X5
Canada

Stina Syrjänen
Department of Pathology
University of Kuopio
PO Box 1627
FIN 70211 Kuopio
Finland

Cyril J. van Gelderen
Department of Obstetrics and Gynaecology
University of the Witwatersrand
Chris Hani Baragwanath Hospital
PO Bertsham, Johannesburg
South Africa, 2013

Preface

Healthy pregnant women are not usually more susceptible to infections than non-pregnant women, but when infections occur during pregnancy there is often considerable concern about the possible adverse effects on the fetus or newborn. Perinatal infections remain a major cause of morbidity and mortality in infants in both the developed and developing world, and the range of infections known to be associated with perinatal infections continues to increase. Diagnosis has improved with new diagnostic techniques, including advanced serological techniques and ultrasonography.

Doctors in obstetrics and paediatrics and their midwifery colleagues need to be aware of recent advances in knowledge with regard to these conditions, which can translate to preventive measures and which have implications for decisions regarding antenatal screening packages. Several exhaustive reference books exist; and this book is not intended to replace these. We hope that it will provide a concise up-to-date review of the field which will provide easily accessible information, with an explanation of the underlying mechanisms and approaches to prevention, for medical practitioners of all disciplines. The authors are all experts in their fields, drawn from both developed and developing countries, which we hope will add to the relevance of this book for all settings.

Marie-Louise Newell and James McIntyre

Part 1

General issues

Infections in pregnancy: introduction

Catherine S. Peckham

Introduction

Infections in pregnancy that can be transmitted from mother to child are of particular concern since congenital or perinatal infections may be associated with adverse sequelae. Maternal infections that have the potential of infecting the fetus or newborn infant are listed in Table 1.1 and include viral, bacterial and protozoal infections. The consequences and management of individual infections are discussed in detail elsewhere in this book. The purpose of the present chapter is to present an overview of the salient features and issues that arise in relation to the detection and management of infections in pregnancy, largely from a population perspective. This epidemiological knowledge is needed to establish a causal relationship between an infection and the outcome, to inform decisions about screening in pregnancy and also to ensure the most appropriate management of a woman with a specific diagnosed infection in pregnancy.

All the infections listed in Table 1.1 can cause fetal or perinatal infection, sometimes associated with an adverse outcome such as fetal loss, stillbirth, prematurity, fetal damage, or acute neonatal infection. For some congenital infections there may be no evidence of symptoms or signs of infection in the neonatal period and it may be weeks, months or even years before damage first becomes apparent (Table 1.2).

Mode of acquisition of infection

The route by which the fetus or newborn acquires the infection has important implications for the management of the infection in pregnancy, or in the neonatal period, and for the development of appropriate intervention programmes to prevent mother-to-child transmission. Infections of the newborn may be acquired in utero (congenital infection), around the time of delivery (intrapartum infection) or in the neonatal period (postpartum infection) (Table 1.3). Intrauterine infection follows systemic blood-borne maternal infection with placental infection and/or transplacental transmission to the fetus. Sometimes the placenta may be

Table 1.1. Infections in pregnancy that can affect the fetus or newborn infant

Rubella	*Toxoplasmosis gondii*
Cytomegalovirus	*Treponema pallidum*
Herpes simplex virus	Group B streptococcus
Varicella-zoster	*Listeria monocytogenes*
Parvovirus B19	
Hepatitis B and C	
Papilloma virus	
Lymphocytic choriomeningitis virus	
HIV-1, 2	
HTLV- 1, 2	

Table 1.2. Possible outcomes of infections in pregnancy

Abortion and stillbirth
Congenital abnormalities
Acute illness or death in neonatal period
Damage – obvious at birth
        – late development or manifestation
Asymptomatic infection

infected without fetal spread. Infection may also be acquired from the genital tract by the cervical amniotic route, or it may be acquired as a result of exposure to infected cervical secretions, maternal blood or faeces during passage through the birth canal. Delayed delivery after rupture of the membranes may therefore increase the risk of infection by increasing the time of exposure. Abrasions of the infant's skin due to birth trauma may also provide a portal of entry, for example in the case of neonatal herpes the risk of infection may be enhanced by the application of invasive procedures such as scalp electrodes. Infection may be acquired by the infant in the postpartum period through breast feeding, transfused blood, by hands or instruments or via the respiratory route from infected contacts such as the mother, other babies, medical attendants or other family members.

Some congenital infections, such as rubella, may cause structural malformations, as a result of interference with organogenesis whereas others, such as cytomegalovirus, cause defects as a result of damage to previously formed organs and tissues. In the case of rubella the gestational age of the fetus at time of exposure will therefore determine the outcome. Malformations are clearly permanent but a number of the effects of damage to normal tissue or organs are not permanent; healing and normal function can result.

The effect of a maternal infection on the fetus may be due to direct actions of

Table 1.3. Routes of transmission

Intrauterine	– transplacental
	– ascending infection
Intrapartum	– contact with infected genital secretions/ blood/ faeces during delivery
Postpartum	– breastfeeding
	– blood transfusion
	– nosocomial

toxins or organisms or they may be indirect and a consequence of interference with placental or uterine function. The effect of a specific infection on fetal development is likely to depend on multiple maternal and fetal factors including genetic make-up, nutritional status, stage of fetal development and anatomical factors such as the site or the structure of the placental vessels. The nature of the infecting organism, its portal of entry, the time of exposure, as well as the dose, are likely to influence outcome.

Although most maternal infections do not cross the placenta or do so rarely, they may affect the mother and result in hyperthermia, biochemical imbalance, hypoxia or nutritional disorder. These effects could be detrimental to the fetus and have long-term effects. In addition, the effect on the developing fetus could be secondary to the treatment or investigation of the mother such as from antibiotics, antipyretics or specific therapeutic agents or radiographic investigations. It has been postulated that the reported increase in malformations associated with the 1957 influenza epidemic could have been due to maternal fever or to the treatment given to the mother rather than to the specific infection. Placental failure secondary to placental infection could affect function as in the case of malaria, or could result in fetal malnutrition. Infection could also cause premature labour and delivery. Long-term effects on the immunological competence of the fetus have also been postulated.

Timing of infection in pregnancy

The gestational age of the pregnancy when infection occurs may influence the risk of vertical transmission and/or the fetal or perinatal consequences. For example, fetal exposure to rubella in the first trimester of pregnancy is associated with a high risk of serious congenital defects including cataracts, heart defects and sensorineural deafness, whereas exposure to infection late in pregnancy or in the postpartum period poses little risk (Miller et al, 1982). On the other hand, exposure of the fetus to a primary cytomegalovirus infection poses a risk of adverse outcome at any stage of pregnancy (Peckham, 1991). The overall rate of fetal infection following exposure to maternal toxoplasmosis infection depends on the time of acquisition of maternal infection: the rate is low (10%) following infection acquired in the first 2 weeks after conception and increases to over 90% following infection in the last 2 weeks of pregnancy (Dunn et al., 1999). In contrast, the risk of serious adverse sequelae following toxoplasma infection is much higher following exposure to infection in early pregnancy than to later exposure.

When genital herpes infection is acquired at the time of delivery, the risk of neonatal herpes infection is considerable and associated with a high risk of neonatal mortality and morbidity. In contrast, maternal genital herpes infection in early pregnancy poses little risk (Prober et al., 1987; Tookey & Peckham, 1996). Varicella at the time of delivery, or just before, may cause overwhelming infection in the newborn, whereas infection acquired in the first and second trimester earlier is associated with a very small risk of congenital varicella syndrome, about 1%, and varicella acquired in the second and third trimester may first present as herpes zoster in infancy or childhood (Enders et al., 1994).

Although congenital cytomegalovirus is associated with a significant risk of adverse sequelae, infection acquired by the infant during birth from exposure to infected cervical secretions, or in the postpartum period from infected breast milk, is not associated with adverse effects, except in the very premature or immune-compromised infant. Some perinatally acquired infections, such as HIV, do not present as acute infections in the newborn period but present subsequently with serious HIV disease.

Primary or recurrent infection

Infections of the fetus or newborn may follow a primary maternal infection, reactivation of a latent maternal infection or result from exposure to infectious agents that constitute part of the lower genital tract flora. A primary infection in pregnancy is likely to present a more serious threat to the fetus or infant than a recurrent or secondary infection. This is related to the mother's immune status and the level of exposure to the organism and is exemplified by the example of perinatal herpes simplex and varicella zoster infection where the presence of maternal antibodies at the time of exposure provides some protection (Miller et al., 1989, Prober et al., 1987).

For some infections such as rubella, it is the primary infection that results in maternal viraemia with subsequent fetal infection and damage. The rationale for the prevention of congenital rubella through immunization is based on this assumption and with the introduction of MMR (measles, mumps and rubella) vaccine, congenital rubella is now a rare condition in the UK (Tookey & Peckham, 1999). However, a few cases of congenital infection have been reported following a reinfection of rubella in pregnancy (Miller, 1990). With the development of a vaccine for cytomegalovirus (CMV) infection, the same assumptions are being made, although CMV is a herpes virus with the characteristic that following a primary genital infection the virus will reactivate intermittently throughout life. For example, cytomegalovirus can be detected in the genital tract of about 10% of women with evidence of past infection and although perinatal infection is common, recurrent infection is rarely associated with adverse problems (Reynolds et al., 1980).

Recurrent genital herpes simplex virus is also common and in the 1970s was considered to be a significant risk to the neonate. In the USA, from the early 1970s until 1988, it was recommended that pregnant women with a history of genital herpes be screened from 35 weeks with weekly genital cultures. For those women with evidence of infection at the time of delivery, or a recent positive culture, caesarean delivery was recommended to avoid fetal contact with an infected site (American College of Obstetricians and Gynecologists, 1988). These recommendations have been withdrawn because most infected neonates have no maternal history of genital herpes and are born to women with a primary genital infection at term and the risk for infants of women with a previous history of genital herpes is low. Similarly, maternal varicella in the last 5 days of pregnancy or in the few days after delivery presents the greatest risk of serious infection as the infant is born with no protective maternal antibodies.

Persistence of infection in the infant

Developmental abnormalities have been associated with specific infections such as rubella, cytomegalovirus and toxoplasmosis whereas other infections, such as herpes simplex virus, result in an acute infection in the newborn associated with a mortality and risk of subsequent morbidity in the survivors. Some infections pose particular problems because the organism persists in the host and continues to replicate and may cause tissue destruction after birth. Other infections, such as measles, mumps and the enteroviruses, may cause intrauterine infection but do not persist. Such chronic infection occurs with rubella, cytomegalovirus, toxoplasmosis, syphilis, HIV and HTLV-1. Exposure to chickenpox in pregnancy may result in subclinical infection with reactivation of the virus in the early months or years of life manifesting as herpes zoster. It has been suggested that the varicella syndrome that occurs following exposure to infection in early gestation is the result of virus reactivation in later pregnancy rather than the result of the initial infection (Higa et al., 1987).

Transplacental transmission of human parvovirus (B19) is well documented (PLHS Working Party on Fifth Disease, 1990), but it is not known whether infection persists as it does with animal parvoviruses. B19 is, however, known to persist in immunocompromised humans who acquire the infection postnatally (Kurtzmann et al., 1988), and there is some evidence of limited prenatal persistence in the fetus and/or placenta in gestational infection.

Long-term effects

Long-term effects are those which become evident or develop after the neonatal period (Table 1.4). They may be caused directly by irreversible damage inflicted at the time of the initial infection or by damage resulting from persistent infection or reactivation of infection during childhood or adult life. Damage may also occur as a result of interference with fetal growth producing disturbances in developmental pattern or structure, as in the case of congenital rubella. There may be a diminution of the normal number or change in the form of fetal cells which interferes with the structure or function of selected organs or whole systems or changes may be very subtle, for example, in the brain they could affect later perception or learning ability. The changes produced may not manifest themselves unless the affected individual meets a specific challenge later in life, possibly many years after the initial infection. Long-term damage associated with congenital or perinatal infection with non-persisting organisms appears to be non-specific and due to prematurity or growth retardation.

As most infants with congenital infections have no clinical illness at birth or history of maternal infection, it is often difficult to establish the link between congenital or perinatal infections and conditions that present in later childhood or adult life. The information needed to establish such a link comes from prospective follow-up of infants with congenital infection diagnosed in the first weeks of life. The phenomenon of long-term effects resulting from congenital infection was first demonstrated in the follow up of children with proven congenital rubella. In one such study, children with no apparent defect, and whose language was developing normally, were later found to have a profound sensorineural hearing loss (Peckham, 1972). Other late onset manifestations of congenital rubella include thyroid disease and diabetes mellitus which presents in late adolescence or early adult life (Forrest et al., 1971). Toxoplasma is another infection where long-term effects, particularly retinochoroidal lesions associated with visual impairment, have been demonstrated and are due to the persistence of the toxoplasmosis cyst (Koppe &

Table 1.4. Possible long term outcomes

Rubella	Diabetes mellitus
	Thyroid disease
	Sensorineural deafness
	Vascular effects
Mumps	Diabetes mellitus
Hepatitis B and C	Liver cirrhosis
	Hepatocellular carcinoma
Non-specific viral infection (herpes viruses)	Malignant disease
Influenza A2	Schizophrenia
HTLV -1	T cell leukaemia
	Tropical spastic paralysis
Toxoplasmosis	Visual impairment

Rothova, 1989). Another example is the immunological defects that result from perinatal HIV infection.

Since long-term effects can only be studied in surviving populations, infections with a high incidence of fetal loss or severe damage in the newborn period are less likely to be implicated than less severe infections. However, it is misleading to extrapolate to the general population the long-term risks derived from the small group of children with obvious and often severe impairment, many of whom are in poor condition at birth. The epidemiological study of long-term effects is therefore fraught with difficulties.

It is often not possible to identify the cause of these late manifestations as children with asymptomatic congenital or perinatal infection are unlikely to be identified, and when late manifestations do occur congenital infection is rarely suspected. If it is, microbiological investigations at this stage are unlikely to be able to distinguish congenital from postnatal infection. This difficulty is often compounded by the non-specific nature of the symptoms. For example, it is not possible to diagnose a congenital infection in a 3-year-old child presenting with global retardation who is excreting CMV in the urine or who has a positive toxoplasma test.

Demonstrating the health impact and causal relationship

The health impact of a maternal infection will clearly depend on the prevalence of maternal infection, the risk of mother-to-child transmission, the mode of transmission, the gestational age at infection and the associated abnormalities. In view

Table 1.5. Information required to assess health impact

Background prevalence
Incidence of infection in pregnancy
Risk of mother-to-child transmission
Timing of mother-to-child transmission
Risk factors for maternal and perinatal infection
Consequences of congenital/ perinatal infection both short term and long term

of the subclinical nature of many of these maternal and perinatal infections, which are often relatively infrequent, this epidemiological information is not easy to acquire.

In order to estimate the burden of disease resulting from a specific infection in pregnancy, detailed epidemiological information is required (Table 1.5). An understanding of the epidemiology of individual infections is also required for counselling women about the risk of adverse effects, the development of appropriate management and prevention strategies and for the evaluation of available interventions. A prospective study is required to estimate the prevalence and gestational effects of an infection that is mild or subclinical. This is no easy task since such a study necessitates the serological follow-up of a large number of women throughout pregnancy to identify those who become infected and to investigate appropriate fetal or neonatal samples for evidence of congenital infection. Where the sensitivity of the laboratory investigation of the neonate is in doubt (as for toxoplasma IgM) or unknown, infants must be followed clinically and serologically for at least their first year of life. The significance of non-specific outcomes such as abortion, prematurity, neurological or sense organ sequelae can only be made by comparison with a control group of pregnancies matched for confounding variables such as age, parity, social class and ethnic background. Large numbers of women have to be studied because even the most common infection, CMV, occurs in only 1% of pregnancies and in only a proportion of these will transplacental infection take place.

When an infection is uncommon in pregnancy and a prospective study is not feasible, it may be difficult, even if the maternal infection is symptomatic, to associate a particular infection with fetal damage. Examples include mumps, chickenpox and measles. The likelihood of an association is increased if the organism can be recovered from the fetus or infant, or if there is serological evidence of infection in the neonate. However, unless a series of cases with similar defects or with a characteristic syndrome is reported, as with congenital varicella, evidence of transplacental transmission does not necessarily confirm that the agent was responsible for the defects.

The role of screening for infections in pregnancy

The diagnosis of a specific infection in pregnancy poses particular problems since many of these maternal infections are asymptomatic or present with non-specific signs and symptoms such as a 'flu-like' illness. It is for this reason that serological testing in pregnancy to screen out those women with a suspected infection in pregnancy has been proposed. If an effective intervention or treatment is available to reduce the risk of vertical transmission and/or its adverse effects, the role of routine testing for the specific infection in pregnancy, or in some situations in the neonatal period, needs to be considered.

The pressure to screen is often considerable in part reflecting the new technological developments, public pressure and the increasing assumption that early detection is beneficial. However, screening is costly and there is always the potential to do more harm than good. Before considering the introduction of a new screening programme to detect a specific maternal infection, for example, CMV, the benefits and risks of such an approach need to be firmly established. Table 1.6 lists the criteria that need to be considered before a new screening programme is implemented. These criteria were first formulated by Wilson and Jugner for the World Health Organization (Wilson & Jugner, 1968) and have since been adapted to respond to contemporary screening issues. Information is required on the prevalence of the infection in the population, the risk of acquiring the infection in pregnancy and the consequences this has for the pregnancy and newborn infant. A suitable and acceptable screening test must be available with a high sensitivity and specificity. In other words, a high proportion of those affected must be identified, and few uninfected individuals wrongly identified, who will need further investigations such as repeat blood samples and amniocentesis.

Even if subsequently shown not to have the infection these women are potentially at risk of anxiety, misdiagnosis and unnecessary interventions. The consequences of a false positive or negative diagnosis must not to be underestimated and have become increasingly important with the increase in litigation. The availability and efficacy of interventions or treatments to reduce the adverse effects of the maternal infection must be known and have been shown to be effective.

In view of the markedly different prevalence of perinatal infections in different parts of the world, and indeed between populations within a country, there will be no single solution to the problem. For example, group B streptococcal infection is more common in the USA than in the UK and there are marked differences in the prevalence of past toxoplasmosis infection in pregnant women with evidence that prevalence in some countries has declined over the past three decades. About 10% of women in the UK and Norway have evidence of past toxoplasmosis infection but over 50% in France and Greece (Gilbert, 1999). The birth prevalence of

Table 6. Characteristics for a successful screening programme

The condition is an important public health problem.

The natural history of the disease is well understood.

The screening test is valid and reliable.

The screening test and its consequences in terms of further diagnostic tests and treatment are acceptable to the population.

There are adequate facilities to confirm the diagnosis and for the treatment of abnormalities detected.

Treatment is of proven effectiveness.

The chances of physical or psychological harm to those screened is less than the chance of benefit.

The objectives of the screening programme justify the costs.

congenital toxoplasmosis also varies from 1–10 per 10 000 newborns. Prevalence may also differ between populations within a country, for example it may be higher in lower socio-economic groups or in women from specific countries of origin. Within the UK, hepatitis B carriage is more prevalent in women from the Far East whereas HIV infection is most prevalent in women from sub-Saharan Africa. Another example is the prevalence of congenital cytomegalovirus, which ranges from 3–4 per 1000 in most European studies to more than 10 per 1000 in the United States (Stagno et al., 1983). Likewise, reported rates of neonatal herpes range from less than 2 per 100 000 in the UK, 6.5 per 100 000 in Sweden to 20–50 per 100 000 in the United States (Forsgren & Malm, this volume). This reflects the proportion of the population with previous evidence of HSV infection as well as the prevalence and distribution of risk factors for genital HSV infection within the population. Geographical variations in patterns of infection highlight the need to base decisions about screening in pregnancy on information available from the target population. For some infections such as syphilis or HIV screening is widely recommended whereas for others, such as the herpes viruses or toxoplasmosis, screening in pregnancy is carried out in some countries or centres but not in others. This depends in part on the different prevalence of the infection, but also on the perceived benefit of screening.

The early diagnosis and management of congenital and perinatal infections in the neonate is important and this will depend on the clinical recognition of the condition. Unfortunately, early diagnosis is problematic. Many of these conditions, such as neonatal herpes, have non-specific manifestations and others like congenital rubella and neonatal syphilis are rare so that clinicians may have a low index of suspicion. This difficulty is exemplified by neonatal herpes infection where early diagnosis and treatment is essential to prevent possible adverse consequences. Neonatal herpes simplex infection is a relatively rare condition and as it often presents with none of the typical skin manifestations (Tookey & Peckham, 1996) diagnosis can be difficult and delayed and early treatment is therefore problematic.

Many of the issues raised in this chapter will be discussed in detail under the headings of individual infections. As the overall incidence of infectious disease among newborn infants in a population and the number of infections in fetuses are unknown, this must be extrapolated from selected studies. In this chapter the broader issues are discussed and the need for good epidemiological information about specific infections emphasized. This is an essential requirement for the understanding of mechanisms of mother-to-child transmission of infection, the development of appropriate interventions and treatments as well as for reaching decisions about the introduction of new antenatal screening programmes.

REFERENCES

American College of Obstetricians and Gynecologists (1988). Perinatal herpes simplex-virus infections. *ACOG Technical Bulletin 122.* Washington, DC: American College of Obstetrics and Gynecologists.

Dunn, D., Wallon, M., Peyron, F., Petersen, E., Peckham, C. & Gilbert, R. (1999). Mother-to-child transmission of toxoplasmosis, risk estimates for clinical counselling. *Lancet,* **353**, 1829–33.

Enders, G., Miller, E., Craddock-Watson, J., Bolley, I. & Ridehalgh, M. (1994). Consequences of varicella and herpes zoster in pregnancy, prospective study of 1739 cases. *Lancet,* **343**, 1548–51.

Forrest, J. M., Menser, M.A. & Burgess, J. A. (1971). High frequency of diabetes mellitus in young adults with congenital rubella. *Lancet,* **ii**, 332–4.

Gilbert, R. (1999). Epidemiology of infection in pregnant women. In *Congenital Toxoplasmosis, Scientific Background, Clinical Management and Control,* ed. E. Pertersen & P. Amboise-Thomas. Paris: Springer-Verlag, France.

Higa, K., Dan, K. & Manabe, H. (1987). Varicella zoster virus infections during pregnancy, hypothesis concerning the mechanisms of congenital malformations. *Obstet. Gynecol.,* **69**, 214–22.

Koppe, J. G. & Rothova, A. (1989). Congenital toxoplasmosis, a long-term follow-up of 20 years. *Int. Ophthalmol.,* **13**, 387–90.

Kurtzman, G. J., Cohen, B. J., Meyers, P., Amunllah, A. & Young, N. S. (1988). Persistent B19 infection as a cause of severe chronic anaemia in children with acute lymphocytic leukaemia. *Lancet,* **ii**, 1159–62.

Miller, E., Craddock-Watson, J. & Ridehalgh, K. S. (1989). Outcome in newborn babies given anti-varicella-zoster immunoglobulin after perinatal maternal infection with varicella-zoster virus. *Lancet,* **ii** ,79–95.

Miller, E., Craddock-Watson, J. E. & Pollock, T. M. (1982). Consequences of confirmed maternal rubella at successive stages of pregnancy. *Lancet,* **ii**, 781–4.

Miller, E. (1990). Rubella reinfection. *Arch. Dis. Child.,* **65**, 820–1.

Peckham, C. S. (1972). A clinical and laboratory study of children exposed in utero to maternal rubella. *Arch. Disease Child.,* **47**, 571–7.

Peckham, C. S. (1991). Cytomegalovirus infection, congenital and neonatal disease. *Scand. J. Infect.,* Suppl. 78, 82–7.

PHLS Working Party on Fifth Disease. (1990). Prospective study of human parvovirus (B19) infection in pregnancy. *B.M.J.,* **300**, 1166–70.

Prober, C. G., Sullender, W. M., Yasukawa, L. L., Au D. S., Yeager, A. S. & Arrin, A. M. (1987). Low risk of herpes simplex virus infections in neonates exposed to the virus at the time of vaginal delivery to mothers with recurrent genital herpes simplex virus infections. *N. Engl. J. Med.,* **316**, 240–4.

Reynolds, D. W., Stagno, S. & Mosty, T. S. (1980). Maternal cytomegalovirus excretion and perinatal infection. *N. Engl. J. Med.,* **302**, 1973–6.

Stagno, S., Pass. R, F., Dworsky, M. E. & Alford, C. A. (1983). Congenital and perinatal cytomegalovirus infections. *Semin. Perinatol.,* **7**, 31–42.

Tookey, P. A. & Peckham, C. (1996). Neonatal herpes simplex virus infection in the British Isles. *Paediatr. Perinat. Epidemiol.,* **10**, 432–42.

Tookey, P. A. & Peckham, C. S. (1999). Surveillance of congenital rubella in Great Britain, 1971–96. *B.M.J.,* **318**, 769–70.

Wilson, J. M. G. & Jungner, G. (1986). *Principles and Practice of Screening for Disease.* Geneva: World Health Organization.

2

Pregnancy, immunity and infection

Cyril J. van Gelderen

BB*: There is at bottom only one genuinely scientific treatment for all diseases, and that is to stimulate the phagocytes.
Stimulate the phagocytes. Drugs are a delusion.

The Doctor's Dilemma, Act I
George Bernard Shaw, 1906

Introduction

Infection, particularly puerperal infection, has been a persistent threat to successful reproduction, and generations of women have lost their lives during and after childbirth as a result of infectious disease. Major epidemics of puerperal sepsis, such as that described by Peu in Paris in 1664, and that which occurred in Lombardy in 1772, left few if any survivors (Graham, 1950), and the vectors of infection were the doctors more often than not. The work of Holmes in 1843 and of Semmelweiss in 1861 led to the recognition of infection as the cause of 'childbed fever', and eventually resulted in a reduction in the role of the obstetrician as the bearer of the causative microorganisms. For this and other reasons, sepsis is no longer an epidemic killer of puerperal women.

Survival in a world surrounded by hostile and potentially harmful organisms depends upon the development of defence mechanisms. Clearly, the first line of defence will be an intact skin, and the employment of physical and chemical measures to enhance its impenetrability.

However, existence also requires that there be interaction with the surrounding environment. The assimilation of nutrients and oxygen dictates that the external defence be breached and, inevitably, microorganisms will accompany whatever is absorbed. When microorganisms have entered the body, defence depends upon the development of an immune response.

The development of immunity concerns the protection of 'self', and the elimination, usually by way of destruction, of 'non-self'. Successful immunity involves the recognition of non-self, followed either by immediate eradication (innate immunity), or by processing the foreign material to render it susceptible to

*Sir Ralph Bloomfield Bonington.

later elimination (adaptive immunity). This is accomplished very effectively by the immune system, a ubiquitous, mobile and heterogeneous collection of cells including phagocytes and lymphocytes which process both the recognition and the removal of foreign elements. The system also incorporates memory, so that reintroduction of an antigen triggers a rapid response.

Pregnancy, in the mammal, involves the tolerance, and indeed the nurturing of a 'non-self' organism within the body of the gravid individual, for periods of time which may extend to a year in some species.

Survival of the species is dependent upon the simultaneous achievement of both objectives for the duration of the pregnancy. The host must remain protected against 'non-self' invasion, but the conceptus must not be rejected. The reconciliation of these divergent aims has been the subject of much speculation (Medawar, 1953), and a great deal of research. Indeed, since organ transplantation has become a reality, extensive effort has gone into the study of the mechanisms whereby tolerance of pregnancy is achieved, in the hope that understanding of the phenomenon would bring with it knowledge which could be applied to the promotion of increased transplant survival.

The tolerance of pregnancy

The effect of pregnancy on the immune system

Many changes affect almost all of maternal physiology as a result of pregnancy, and the immune system is not exempt. Most, if not all of the changes influencing the immune system are concerned with the maintenance of the pregnancy, and failure of adaptive changes may lead to reproductive failure. In some cases of recurrent abortion, for example, the mechanism has been attributed to a deficit in blocking antibody, which in turn has been consequent upon a failure of immunization of the mother to paternal antigens. Treatment by means of immunization to paternal lymphocyte antigens has been attempted, and some success has been achieved (van Iddekinge et al., 1993). The evidence, however, is contradictory, and meta-analysis of some 16 trials of immunotherapy has demonstrated little benefit (Scott, 1999). It may be that accurate tests to identify the subgroups which may benefit from specific therapy remain to be developed.

Understanding of why pregnancy is tolerated remains sketchy, and therefore it is not realistic to expect to understand what has happened when this tolerance has failed.

Factors involved in tolerance of pregnancy

Medawar (1953) speculated that the conceptus might not be immunogenic, that the maternal immune response might be altered by pregnancy, that the uterus might be a privileged site, protected against immune attack, or that the placenta might be an efficient immune barrier. None of these attractive hypotheses has been shown to play more than a minor role in the tolerance of pregnancy.

Some factors which are important, include the following.

Semen and spermatozoa

These seldom elicit an antibody reaction. On those occasions when they do, a form of infertility which is particularly difficult to treat, may result. This freedom from immune response, however, does not endure in the conceptus, which does express major histocompatibility complex (MHC) antigens, and does elicit maternal antifetal HLA (human leukocyte antigen) antibody production (Johnson, 1995).

Trophoblast

After implantation, direct vascular connection between mother and fetus is not present, and this is a very important part of the protection of the fetus from maternal attack.

Interaction occurs through the trophoblast. Trophoblast is of fetal origin, and has certain immunological characteristics.

(i) Syncitiotrophoblast lacks major HLA antigens (Hunt & Hsi, 1990). The position is as yet unclear with regard to cytotrophoblast or other trophoblastic tissue. Indeed, extravillous cytotrophoblast does exhibit the HLA molecule HLA-G, which is thought to have protective properties (Iwatani & Watanabe, 1998; Rouas-Freis et al., 1997).

(ii) Human trophoblast produces at least three membrane-bound proteins which, by means of complement regulation, appear to render the tissue resistant to immune lysis (Holmes & Simpson, 1992). They are decay accelerating factor (DAF), which carries the CD55 antigen, membrane cofactor protein (MCP) with the CD46 marker, and membrane attack complex (MAC), bearing CD59. It is believed that derangement in the structure or function of these proteins may lead to problems in the maintenance of the pregnancy.

(iii) Certain placental products have an immune function. Human placental protein 14 (PP14), produced in response to progesterone stimulation, has been shown to suppress natural killer (NK) cell activity (Okamoto et al., 1991). Less specific earlier studies (Toder et al., 1984) indicated that some substances produced during pregnancy had a suppressor effect on NK activity. The effect certainly appears to be localized to the placental site; Opsahl et al. (1994) found no intrinsic difference between peripheral NK cells in early pregnancy, and those obtained from non-pregnant subjects.

The decidua

The endometrium of pregnancy is unique. Granulated lymphocytes make up three-quarters of the leukocyte population in the first trimester and decline in number after mid-pregnancy. They do not express the antigens CD3, CD4 and CD8. CD56 is abundant, but its role is not clear (Bulmer,1992). Macrophages expressing CD45, CD14 and CD68 constitute a third to a half of the leukocyte community, and appear to play a regulatory role (Bulmer et al., 1991). T cells, constituting around one-fifth of the population, are present at all levels, and are mostly CD8 positive suppressor/cytotoxic in function (Pace et al., 1991). The decidua is thus immunologically competent, but in a modified way, and the significance of the modifications is uncertain. The changes may be related to tolerance of pregnancy, or even to the protection of the conceptus from infection.

General maternal response

The maternal response to MHC antigens appears to be down-regulated, and such antibodies as are produced may be masked by their forming complexes with soluble HLA antigens. These may result in the production of anti–anti-HLA (anti-idiotype), which would protect the fetal antigens from immune attack. The source of the antigenic stimulus would seem to be the almost universal leakage of small numbers of fetal leukocytes into the maternal circulation. Antifetal antibodies can be produced, and are found to be present, but not consistently, and not in all cases (Billington, 1992). Antiviral antibodies are generated, and their concentrations are also inconsistent. In general, it is believed that humoral immunity remains intact during pregnancy (Baboonian & Griffiths, 1983).

Cytokine production

One of the most important changes affecting the immune system in pregnancy is the shift from T helper type 1 (Th1) cells to T helper type 2 (Th2) cells (Piccinni et al., 1998; Stirrat, 1994). Th1 cells produce the cytokines Interleukin 2 (IL-2) and Interferon gamma (Ifn-γ), while Th2 cells secrete IL-4, IL-5 and IL-10. The latter facilitate humoral immunity, while the former are associated with cell-mediated response. It has been noted that this shift does not occur in pregnancies fated to end in spontaneous abortion (Raghupathy, 1997). Progesterone is known to have immunosuppressive properties (Spina et al., 1998), and this may be one mechanism by which this is effected.

Non-specific immunity

There is some evidence that, in pregnant women, the non-specific response to infections, particularly that mediated by monocytes, may be enhanced (Davis et al., 1998).

Endocrine effects

The endocrine milieu has a profound effect upon most physiological functions. Immune response is altered, but the specific effects of the pregnancy hormone changes on immunity are not clearly understood. Apart from the possible progesterone mediation of both PP14 production and the Th1-Th2 shift, estrogen has been noted to suppress immunity in autoimmune disease (Jansson & Holmdahl, 1998), and this effect may apply in pregnancy as well. It has also been suggested that human chorionic gonadotrophin (hCG) may promote increased non-specific immune responses (Shibuya et al., 1987).

The genital tract flora

The lower genital tract is inhabited by many species of microorganisms, living in an ecological balance, and in a symbiotic relationship with the host. The healthy balance is part of the defence mechanism which keeps the region free of pathogens. When the balance is disturbed, even the normally commensal organisms are capable of causing disease. The changes of pregnancy, including the changes in immune response, may result in such a disturbance. This mechanism of disease is exemplified by the increased incidence of *Candida albicans* during pregnancy.

The bottom line seems to be that the immune response is modified in pregnancy, the net effect being that rejection of the fetus is rare. The maternal organism almost certainly remains competent to defend itself and the pregnancy against pathogenic invasion. Cell-mediated immunity is probably down-regulated, and humoral immunity is either unchanged or augmented.

Perinatal infections

The effect of the endocrine alterations

Glucocorticoid production is vastly increased during pregnancy. Most of the cortisol is bound, but can be displaced from transcortin by progesterone, which is also abundant at this time (McFadyen, 1995). Although little is known concerning the effect of corticosteroid on either pregnancy maintenance or the response to infection during pregnancy, the presence of large amounts of such a very immuno-active hormone must be significant. Certainly a loss of immunity against malaria during the time of corticosterone peak has been demonstrated in the mouse model under laboratory circumstances (van Zon et al., 1982), and this mechanism might be applicable to human pregnancy in a malaria-infested environment.

Oestrogens, with their proliferative effect on the female genital tract, are generally considered to be protective. There is some evidence, however, of a direct effect on the virulence of certain fungi (Styrt & Sugarman, 1991) and an oestrogen-binding protein (of uncertain significance) has been identified in *Pseudomonas aeruginosa* (Rowland et al., 1992).The changes in the production of cortisol, progesterone and oestrogen may be important in modulating the critical Th1/Th2 balance (Wilder, 1998)

The effect of the changes in the immune system

There is no increased incidence of the common infections in the perinatal period. Concern is heightened by the following questions which this chapter will address from an immunity-related viewpoint.

  (i) Will the pregnancy, in particular the changes in the endocrine and the immune milieux, alter the normal course of the infection?

 (ii) What defence mechanisms are available?

(iii) Will the infection be transmitted to the fetus or to the placenta?

(iv) Can the fetus mount an immune defence?

There are some infections that cannot occur in the absence of pregnancy. This chapter will discuss infections which are not unique to the gravid state, but which may be altered in frequency or in severity by the changes which accompany pregnancy.

Alteration of the course of disease

Clearly, progression of infectious disease is directly affected by the immune status of the host organism. It is still uncertain to what extent the changes which accompany pregnancy constitute immunosuppression. It is accepted that altered immunoregulation occurs, but the effects upon infections and defence are inconsistent and unpredictable. The majority of infectious diseases will follow a course similar to that which occurs in the non-pregnant woman, and the management will not be different. Infectious diseases in pregnancy may assume more significance if:

  (i) they are acquired more frequently in pregnancy;

 (ii) they tend to be more severe;

(iii) they are frequently transmitted to the fetus;

(iv) they frequently lead to an adverse outcome for mother, fetus or both.

Common acute infections

Community-acquired pneumonia may serve as an example. This condition is not particularly common in pregnant women, having an incidence of around 1:1400, nor is the spectrum of microorganisms involved any different from any other group of young adults (Bartlett, 1993). Pneumonia becomes important in the context of pregnancy because it poses serious maternal and fetal hazards

(Rodrigues & Niederman, 1992). Most acute infections might be considered in the same way, and need not be discussed in the context of immunity or endocrinology. Similarly, the immune and endocrine frameworks are not necessary for consideration of those infections which occur purely because of the anatomical variations associated with pregnancy. Conditions such as puerperal sepsis, mastitis, and infection related to caesarean section or to ruptured fetal membranes are consequent on alterations in host anatomy and physiology, and largely independent of changes in immunity. These will be discussed in their own settings. Infection with the human immunodeficiency virus (HIV), which clearly has profound implications for immunity, will be discussed in great detail elsewhere. The altered immune status of pregnancy, even if we do believe that it is no less efficient than that of non-pregnant women, may still account for some of the infections which occur with a greater frequency, and some which progress with a greater severity, during and around the time of gestation.

Infections which increase in frequency or severity at the time of pregnancy

A summary of some of the more important of these infections may be seen in Table 2.1.

Bacterial infections

Urinary tract infection (UTI)

The evidence seems to be that the increased rate of urinary tract infection, as well as asymptomatic bacteriuria is probably related to the factors of site (adjacent to the increasingly large uterus) and hormonal effect (smooth muscle relaxation engendered by progesterone). There is considerable research to indicate that both parasite and host factors are important in the establishment of UTI. Normal resistance on the part of the host requires increased virulence on the part of the microorganism, *Escherichia coli* in the vast majority of cases. This virulence is dependent upon the ability to attach to uroepithelial cells (Svanborg-Eden et al., 1987). Diminished host resistance, particularly cellular immunity, will lessen the need for multiple virulence factors. Pregnancy may provide this reduction in local immunity.

Septic shock

Septic shock is uncommon, but deadly, and is seldom seen in young healthy people, except in association with pregnancy. The prevalence remains low, however. It has been suggested that the response to bacterial endotoxin is more severe in the pregnant than in the non-pregnant state (Beller et al., 1985). The reason is not clear, and no immunological mechanism has been imputed. Severe infections

Table 2.1. Infections which increase in frequency or severity in pregnancy

Micro-organism	Increased prevalence	Increased severity (maternal)	Transmission to fetus/ neonate	Placental lesions
C. trachomatis	+		+	
M. hominis			+	
T. pallidum			+	+
L. monocytogenes			+	+
S. agalactiae			+	
'Septic shock'	+	+		
T. gondii			+	+
P. falciparum	+	+	□	+
C. albicans	+			
HIV	+		+	
Influenza		+		
CMV			+	+
Poliovirus	+	+		
Varicella	□	+	+	□
Rubella			+	+
Hepatitis			+	

□: variable.

in pregnancy, consequent upon abortion or intrauterine infections, need particular care, as the mortality rate remains high.

Sexually transmitted infections
Treponema pallidum, *Chlamydia trachomatis* and *Mycoplasma hominis* appear to have an increased prevalence in pregnancy. *C. trachomatis* occurs in up to 40% of sexually active women whether pregnant or not (Walker & Sweet, 1993). The perceived increased prevalence in pregnancy may simply be because it is actively sought in view of its possible deleterious effects on pregnancy outcome. Screening for *T. pallidum* is almost universal, for in cases of syphilis the effects are severe, and treatment is effective. There is no good evidence of increased susceptibility to either of these microorganisms in pregnancy, other than the obvious detail that pregnant women are by definition relatively young and sexually active, and so fall into a high-risk group.

The genital mycoplasmas, *Mycoplasma hominis* and *Ureaplasma urealyticum*, are peculiar microbes with no cell walls, making them resistant to cell wall antibiotics like the penicillins (Cummings & McCormack, 1993), and perhaps affecting their antigenicity. Immunity to these organisms is deficient, either reflecting a poor response, or multiple serotypes. There is no obvious reason for increased prevalence in pregnancy, other than that, like *T. pallidum* and *C. trachomatis*, they are actively sought in the perinatal period.

Listeria monocytogenes

This usually causes mild disease outside pregnancy, but can cause severe sequelae in the newborn (Hurley, 1995). It does appear to have a predilection for the feto-placental unit, and there is clear evidence that immunity to this organism, which is an intracellular parasite, is depressed (Sano et al., 1986; Charles, 1993). Weinberg (1984) has related this to increased T-suppressor activity, and Issekutz et al. (1984) demonstrated poor immune response in infants who had been infected as neonates. Although *L. monocytogenes* is a very widespread organism, sporadic cases of infection are uncommon, and symptoms are generally mild and non-specific, so the diagnosis is often not considered until the fetal effects become evident.

Streptococcus agalactiae (Group B streptococcus, or GBS)

These are recognized as members of the vaginal flora in many adult women, and the carriers are generally asymptomatic. Three cases of puerperal sepsis reported by Fry (1938) provided the first evidence that this organism could cause severe disease. The important problems arise with transmission to the fetus or neonate. GBS is characterized by variable virulence, and it is uncertain what part immunity in the adult host plays. It appears that C3-dependent binding is an important factor in clearing the organism (Noel et al., 1991). Attempts to produce a vaccine have met with little success so far.

Mycobacterium tuberculosis

Isolated reports of reactivation of tuberculosis have surfaced, and authors have suggested that suppressed cell-mediated immunity is responsible (Warner et al., 1992). Interestingly, it has been reported (Howard & Zwilling, 1999) that reactivation of tuberculosis is associated with a shift from Type 1 to Type 2 cytokines – as is pregnancy!

Fungal infection

Candida albicans

This is present in up to 36% of pregnant, and in 16% of non-pregnant women (Hurley, 1995), so clearly the circumstances of pregnancy favour colonization with this microorganism. *C. albicans* is also found more frequently in cases of diabetes mellitus, after administration of broad-spectrum antibiotics, and in cases of immune deficiency such as HIV infection. An important factor in pregnancy which promotes candidiasis is the high level of oestrogen, with consequent increased levels of glycogen in the vaginal epithelium, and increased acidity in the lower genital tract. This is probably only one of several factors, however. It has also been suggested that progesterone suppresses anti-candida activity (Nohmi et al., 1995). Levy et al. (1990) indicated that monocyte dependent killing, which forms the main basis of defence against *C. albicans*, was deficient during pregnancy.

Protozoal infections

Toxoplasma gondii

This infection is widespread and common, and the risk of infection depends upon the local prevalence, and the individual's immune status with regard to the microorganism. The importance of the infection lies with the severe fetal deformities that may follow. Although *T. gondii* crosses the placenta with relative ease during primary infection, and although it is an intracellular parasite, thus requiring to be dealt with by means of cell-mediated immunity, pregnant women do not appear to have any difficulty in mounting a defence against the organism. The infection tends to remain chronic and latent, and may be reactivated in states of immunosuppression. Such reactivation does not occur in pregnancy (Biedermann et al., 1995).

Malaria

Most investigators are agreed that malaria has both an increased incidence and a more serious prognosis when contracted during pregnancy. This applies especially to malaria caused by *Plasmodium falciparum*, and particularly to young primigravidae who have had no prior exposure (Nthwani et al., 1992). The increased severity of malaria is not well understood, but there has been work indicating that the poor outcome can be correlated to some extent by measuring placental cytokines. A shift toward Th1 cytokines was demonstrated (Fried et al., 1998), but there have been conflicting views (Moore et al., 1999). The increasing concentration of cortisol mentioned earlier, may also be important.

Viral infections

Viral infections have become important since the work of Gregg (1941) reporting the association of congenital defects, specifically cataracts, in the infants of mothers who had developed German measles during pregnancy. The effect on the mother of viral infection is often minor, although on occasion serious illness develops. Transplacental transmission, however, is common, and fetal or neonatal disease is frequently the result, and constitutes the chief cause for concern in pregnancy. Immunological response in pregnancy in most cases does not vary from that in the non-pregnant woman, but is poorly understood.

Rubella

German measles is typically a mild infection, and may be clinically imperceptible. Immunity is good, and this forms the basis for the drive towards immunization. In a primary infection, however, transplacental infection of the fetus may occur in more than 65% of cases during the first trimester of pregnancy (Miller et al., 1982)

Cytomegalovirus (CMV)

Infection with this virus also endangers the fetus more than the mother, and is associated with birth defects. There is some suggestion that the virus may exert some immunosuppressive effects during infection (Ho, 1984), a characteristic shared by a number of the herpesvirus types.

Varicella-zoster

This is an uncommon infection during pregnancy, as most adults have established immunity during childhood. Severe maternal disease has been described in pregnant women who do acquire the infection (Stagno & Whitley, 1985), and hospital admission is advisable. Current opinion is that the incidence of this complication is not high (Baren et al., 1996), but that there is a significant mortality when it does occur. The exception to this is in HIV-positive pregnant women, where *Herpes zoster* may occur at a relatively early stage of the disease and before other opportunistic infections. The virus crosses the placenta, and may result in fetal anomalies.

Poliovirus

Since widespread immunization has been implemented, poliomyelitis during pregnancy has become uncommon, but this condition has always had the reputation of being worse when contracted during pregnancy. In the 1950s it was demonstrated that the incidence of the disease, as well as the mortality, was increased during pregnancy (Siegel & Goldberg, 1955). An immune-related mechanism has frequently been postulated, but not demonstrated. In general, in the absence of pre-existing immunity, protection against virus is poor.

Fetal immunity

It is well known that maternal immunoglobulin G (IgG) is able to cross the placenta. This passage, which commences at around 16 weeks' gestation is not effected by simple diffusion of a small molecule, as it needs to be selective. Some maternal IgG must be stopped at the placental level. This is achieved by means of high avidity Fcγ receptors on non-trophoblastic cells within the placental villous stroma (Johnson, 1995). These receptors act as a trap for IgG which might otherwise be directed at fetal antigens. Most of the maternal IgG is transferred in the last four weeks of pregnancy, thus providing valuable passive immunity for protection during the first weeks of extrauterine life. Clearly, then, preterm infants will have proportionally less, and be more susceptible to infections to which the mother may well have been immune. Transport is selective, and involves recognition of the molecule by specific receptors on the syncitiotrophoblast.

The development of the immune system begins early, and B lymphocytes are found in fetal liver by 9 weeks' gestation (Hayward, 1983). By 14 weeks T- and B-cells capable of responding to protein antigens are present in the fetal circulation. However, actual antibody response by the fetus to antigen, and especially to polysaccharide antigen, remains immature well into postnatal life. This may be partially but not completely explained by passively acquired antibodies of maternal origin. There is divergent opinion as to whether passively acquired maternal IgG inhibits immune response or not (Glezen & Alpers, 1999; Siegrist & Lambert, 1998). Immunization of the mother remains an effective means of preventing neonatal infectious diseases like tetanus. A further explanation for the poor response involves the lack of previous antigen exposure, and therefore an absence of specific clones of T-cells. Having said this, the fetus is considered capable of responding to in utero infection in a sophisticated way (Nahmias & Kourtis, 1997).

Immunoglobulin M (IgM) does not cross the placenta, and any IgM present in the fetus indicates a fetal response to infection. This is seen in cases of congenital infection with rubella, cytomegalovirus and *T. gondii* (Cunningham et al., 1997).

Antibiotic therapy

For practical purposes it can be assumed that any medication administered to the mother will be transferred to the fetus. A significant number of pregnant women, and consequently their fetuses, will be exposed to antibiotics. It is not the purpose of this chapter to discuss the selection of antimicrobial agents, their risks or hazards, and their effects upon the fetus.

It should be noted, however, that the use of antibiotics will inevitably alter the ecology of both mother and fetus. There is no evidence that the commonly used antibiotics have a deleterious effect upon immunity. Erythromycin, commonly used and reasonably safe during pregnancy, is known to stimulate phagocyte activity in both healthy and immunosuppressed individuals (Sakaeva & Lazareva, 1999), and beta-lactamase inhibitors, commonly combined with the broad-spectrum penicillins, do not interfere with immune response (Tawfik et al., 1996).

Almost all drugs will result in some degree of immunomodulation, but in the case of most antibiotics, this does not appear to be damaging.

Prevention strategies

There is no magic formula for the prevention of infection during pregnancy, other than the application of common sense and trusted principles. Clearly, immunization prior to pregnancy is a tactic that merits application. Successfully applied in the case of rubella, this strategy is under intensive investigation for other viral infections, including HIV, and for *Streptococcus agalactiae*. In times of epidemic exacerbation of particular viral infections such as measles or varicella, it would be prudent for pregnant women to avoid exposure in so far as it was possible. Bacterial infections remain preventable by the adoption of simple precautions such as hand-washing and surgical asepsis (Iffy & Ganesh, 1993). In this age of ever more effective antibiotics, it is easy to become blasé about basic techniques, and to neglect to apply them properly, but simple measures continue to be effective and safe, and do not have unforeseen effects on the environment. Immune manipulation is not a realistic prospect in the immediate future, but research is being conducted at many centres, and may produce results.

The response of the parasite

The parasite population is also altered by the encounter with the host. Selection by the immune system, as well as by antibiotic treatment results in evolution of the organism (Anderson, 1994). Antibiotics will select organisms with resistance characteristics, and allow preferential multiplication. The objective, like that of any living organism, is completion of the life cycle (Locksley, 1997). Contact with the immune system of the host promotes transformation of parasite and host, and both will change (Soler et al., 1998). The altered immune state of pregnancy will therefore initiate adaptation. This will add to the diversity of microbiological populations.

Conclusion

Infection is no longer the epidemic killer of large numbers of pregnant women that it was in the nineteenth century, but it remains an ever-present threat. Understanding of the nature of the immune response, and of the alterations which accompany pregnancy, is essential for ensuring that prevention and management strategies are logical and effective.

REFERENCES

Anderson, R. M. (1994). The Croonian Lecture, 1994. Populations, infectious disease and immunity: a very nonlinear world. *Phil. Trans. R. Soc. Lond. B. Biol. Sci.*, **29**, 457–505.

Baboonian, C. & Griffiths, P. (1983). Is pregnancy immunosuppressive? Humoral immunity against viruses. *Br. J. Obstet. Gynaecol.*, **90**, 168–75.

Baren, J. M., Henneman, P. L. & Lewis, R. J. (1996). Primary varicella in adults: pneumonia, pregnancy, and hospital admission. *Ann. Emerg. Med.*, **28**, 165–9.

Bartlett, J. G. (1993). Pneumonia. In *Obstetric and Perinatal Infections*, ed. D. Charles, pp. 29–35. St Louis: Mosby Year Book Inc.

Beller, F. K., Schmidt, E. H., Holzgreve, W. & Hauss, J. (1985). Septicemia during pregnancy: a study in different species of experimental animals. *Am. J. Obstet. Gynecol.*, **151**, 967–75.

Biedermann, K., Flepp, M., Fierz, W., Joller-Jemelka, H. & Kleihues, P. (1995). Pregnancy, immunosuppression and reactivation of latent toxoplasmosis. *J. Perinat. Med.*, **23**, 191–203.

Billington, W. D. (1992). The normal fetomaternal relationship. *Baillières Clin. Obstet. Gynaecol.*, **6**, 417–38.

Bulmer, J. N. (1992). Immune aspects of pathology of the placental bed contributing to pregnancy pathology. *Baillières Clin. Obstet. Gynaecol.*, **6**, 461–88.

Bulmer, J. N., Morrison, L., Longfellow, M., Ritson, A. & Pace, D. (1991). Granulated lymphocytes in human endometrium, histochemical and immunohistochemical studies. *Hum. Reprod.*, **6**, 791–8.

Charles, D. (1993). Listeriosis. In *Obstetric and Perinatal Infections*, ed. D. Charles, pp. 193–209. St Louis: Mosby Year Book Inc.

Cummings, M. C. & McCormack, W. M. (1993). Genital mycoplasmas. In *Obstetric and Perinatal Infections*, ed. D. Charles, pp. 188–92. St Louis: Mosby Year Book Inc.

Cunningham, F. G., MacDonald, P. C., Gant, N. F., Leveno, K. J., Gilstrap, L. C., Hankins, G. D. V. et al. (1997). The morphological and functional development of the fetus. In *Williams Obstetrics*, 20th edn, ed. F. C. Cunningham, P. C. MacDonald, N. F. Gant, K. J. Leveno, L. C. Gilstrap, G. D. V. Hankins et al., pp. 151–90. Stamford, CT: Appleton & Lange.

Davis, D., Kaufmann, R. & Moticka, E. J. (1998). Nonspecific immunity in pregnancy, monocyte surface Fcgamma receptor expression and function. *J. Reprod. Immunol.*, **40**, 119–28.

Fried, M., Muga, R. O., Misore, A. O. & Duffy, P. E. (1998). Malaria elicits type 1 cytokines in the human placenta, IFN-gamma and TNF-alpha associated with pregnancy outcomes. *J. Immunol.*, **160**, 2523–30.

Fry, R. M. (1938). Fatal infections by haemolytic streptococcus group B. *Lancet*, **i**, 199–201.

Glezen, W. P. & Alpers, M. (1999). Maternal immunization. *Clin. Infect. Dis.*, **28**, 219–24.

Graham, H. P. (1950). *Eternal Eve*. London: Heinemann.

Gregg, N. M. (1941). Congenital cataract following German measles in the mother. *Trans. Ophthalmol. Soc. Aust.*, **3**, 35–41.

Hayward, A. R. (1983). The human fetus and newborn, development of the immune response. *Birth Defects Orig. Artic. Ser.*, **19**, 289–94.

Ho, M. (1984). Immunology of cytomegalovirus, immunosuppressive effects during infection. *Birth Defects Orig. Artic. Ser.*, **20**, 131–47.

Holmes, C. H. & Simpson, K. L. (1992). Complement and pregnancy: new insights into the immunobiology of the fetomaternal relationship. *Baillière's Clin. Obstet. Gynaecol.*, **6**, 439–60.

Holmes, O. W. (1843). The contagiousness of puerperal fever. *N. Engl. Quart. J. Med. Surg.* 1842–1843, **1**, 503–50.

Howard, A. D. & Zwilling, B. S. (1999). Reactivation of tuberculosis is associated with a shift from type 1 to type 2 cytokines. *Clin. Exp. Immunol.*, **115**, 428–34.

Hunt, J. S. & Hsi, B-L. (1990). Evasive strategies of trophoblast cells, selective expression of membrane antigens. *Am. J. Reprod. Immunol.*, **23**, 57–63.

Hurley, R. (1995). Infections in pregnancy. In *Turnbull's Obstetrics*, 2nd edn, ed. G. Chamberlain, pp. 471–88. Edinburgh: Churchill Livingstone.

Iffy, L. & Ganesh, V. (1993). Epidemiology of obstetric infections. In *Obstetric and Perinatal Infections*, ed. D. Charles, pp. 10–28. St Louis: Mosby Year Book Inc.

Issekutz, T. B., Evans, J. & Bortolussi, R. (1984). The immune response of human neonates to *Listeria monocytogenes* infection. *Clin. Invest. Med.*, **7**, 281–6.

Iwatani, Y. & Watanabe, M. (1998). The maternal immune system in health and disease. *Curr. Opin. Obstet. Gynecol.*, **10**, 453–8.

Jansson, L. & Holmdahl, R. (1998). Estrogen-mediated immunosuppression in autoimmune diseases. *Inflamm. Res.*, **47**, 290–301.

Johnson, P. M. (1995). Immunology of pregnancy. In *Turnbull's Obstetrics*. 2nd edn, ed. G. Chamberlain, pp. 143–59. Edinburgh: Churchill Livingstone.

Kaushic, C., Murdin, A. D., Underdown, B. J. & Wira, C. R. (1998). *Chlamydia trachomatis* infection in the female reproductive tract of the rat, influence of progesterone on infectivity and immune response. *Infect. Immun.*, **66**, 893–8.

Levin, B. R., Lipsitch, M. & Bonhoeffer, S. (1999). Population biology, evolution, and infectious disease, convergence and synthesis. *Science*, **283**, 806–9.

Levy, R., Latzer, S., Sachs, J., Insler, V. & Alkan, M. (1990). Host defense during pregnancy, monocyte adherence and killing. *Isr. J. Med. Sci.*, **26**, 361–6.

Locksley, R. M. (1997). Exploitation of immune and other defences by parasites, an overview. *Parasitology*, **115**, Suppl., S5–7.

McFadyen, I. R. (1995). Maternal physiology in pregnancy. In *Turnbull's Obstetrics*, 2nd edn, ed. G. Chamberlain, pp. 115–41. Edinburgh: Churchill Livingstone.

Medawar, P. B. (1953). Some immunological and endocrinological problems raised by the evolution of viviparity in vertebrates. *Symp. Soc. Exp. Biol.*, **7**, 320–8.

Miller, E., Cradock-Watson, J. E. & Pollock, T. M. (1982). Consequences of confirmed maternal rubella at successive stages of pregnancy. *Lancet*, **ii**, 781–4.

Moore, J. M., Nahlen, B. L., Misore, A., Lal, A. A. & Udhayakumar, V. (1999). Immunity to placental malaria. I. Elevated production of interferon-gamma by placental blood mononuclear cells is associated with protection in an area with high transmission of malaria. *J. Infect. Dis.*, **179**, 1218–25.

Nahmias, A. J. & Kourtis, A. P. (1997). The great balancing acts. The pregnant woman, placenta, fetus, and infectious agents. *Clin. Perinatol.*, **24**, 497–521.

Noel. G. J., Katz, S. L. & Edelson, P. J. (1991). The role of C3 in mediating binding and ingestion of group B streptococcus serotype III by murine macrophages. *Pediatr. Res.*, **30**, 118–23.

Nohmi, T., Abe, S., Dobashi, K., Tansho, S. & Yamaguchi, H. (1995). Suppression of anti-*Candida* activity of murine neutrophils by progesterone in vitro, a possible mechanism in pregnant women's vulnerability to vaginal candidiasis. *Microbiol. Immunol.*, **39**, 405–9.

Nthwani, D., Currie, P. F., Douglas, J. G., Green, S. T. & Smith, N. C. (1992). *Plasmodium falciparum* malaria in pregnancy, a review. *Br. J. Obstet. Gynaecol.*, **99**, 118.

Okamoto, N., Uchida, A., Takakura, K., Kariya, Y., Kanzaki, H., Riitinen, L. et al. (1991). Suppression by human placental protein 14 of natural killer cell activity. *Am. J. Reprod. Immunol.*, **26**, 137–42.

Opsahl, M., Hansen, K., Klein, T. & Cunningham, D. (1994). Natural killer cell activity in early human pregnancy. *Gynecol. Obstet. Invest.*, **37**, 226–8.

Pace, D. P., Longfellow, M. & Bulmer, J. N. (1991). Intraepithelial lymphocytes in human endometrium. *J. Reprod. Fertil.*, **91**, 165–74.

Piccinni. M-P,, Beloni, L., Livi, C., Maggi, E., Scarselli, G. & Romagnani, S. (1998). Defective production of both leukemia inhibitory factor and type 2 T-helper cytokines by decidual T cells in unexplained recurrent abortions. *Nature Med.*, **4**, 1020–4.

Raghupathy, R. (1997). Maternal anti-placental cell-mediated reactivity and spontaneous abortions. *Am. J. Reprod. Immunol.*, **37**, 478–84.

Rodrigues, J. & Niederman, M. S. (1992). Pneumonia complicating pregnancy. *Clin. Chest Med.*, **13**, 679–91.

Rouas-Freis, N., Goncalves, R. M., Menier, C., Dausset, J., & Carosella, E. D. (1997). Direct evidence to support the role of HLA-G in protecting the fetus from maternal uterine natural killer cytolysis. *Proc. Natl Acad. Sci. USA*, **14**, 11520–5.

Rowland, S. S., Falkler, W. A. J. & Bashirelahi, N. (1992). Identification of an estrogen-binding protein in *Pseudomonas aeruginosa*. *J. Steroid Biochem. Mol. Biol.*, **42**, 721–7.

Sakaeva, D. D. & Lazareva, D. N. (1999). The effect of erythromycin on immunity in immunodeficiency. *Eksp. Klin. Farmakol.*, **62**, 50–2.

Sano, M., Mitsuyama, M., Watanabe, Y. & Nomoto, K. (1986). Impairment of cell-mediated immunity to *Listeria monocytogenes* in pregnant mice. *Microbiol. Immunol.*, **30**, 165–76.

Scott, J. R. (1999). Immunotherapy for recurrent miscarriage (Cochrane review). In *The Cochrane Library*, Issue 4. Oxford: Update Software.

Semmelweiss, I. P. (1861). Die Aetiologie, der Begriff und der Prophylaxis des Kindbettfiebers. Pest, Wien und Leipzig: CA Hartleben Verlag.

Shibuya, T., Izuchi, K., Kuroiwa, A., Okabe, N. & Shirakawa, K. (1987). Study on nonspecific immunity in pregnant women; increased chemiluminescence response of peripheral blood phagocytes. *Am. J. Reprod. Immunol.*, **15**, 19–23.

Siegel, M. & Goldberg, M. (1955). Incidence of poliomyelitis in pregnancy. *N. Engl. J. Med.*, **253**, 841–7.

Siegrist, C. A. & Lambert, P. H. (1998). Maternal immunity and infant responses to immunization; factors influencing infant responses. *Dev. Biol. Stand*, **95**, 133–9.

Soler, J. J., Moller, A. P. & Soler, M. (1998). Mafia behaviour and the evolution of facultative virulence. *J. Theor. Biol.*, **191**, 267–77.

Spina, V., Aleandri, V., Pacchiarotti, A. & Salvi, M. (1998). Immune tolerance in pregnancy. Maternal–fetal interactions. *Minerva Ginekol.*, **50**, 533–7.

Stagno, S. & Whitley, R. J. (1985). Herpesvirus infections of pregnancy. Part II: Herpes simplex virus and varicella-zoster virus infections. *N. Engl. J. Med.*, **313**, 1327–30.

Stirrat, G. M. (1994). Pregnancy and immunity. *Br. Med. J.*, **308**, 1385–6.

Styrt, B. & Sugarman, B. (1991). Estrogens and infection. *Rev. Infect. Dis*, **13**, 1139–50.

Svanborg-Eden, C., de Man, P., Jodal, U., Linder, H. & Lomberg, H. (1987). Host parasite interaction in urinary tract infection. *Pediatr. Nephrol.*, **1**, 623–31.

Tawfik, A. F., Al-Zamil, F. A., Ramadan, M. A. & Shibl, A. M. (1996). Effect of beta-lactamase inhibitors on normal immune capabilities and their interactions with staphylococcal pathogenicity. *J. Chemother.*, **8**, 102–6.

Toder, V., Nebel, L., Elrad, H., Blank, M., Durdana, A. & Gleicher, N. (1984). Studies of natural killer cells in pregnancy. II. The immunoregulatory effect of pregnancy substances. *J. Clin. Lab. Immunol.*, **14**, 129–33.

van Iddekinge, B., Hofmeyr, G. J., Bezwoda, W. R., Wadee, A. A. & van Rooy, P. (1993). Recurrent spontaneous abortion, histocompatability between partners, response to immune therapy, and subsequent reproductive performance. *Am. J. Reprod. Immunol.*, **30**, 37–44.

van Zon, A. A., Eling, W. M., Hermsen, C. C. & Koekkoek, A. A. (1982). Corticosterone regulation of the effector function of malaria immunity during pregnancy. *Infect. Immun.*, **36**, 484–91.

Walker, C. K. & Sweet, R. L. (1993). Perinatal chlamydial infections. In *Obstetric and Perinatal Infections*, ed. D. Charles, pp. 181–7. St Louis: Mosby Year Book Inc.

Warner, T. T., Khoo, S. H. & Wilkins, E. G. (1992). Reactivation of tuberculous lymphadenitis during pregnancy. *J. Infect.*, **24**, 181–4.

Weinberg, E. D. (1984). Pregnancy-associated depression of cell-mediated immunity. *Rev. Infect. Dis.*, **6**, 814–21.

Wilder, R. L. (1998). Hormones, pregnancy, and autoimmune diseases. *Ann. N. Y. Acad. Sci.*, **840**, 45–50.

3

Maternal infections and their consequences

Patrick S. Ramsey and Robert L. Goldenberg

Introduction

Pregnancy is a vulnerable period for the acquisition of infections and infectious diseases. Not only can the pregnant woman herself become infected, but fetal and/or neonatal transmission may also occur. Although pregnancy does not usually affect the incidence and severity of infections, some physiological adaptations of pregnancy can result in increased risk for some infections particularly urinary tract infections, pneumonia and chorioamnionitis. In addition to maternal sequelae, the developing fetus is often placed at risk secondary to hyperpyrexia, hypoxia, preterm labour and congenital infection. The number of maternal infections known to be associated with adverse pregnancy outcomes continues to increase. Adverse pregnancy outcomes can be a direct consequence of fetal or neonatal infection or an indirect effect secondary to vaginal, cervical or intrauterine infections. Specific fetal risks are highly dependent on the causal organism, potential for transplacental passage, timing of exposure and maternal/fetal immune status. Adverse outcomes associated with maternal infection during pregnancy are varied and include infertility, ectopic pregnancy, miscarriage, congenital anomalies, stillbirth, intrauterine growth retardation, preterm delivery, neonatal death, and long-term disability of the infant.

Maternal infection and pregnancy

Infections are common during pregnancy, but the risks associated with infections vary by pathogen and disease site (Alexander, 1984). Infections such as acute cystitis, upper respiratory viral infections and trichomoniasis are generally of concern for maternal health but pose less risk to the fetus. In contrast, infections such as cytomegalovirus (CMV), genital herpes simplex virus (HSV), parvovirus, and rubella can lead to significant fetal morbidity/mortality but have little or no maternal sequelae. Similarly, relatively innocuous constituents of the genital and rectal flora, such as group B streptococcus (*Streptococcus agalactica*) and *Escherichia coli*, may represent benign maternal colonization. However, intrapartum exposure of a susceptible preterm neonate to these pathogens can result in neonatal pneumonia, sepsis, and even death. Bacterial vaginosis also poses little direct risk to the mother and neonate, but through increased risk of preterm delivery, bacterial vaginosis may result in significant neonatal morbidity and mortality. Other infections can result in significant morbidity and mortality in both mother and infant.

Acute maternal infection may result from exposure to contaminated air, animal or human waste, food, blood products, and other biological fluids (Wendel & Wendel, 1993). Varicella, rubella, measles, influenza, parvovirus, and tuberculosis are typically acquired through the respiratory system or mucosal membrane contact, while hepatitis B and C transmission in adults usually occurs through exposure to blood products, human waste, and semen. Toxoplasmosis and listeriosis generally follow exposure to contaminated uncooked foods. Syphilis, gonorrhoea, HIV, HSV, trichomonas and chlamydia, are nearly universally transmitted through sexual contact. In contrast, the agents responsible for Lyme borreliosis (*Borrelia burgdorferi*) and malaria (*Plasmodium* sp.) are transmitted to humans though the arthropod vectors, deer tick (*Ixodes daamini*) and mosquito (*Anopheles* sp.), respectively. In other instances, the pathogen of interest may represent a chronic infection (e.g. hepatitis B virus, hepatitis C virus, cytomegalovirus), benign colonization (group B streptococcus, *E. coli*), or abnormal colonization secondary to bacterial overgrowth (bacterial vaginosis). While exposure to many of these pathogens during pregnancy can result in adverse outcomes, the majority of women, and their infants when exposed to these infections, will not be affected.

Before focusing specifically on those infections that pose significant fetal/neonatal risk, we will briefly address several important maternal infections encountered during pregnancy. While any infection may result in maternal sequelae, we will limit our discussion here to those infections which commonly complicate pregnancy and which are associated with significant maternal morbidity or mortality.

Respiratory infections

In general, upper respiratory tract infections pose little concern for maternal well being, apart from the common discomforts of rhinorrhea, sinus congestion, and cough. Typically, upper respiratory infections result from a variety of viral and bacterial pathogens, including rhinovirus, adenovirus, coronavirus, and coxsackie A virus infections. Few, if any, of these infections are significantly associated with adverse maternal/neonatal outcomes. Infections of the lower respiratory tract, however, pose a significant threat to maternal health and secondarily to the fetus *in situ*. Physiological pulmonary adaptations of pregnancy result in increased oxygen consumption, increased tidal volume, and decreased residual lung volume. These changes increase maternal susceptibility to pulmonary compromise during infection. Pneumonia complicates up to 1% of all pregnancies and may be caused by a variety of bacterial and viral pathogens (Hopwood, 1965). Prior to the advent of antibiotics, pneumonia in pregnancy was associated with a high risk of preterm labour (70%) and maternal mortality (20%) (Oxorn, 1955). With modern antibiotics these risks are markedly reduced and preterm labour complications are now found in only approximately 8% of cases (Benedetti et al., 1982).

While the clinical course of bacterial pneumonia does not appear to be modified by pregnancy, viral pneumonia, especially when caused by varicella, measles (rubeola), and influenza, can be severe and may result in acute respiratory decompensation, respiratory failure, and adult respiratory distress syndrome (ARDS). Development of ARDS can lead to maternal/fetal hypoxia, preterm labour, and multisystem organ failure. Varicella infection, or chicken-pox, is an uncommon but potentially devastating infection during pregnancy (Luby, 1987). Varicella encephalitis occurs in approximately 1% of infected pregnant women. More important, however, varicella pneumonia develops in up to 20% of varicella infected pregnant women and, in the absence of acyclovir therapy, may be associated with a mortality rate as high as 40% (Chapman & Duff, 1993; Smego & Asperilla, 1991). Significant pulmonary involvement (50%) can also occur in measles infection. Unlike varicella pneumonia, measles pneumonia is more often associated with bacterial super-infection with *Staphylococcus aureus* or *Streptococcus pneumoniae*. Fortunately, where active immunization programmes are in place, these viral pathogens are now less frequently encountered. Influenza, however, remains a major respiratory pathogen globally. In contrast to the general population, pregnant women appear to be at higher risk for developing influenza pneumonia (Kort et al., 1986, Mullooly et al., 1986). Data from the 1918–19 influenza A pandemic revealed a 50% increase in maternal mortality due to influenza pneumonia (Harris, 1919). In addition to maternal outcomes secondary to viral infections, we will later discuss fetal/neonatal outcomes related to exposure to these pathogens.

Tuberculosis remains an important respiratory pathogen. Recent epidemiological data suggests an increasing prevalence of tuberculosis worldwide. An estimated 1–2 % of all pregnant women in the USA exhibit tuberculin skin test reactivity, but less than 10% of these have active tuberculosis lesions (Sever et al., 1989). Pregnant women with tuberculosis are usually symptomatic with cough, weight loss, fever, fatigue and haemoptysis (Good et al., 1981). Pregnancy does not appear to affect the clinical course of tuberculosis. Haematogenous spread of *Mycobacterium tuberculosis* may result in congenital tuberculosis (Nemir & O'Hare, 1985).

Gastrointestinal infections

Gastrointestinal infections frequently occur during pregnancy. Of the bacterial pathogens, *Salmonella typhi* (typhoid fever) poses the greatest maternal and fetal risk. Patients may have severe diarrhoea, abdominal pain, fever, nausea and vomiting. Abortion and preterm birth rates have been reported to occur in up to 80% of cases, with fetal mortality approaching 60% and maternal mortality 25% (Dildy et al., 1990). Viral causes of gastroenteritis are many, and include rotavirus, pararotavirus, Norwalk agent, adenoviruses, and calicivirus. These infections are usually self-limited and with minimal maternal/fetal risk. Protozoal infestations, for example giardiasis or amoebiasis, can lead to severe diarrhoea. Severe dehydration, bowel malabsorption and electrolyte imbalances are the primary maternal risks. Neither maternal giardiasis (*Giardia lamblia*) nor amoebiasis (*Entamoeba histolytica*) directly affects the fetus, but severe dehydration/malnutrition could result in intrauterine growth restriction.

Urinary tract infections

Between 5% and 10% of all pregnant women present with asymptomatic bacteriuria (defined as 1×10^5 colonies/ml urine on two consecutive, clean-catch, mid-stream collections), however acute cystitis occurs in only 1–3% of all pregnancies. Acute cystitis may develop *de novo* or as the result of a previously unrecognised and untreated asymptomatic bacteriuria. Adequate treatment is important to prevent development of upper urinary tract infection, or pyelonephritis. Pyelonephritis occurs in 1–2% of all pregnancies (Duff, 1984). The relatively high rate of pyelonephritis during pregnancy results from elevated progesterone levels which decrease smooth muscle contractility and ureteral peristalsis. Additionally, the gravid uterus directly or indirectly causes ureteral compression, particularly on the right side. The combination effect of these factors results in relative urinary stasis and facilitates migration of bacterial pathogens, primarily *E. coli*, *Klebsiella* sp., and *Proteus* sp., into the bladder, ureters or kidneys. Pyelonephritis in pregnancy may result in preterm labour, septic shock, and ARDS (Cunningham et al., 1973). Hence, prompt treatment with intravenous antibiotics is essential. Approximately 20–30% of patients who develop pyelonephritis will develop recurrent urinary tract infection during the pregnancy. In light of this potential risk, prophylactic antibiotic treatment is usually recommended.

Genital tract infections

Perhaps the most important category of maternal infection which may result in maternal morbidity and mortality, as well as fetal or neonatal complications, are those of the upper genital tract (chorioamnionitis) and lower genital tract (bacterial vaginosis, chlamydia, gonorrhoea, HSV, human papilloma virus (HPV), syphilis, trichomoniasis). Bacterial vaginosis is a common lower genital tract infection found in approximately 20–40% of African–American women and 10–15% of Caucasian women in the USA (Eschenbach, 1993; Goldenberg et al., 1996; Meis et al., 1995). Bacterial vaginosis is a clinical syndrome characterized by alteration of the normal vaginal lactobacilli dominant microflora resulting in a predominance of bacteria such as *Gardnerella vaginalis, Prevotella* sp., *Bacteroides* sp., *Peptostreptococcus, Mobiluncus, Mycoplasma hominis,* and *Ureaplasma urealyticum* (Hill, 1993; Hillier, 1993). Characteristically, patients with symptomatic bacterial vaginosis will complain of a watery, homogenous greyish discharge with a fishy amine odour. Bacterial vaginosis has been associated with increased risk for preterm labour and delivery (Eschenbach et al., 1984; Krohn et al., 1991; Kurki et al., 1992; McDonald et al., 1991, 1992; Riduan et al., 1993). In the USA, nearly 40% of early spontaneous preterm births, especially in African–American women, have been attributed to bacterial vaginosis (Fiscella, 1996a, b). Bacterial vaginosis seems to be more associated with early preterm birth rather than late preterm birth. The results from two randomized clinical trials demonstrate that treatment of bacterial vaginosis in patients at high risk for preterm delivery results in substantial reductions of the preterm birth rates (Hauth et al., 1995; Morales et al., 1994). An important point to emphasize is that, based on the present data available, treatment of bacterial vaginosis appears to only be effective in preventing preterm birth in high-risk populations. Data from a study of low-risk women with bacterial vaginosis in Australia and a recently completed NICHD/MFM network study in the United States, evaluating and treating asymptomatic women with bacterial vaginosis, failed to demonstrate a reduction in preterm delivery (Klebanoff et al., 1999; McDonald et al., 1997).

The majority of women with bacterial vaginosis never manifest any signs or adverse outcomes related to the colonization and it is likely that bacterial vaginosis is only a surrogate marker for a more important, currently unrecognized condition which may cause the preterm birth (Romero et al., 1989). One compelling theory is that bacterial vaginosis is a marker for occult upper genital tract infection (Andrews et al., 1995; Gray et al., 1992; Hammed et al., 1984; Hillier et al., 1988; Krohn et al., 1995; Korn et al., 1995). Therefore, premature births, attributed to bacterial vaginosis or prevented by its treatment, may instead be related to an associated upper genital tract infection.

Other lower genital tract infections, such as chlamydia, gonorrhoea, human papilloma virus (HPV), HSV, syphilis, and trichomoniasis, are of clinical importance. Chlamydia and gonorrhoea can result in cervicitis, pelvic inflammatory disease, infertility, chorioamnionitis, and preterm delivery. Human papilloma virus (HPV) infection of the lower genital tract can result in a spectrum of clinical disease ranging from benign condylomata to cervical dysplasia to frank malignant transformation, depending on the type. Herpes simplex virus (HSV) infection is typically a self-limited chronic disease with minimal risk for maternal sequelae. Syphilis is an indolent systemic infection, which can eventually result in cardiovascular, dermatological and neurological manifestations if left untreated. Trichomoniasis may result in a relatively innocuous vaginal discharge, however, infection during pregnancy may increase the risk of preterm delivery. In addition to the maternal morbidity associated with the above infections, transmission of these infections to the fetus/neonate may result in significant morbidity and/or mortality.

Chorioamnionitis, or intra-amniotic infection, is a common complication of both term and preterm pregnancies with the potential for serious maternal and fetal morbidity and mortality. Chorioamnionitis occurs in 1 to 5% of term pregnancies and nearly 25% of patients with preterm delivery (Armer & Duff, 1991). It most commonly represents an ascending infection of organisms, which are usually part of the normal vaginal flora. Typical pathogens include *Bacteroides* sp. and *Prevotella* sp., anaerobic streptococci, group B streptococci, and *E. coli*. Risk factors for chorioamnionitis include low socio-economic status, nulliparity, prolonged rupture of membranes, protracted labour, multiple vaginal exams, and lower genital tract infection (Gibbs & Duff, 1991). Bacteraemia can occur in 3–12% of patients with chorioamnionitis. Additionally, infants born in the presence of chorioamnionitis have a 5–10% risk of becoming bacteraemic or of developing pneumonia.

Periodontal infections

Periodontal disease typically results from gram-negative anaerobic colonization of the gingiva. Opportunistic oral pathogens and/or their inflammatory products may play a role in premature birth and evidence for this comes from two sources. First, amniotic fluid cultures from women with preterm labour and intact membranes have occasionally produced mouth organisms commonly associated with periodontal disease (Hill, 1998). Secondly, recent investigations have demonstrated that periodontal disease may be associated with prematurity or low birth weight (Offenbacher et al., 1996). Further research is needed to explore and confirm these findings.

Transmission of organisms to the fetus and newborn

Risks associated with maternal infection are dependent upon the specific pathogen, the prevalence of the disease in the population, the timing of exposure, and the risk of fetal/neonatal transmission. Table 3.1 shows these factors for many common human pathogens. Data for this table are derived from a wide range of

Table 3.1. Perinatal transmission of major human pathogens[a]

Maternal infection/organism	Approximate maternal prevalence (%) in the USA	Usual timing of transmission		Neonates infected/colonized (%) when mother colonized
		Prenatal	Intrapartum	
Bacterial vaginosis	20.0	–	–	0
Chlamydia	5.0	–	+	50.0
Coxsackievirus	Unknown	+	–	±
Cytomegalovirus	33.0	+	+	3.0
Echovirus	Unknown	–	+	±
Gonorrhoea	1.0	–	+	50.0
Group B Strep	20.0	–	+	50.0
Hepatitis A	0.1	–	–	–
Hepatitis B	1.0	–	+	30.0
Hepatitis C	2.0	–	+	20.0
Herpes simplex	20.0	±	+	50.0
HIV	0.2	+	+	25.0
HPV	5.0	–	+	5.0
Influenza	10.0	+	–	±
Listeria	5.0	+	–	±
Lyme borreliosis	0.08	+	–	±
Malaria	±	+	–	4.0
Measles (rubeola)	0.04	+	–	±
Mumps	0.1	+	–	±
Parvovirus	1.0	+	–	20.0
Rubella	±	+	–	50.0
Syphilis	0.2	+	±	40.0
Toxoplasmosis	1.0	+	–	30.0
Trichomonas	2.0	–	–	0
Tuberculosis	0.1	+	–	±
Varicella	0.05	+	+	2.0

± May occur, uncommon.

– Occurs rarely, if at all.

[a] Adapted from Goldenberg et al., 1997, 1999

sources including many on the accompanying reference (Sever et al., 1989; Remington & Klein, 1995). Estimates in these resources are often widely discrepant (Goldenberg et al., 1997). These differences are, in part, due to racial and socio-economic differences in study populations, relative population size, and ascertainment bias. Estimates of disease prevalence are based on data from the USA unless otherwise specified.

The prevalence of certain maternal diseases has changed substantially over time. Improved public health prevention and screening strategies, immunization campaigns, and improved treatment modalities influence disease prevalence. For example, rubella and measles immunization programmes have led to a marked reduction in the prevalence of these diseases. Chicken-pox, which currently affects 0.05% of pregnant women per year in the USA, is likely to decrease as vaccination is introduced. Universal newborn hepatitis B vaccination in the United States is likely to result in a similar reduction in the prevalence of chronic hepatitis B (Centers for Disease Control and Prevention, 1990, 1991). Syphilis and HIV infections currently complicate approximately 0.15% to 0.2% of pregnancies in the United States (Gwinn et al., 1991; Davis et al., 1995). Additionally, parvovirus and *Toxoplasma gondii* infections affect approximately 1% of pregnant women in the United States. *Listeria monocytogenes* colonizes the gastrointestinal tract of up to 5% of humans; however, fetal/neonatal infection is infrequent (Sever et al., 1989). Gonorrhoea, hepatitis B virus, and *Trichomonas* infections are found in 1% to 2% of all pregnant women, with chlamydial infections found in about 5% (Mason & Brown, 1980; McGregor & French, 1991; Judson, 1985). Maternal colonization with HSV, group B streptococcus, or bacterial vaginosis is found in approximately 20% of pregnant women (American College of Obstetricians and Gynecologists, 1992; Lewin & Amstey, 1981; Regan at al., 1991; Stone et al., 1989). Although primary CMV infection occurs in only 1–2% of pregnant women, latent cytomegalovirus colonization, as determined by antibody positivity, is estimated to occur in about one-third of all pregnant women (Stagno et al., 1986). Subpopulations of women who have markedly higher and lower prevalences have been described. Influenza epidemics typically occur in the autumn or winter and can result in infection rates as high as 50% in urban populations. Although a minor cause of maternal/neonatal morbidity and mortality in the United States, malaria is a major global health concern with over 100 million cases of malaria reported annually. In areas where malaria is endemic, the prevalence of malaria infection in pregnancy can be as high as 75%.

Clearly, maternal/fetal infection and subsequent sequelae are highly dependent upon the timing of the exposure to the infectious agent. It is common to subdivide pregnancy into periods to better delineate timing of exposure. Commonly used terms include 'prenatal', 'perinatal' and 'intrapartum'. While definitions may vary, the prenatal period typically refers to the time between conception and the onset of labour. In contrast, the perinatal period usually encompasses the time from the onset of labour until the 28th day of life. The intrapartum period refers to the period between the onset of labour and delivery. These distinctions are important as not all maternal infections result in fetal/neonatal infection by the same mechanism.

Infections which may be transmitted prenatally include CMV, HIV, HCV, parvovirus, toxoplasmosis, rubella, measles, syphilis, listeriosis, Lyme borreliosis, malaria, influenza, varicella, and tuberculosis (Table 3.1). Cytomegalovirus transmission typically occurs prenatally, with vertical transmission rates increasing with gestational age (Hagay et al., 1996; Hanshaw, 1994; Sever et al., 1989). Parvovirus may infect the fetus throughout pregnancy, although fetal hydrops, resulting from aplastic crisis, is usually limited to those infections occurring in the late first or second trimester (Valeur-Jensen et al., 1999). Transmission of toxoplasmosis with acute maternal infection is less frequent earlier in pregnancy and more common in the third (Foulon et al., 1999; Sever et al., 1989). Early fetal infection is more likely to result in severe fetal sequelae, which may result in abortion and fetal death. Varicella can be transmitted throughout gestation. First trimester exposure has been associated with congenital malformations whereas infection in the second and third trimester typically is not. However, intrapartum transmission of varicella can result in a devastating neonatal infection. Rubella transmission classically occurs prenatally, with fetal sequelae dependent upon the gestational age of exposure. Fetal infection prior to the eighth week of gestation often results in development of congenital heart disease and cataracts, while infection between 8 and 16 weeks' gestation is more commonly associated with congenital deafness. Infection later in pregnancy appears to result in few adverse effects. Syphilis can be acquired at any time during the pregnancy and may result in intrauterine growth restriction, non-immune hydrops fetalis, stillbirth, preterm delivery, and congenital infection (Vaules et al., 2000). Similarly, the spirochete *Borrelia burgdorferi* has been shown to infect the fetus in utero (Nadel et al., 1989; Strobino et al., 1993; Schlesinger et al., 1985). Neonatal HIV infection may be acquired prenatally; however, studies of second trimester abortuses suggest that early in utero infection is rare (Luzuriaga & Sullivan, 1994; Mandelbrot et al., 1996, Mayaux et al., 1995). About two-thirds of all HIV perinatal transmission occurs in the intrapartum period, with the remaining 33% occurring prenatally, usually in the last few weeks of pregnancy (Rouzioux et.al., 1995; Minkoff et al., 1995; Newell et al., 1994; DeRossi et al., 1992). Additionally, HIV transmission may occur through breastfeeding.

Examples of intrapartum transmission include chlamydia, gonorrhoea, group B streptococcus, HPV, HSV, varicella, hepatitis B virus, and hepatitis C virus infections. These infections are generally transmitted as the infant passes through the birth canal, and rarely occur before rupture of the membranes (Alger et al., 1988). Intrapartum transmission of *Chlamydia trachomatis* is responsible for inclusion conjunctivitis, a leading cause of blindness in developing countries (Alexander & Harrison *et al.*, 1983). Similarly, *Neisseria gonorrhoeae* may be transmitted in the intrapartum period and can cause serious ophthalmological injury (American College of Obstetricians and Gynecologists, 1994, Edwards et al., 1978). If routine ophthalmological prophylaxis is not used, approximately 50% of the infants of colonized mothers will acquire gonorrhoea or chlamydia eye infections. Intrapartum exposure to varicella and HSV can lead to severe neonatal infection resulting in morbidity and mortality. Intrapartum transmission of HPV occurs in approximately 5% of patients with lower genital tract HPV infection (Watts et al., 1998). Laryngeal papillomatosis, secondary to neonatal HPV infection, however, only complicates 1 in 400 exposed patients. Group B streptococcus is a major cause of neonatal infection. Neonatal group B streptococcal infection, which often presents as pneumonia or systemic infection and later as meningitis, may result from colonization acquired in utero following membrane rupture or during passage through the birth canal (American College of Obstetricians and Gynecologists, 1992). Nearly 50% of neonates born to colonized mothers become colonized soon after birth. Preterm infants appear to be more susceptible to this pathogen. In addition to neonatal infection, ascending group B streptococcus infection following premature preterm rupture of membranes can result in fetal demise and/or chorioamnionitis. Neonatal infections with *Ureaplasma urealyticum*, *Mycoplasma hominis*, *Bacterioides* sp., *Gardnerella* sp., or other bacterial vaginosis-related organisms have been reported (Harrison et al., 1983). Infants are virtually never colonized with *Trichomonas vaginalis*.

Not only is the timing and route of pathogen transmission a critical factor in the potential for adverse outcome, the specific stage of infection is important as well. For example, although prenatal vertical transmission can occur at any stage of syphilis, risk of transmission correlates with the degree of spirochetemia (Harter & Benirschke, 1976; Ray, 1995; Reyes et al., 1993; Vaules et al., 2000). Hence, vertical transmission of *Treponema pallidum*, the etiologic agent responsible for syphilis, is more common with primary (50%) and secondary syphilis (50%), as compared to early latent (40%), late latent (10%), and tertiary syphilis (10%) (Fiumara et al., 1952).

Immune status and perinatal transmission

Although timing of exposure to specific infectious agents is important with regard to potential for adverse outcome, the status of the maternal/fetal immune system may be equally or more important. Both the maternal and fetal immune systems are instrumental in protecting against, modifying the disease process, and in eradicating infection when it occurs. In general, previous exposure to a given infectious agent provides immunity to prevent future reinfection. Additionally, active immunization has significantly enhanced immunity to a variety of infectious agents that once were a major cause of maternal and neonatal morbidity and mortality. The incidence of diseases such as rubella, measles, mumps, and polio, has been reduced significantly through these public health efforts.

The importance of the immune system is evident as we observe the outcome of HIV infection. The array of opportunistic infection seen in mothers and neonates with acquired immunodeficiency syndrome (AIDS) is the direct result of immune system impairment. Infection and destruction of the helper T-lymphocytes (CD4 +) by HIV, results in compromise of both cellular and humoral immunity. Maternal HIV infection and host immunity is also evident as we evaluate vertical transmission. As previously discussed, vertical HIV transmission usually occurs in the intrapartum period. Chorioamnionitis represents an important risk factor (European Collaborative Study, 1992; Minkoff et al. 1995; St. Louis et al., 1993). Host response to intra-amniotic/intrauterine infection results in the recruitment of neutrophils, macrophages, and lymphocytes. Activation of these immune mediators increases the production and release of a variety of pro-inflammatory and chemotactic cytokines, and vasoactive substances. The resulting cascade leads to an intense inflammatory response as the host counters the bacterial invasion. Ironically, the resultant increase in vascular permeability, vascular injury, and tissue destruction, is likely to lead to an increased risk for vertical transmission of HIV (Goldenberg et al., 1998). Presence of chorioamnionitis with prolonged rupture of membranes has been suggested to substantially increase the risk of perinatal transmission of HIV.

Humoral immunity is not only protective against acquisition of maternal infection, but immunity may modify perinatal transmission. Malarial and HSV infections are classic examples of this protection. Antimalarial IgG antibodies are actively transported across the placenta. The protective value of these antibodies is demonstrated through epidemiological studies of congenital malaria in immune and non-immune pregnant women. In pregnant women living in areas where malaria is endemic (high level of maternal immunity), congenital malaria complicates 0.3% of live births from infected mothers (Covell, 1950). In contrast, non-immune women experiencing a primary attack of malaria during pregnancy have a 7% risk of congenital malaria (Hulbert, 1992). Transfer of antimalarial IgG antibodies confers protection to the exposed neonate. Studies of humoral immunity in acquired neonatal malaria infection demonstrated that the presence of antimalarial antibodies was associated with a greater proportion of neonates with asymptomatic malarial infection (Sehgal et al., 1989). By 4–7 months of age, 96 % of neonates lost this protective passive immunity. Similar to malaria, humoral immunity to HSV is protective. Primary HSV infection is associated with a 50% risk of neonatal infection. In contrast, with recurrent HSV infection, the risk of intrapartum transmission is approximately 5–8% (Hutto et al., 1987; Overall, 1994; Prober et al., 1987; Whitley & Hutto, 1985; Whitley et al., 1991).

For some infections, however, previous exposure or immunization does not provide sufficient protection from reinfection and/or risk for fetal transmission during pregnancy. Cytomegalovirus infection is an example of this phenomenon (Fowler et al., 1992). An estimated 30–60% of pregnant women demonstrate anti-CMV IgG antibodies. These antibodies, however, do not eradicate or prevent recurrent CMV infection, and therefore the fetus is at risk for perinatal transmission. The risk of perinatal transmission of CMV is similar in patients with a primary or recurrent infection (Reynolds et al., 1973; Stagno et al., 1986). In spite of the equal frequency of congenital infection with primary and recurrent infections, nearly all cases of clinically apparent disease are seen in infants of women with primary CMV infection.

Thus far we have focused on the maternal immune system. In some instances, the fetal immune system plays an important role in the pathogenesis of some congenital infections. Perhaps the most classic example, demonstrating the role of fetal immunity in the pathogenesis of fetal/neonatal sequelae, is seen with syphilis. *Treponema pallidum* can readily pass transplacentally at any gestational age. Seventy to 100% of infants born to untreated infected mothers are infected (Wendel, 1988; Ricci et al., 1989; Vaules et al., 2000). If maternal therapy is implemented prior to 18–20 weeks' gestation, fetal infection typically results in few clinical manifestations because of relative fetal immunocompetence (Harter & Benirschke, 1976; Wendel, 1988). Immaturity of the fetal immune system early in pregnancy prevents development of the chronic inflammatory response which results in the histologic/pathologic findings associated with congenital syphilis (Silverstein, 1962).

Timing of onset of disease

Neonatal infection resulting from prenatal or intrapartum transmission usually becomes apparent during the neonatal period. Examples include most of the infants infected with rubella, varicella, *L. monocytogenes*, parvovirus, HSV, group B streptococcus, syphilis, chlamydia, and gonorrhoea. In other instances, however, sequelae may not become apparent for months or years. For example, while the ophthalmologic damage caused by *N. gonorrhoeae* and *C. trachomatis* becomes apparent within several days or weeks after birth, the pneumonia associated with chlamydia infection generally occurs months after delivery (Cohen et al., 1990; Schachter et al., 1986). Neonatal listeriosis and group B streptococcal infection may present either as early disease (within first 2 weeks of life), characterized by pneumonia and/or sepsis, or as late disease, characterized by meningitis. Deafness associated with congenital cytomegalovirus, toxoplasmosis, syphilis, or rubella infection is often not apparent until later in childhood. Similarly, the neurological

Table 3.2. Adverse reproductive outcomes associated with maternal infection[a]

Maternal colonization/organism	Infertility	Abortion	Congenital anomalies	Stillbirth	IUGR	Preterm birth	Neonatal death	Postnatal death	Long-term disability		
									Deafness	Eye disease	Neurologic
Bacterial vaginosis	–	–	–	–	–	+	–	–	–	–	–
Chlamydia	+	–	–	–	–	+	–	–	–	+	–
Coxsackievirus	–	–	–	–	–	–	–	–	–	–	–
Cytomegalovirus	–	–	–	–	+	+	+	+	+	+	+
Echovirus	–	–	–	–	–	+	+	–	–	–	–
Gonorrhoea	+	–	–	–	–	+	–	–	–	+	–
Group B Strep	–	–	–	+	–	+	+	+	–	–	+
Hepatitis A	–	–	–	–	–	–	–	–	–	–	–
Hepatitis B	–	–	–	–	–	–	–	+[b]	–	–	–
Hepatitis C	–	–	–	–	–	–	–	+[b]	–	–	–
Herpes simplex	–	–	–	–	–	+	+	+	–	+	+
HIV	–	–	–	–	±	–	–	+[b]	–	–	±[b]
HPV	–	–	–	–	–	–	–	–	–	–	–
Influenza	–	–	–	–	–	–	–	–	–	–	–
Listeria	–	+	–	+	+	+	+	+	–	–	+
Lyme borreliosis	–	–	–	+	+	±	–	–	–	–	±[b]
Malaria	–	+	–	+	+	+	+	–	–	–	–
Measles	–	–	–	–	+	+	+	+	–	–	–
Mumps	+	±	–	–	–	–	–	–	–	–	–
Parvovirus	–	+	–	+	–	–	–	–	–	–	–
Rubella	–	±	+	+	+	+	+	+	+	+	+
Syphilis	–	+	+	+	+	+	+	+	+	+	+
Toxoplasmosis	–	+	–	+	+	+	–	–	–	+	+
Trichomonas	–	–	–	–	–	+	–	–	–	–	–
Tuberculosis	–	–	–	–	–	–	+	+	–	–	–
Varicella	–	–	+	–	+	+	+	+	–	+	+

± May occur, uncommon.

– Occurs rarely, if at all.

[a] Adapted from Goldenberg et al., 1997, 1999.

[b] Late sequelae (> 1 year of age).

sequelae of fetal/neonatal infections with toxoplasmosis, cytomegalovirus, rubella, herpes virus, group B streptococcus and syphilis are usually not apparent until later in life (Hardy et al., 1984). The most important outcome in HIV-infected neonates, childhood AIDS, does not appear until well after the perinatal period. Perinatal hepatitis B and hepatitis C virus transmission may result in an initial infection, however, chronic hepatitis develops later. Additionally, late sequelae of perinatal hepatitis B infection (cirrhosis and hepatocellular carcinoma) may occur decades later (Sweet, 1990; Snydman, 1985).

Adverse outcome associated with vertical transmission

Many adverse outcomes of pregnancy have been attributed to maternal infection (Table 3.2). Specific definitions of the most important adverse pregnancy outcomes are indicated below for reference. Abortion is defined as removal or expulsion of the fetus from the uterus before the 20th week of gestation. In contrast, a stillbirth is defined as a fetus born at (≥ 20 weeks' gestation with no signs of life present at birth. A live born infant is generally defined as an infant born at any gestational age with a heartbeat or respiratory effort. Death of a live born infant can occur during the neonatal period (in the first 28 days of life, neonatal death) or in the post neonatal period (between 28 days and one year of age, postneonatal death). Infant mortality is defined as the death of a live born baby occurring between birth and one year of age (i.e. sum of neonatal and postneonatal deaths). Perinatal mortality is frequently defined as the sum of stillbirths and neonatal deaths, although other definitions are used. There are many definitions of morbidity, but handicap frequently includes those children with blindness, deafness, cerebral palsy or mental retardation. Mental retardation is usually defined by an IQ cut-off less than 70 or 75 (Allen, 1984).

Infertility/ectopic pregnancy

Reproductive sequelae of maternal infection are not limited to adverse pregnancy outcome. Specifically, gonorrhoeal and chlamydial infections have been associated with both female infertility and ectopic pregnancy. These organisms typically cause localized infection of the urethra, endocervix, and rectum. Infection of the upper genital tract may occur resulting in pelvic inflammatory disease with subsequent fallopian tube damage. Tubal damage in turn results in increased risk for infertility and ectopic pregnancy. The incidence of tubal infertility following one episode of pelvic infection is approximately 12%, with the rate increasing to 23% following two episodes, and 54% after three episodes (Westrom, 1980). Additionally, fallopian tube damage secondary to chlamydia and gonorrhoea infection frequently results in ectopic pregnancy, which complicates nearly

100 000 pregnancies in the USA each year (Lawson et al., 1988). The risk of ectopic pregnancy is increased 6–7 fold in patients with a previous history of pelvic inflammatory disease. In males, mumps infection can result in male infertility. Bacterial vaginosis has also been implicated as a precursor of pelvic inflammatory disease, infertility, and ectopic pregnancy.

Early pregnancy loss

First trimester spontaneous abortion, defined as a spontaneous pregnancy loss before 12 weeks' gestation, complicates an estimated 15–20% of confirmed pregnancies. The majority of pregnancy losses in the first trimester are secondary to chromosomal abnormalities. Spontaneous abortion of a normally developed fetus is rare in the first trimester. Maternal infections such as toxoplasmosis, syphilis, malaria, mumps, listeriosis, and parvovirus have been reported to cause early spontaneous abortion. However, conclusive evidence to support these associations is lacking.

Second trimester abortion ($\geq$ 12–20 weeks' gestation) is a much less common occurrence, complicating only 1–2% of all pregnancies. In contrast to first trimester abortion, second trimester pregnancy loss often occurs in the face of a normally developed fetus. Although second trimester pregnancy losses may be associated with a previous history of second trimester abortion, fetal anomalies, fetal aneuploidy, uterine malformations, incompetent cervix, and uterine leiomyomata, most cases occur secondary to either spontaneous preterm labour, previable rupture of membranes, or fetal demise with subsequent spontaneous delivery. Additional obstetric complications such as twin gestation, placental abruption, antiphospholipid antibody syndrome, and intrauterine growth restriction have also been associated with spontaneous second trimester pregnancy losses. The relative contribution of these aetiologies is not well quantified.

Occult intrauterine infection has been suggested as one possible cause of second trimester pregnancy loss. As mentioned above, preterm labour has been associated with occult upper genital tract infection. Support for this hypothesis comes from the observation that products of conception from spontaneous second trimester pregnancy losses are more frequently found to have histological chorioamnionitis or to be colonized with microorganisms, than comparable material from women with induced abortions. Further research in this area is needed to firmly establish causality.

Congenital anomalies

The baseline rate for congenital anomalies in the general population ranges from 1–3%. Many infections have been associated with congenital anomalies, however, for the majority little conclusive evidence exists to establish causality. Of the organisms listed in Table 3.2, only syphilis, varicella, and rubella have been shown to be associated with increased rates of congenital anomalies. Varicella embryopathy, characterized by skin-scarring, muscle atrophy, hypoplastic extremities, and cortical atrophy, has been reported to complicate approximately 3% of patients with acute varicella infection (≤ 20 weeks' gestation). Congenital rubella, although less common now in areas with routine immunization programmes, formerly was the most common cause of congenital heart disease, and deafness. Congenital syphilis, characterized by skeletal abnormalities, pneumonia, anaemia, hydrops, etc., may develop in 10–50% of infected pregnant women, depending upon the stage of maternal syphilis infection (Vaules et al., 2000).

Stillbirth

Stillbirth complicates approximately 1% of all births in the USA. For women of all ethnic groups, the stillbirth rate has been slowly decreasing over the last three decades, but remains nearly twice as high in African–American than in Caucasian women in the USA. Improvements in prenatal care, medical therapy for hypertension and diabetes mellitus, the use of RhoGam in Rh-negative women, and improved fetal surveillance have led to a significant reduction in term fetal deaths in the last two decades. Because of the reduction in term stillbirths over the last several decades, most stillbirths now occur in the preterm gestational ages. In fact, approximately 80% of stillbirths occur prior to 37 weeks' gestation, with half occurring prior to 28 weeks' gestation (Copper et al., 1994). The aetiology of stillbirth, however, is not always clear. Many of the early gestational age fetuses died in conjunction with spontaneous preterm labour or rupture of the membranes. Placental histologic changes consistent with chorioamnionitis are frequently found in association with early stillbirth. Additionally, patients delivering stillborn fetuses are at higher risk for postpartum endometritis. These findings suggest that intrauterine infection may be a contributing factor in many stillbirths, either through initiating preterm labour, or ruptured membranes, or causing fetal death that ultimately leads to the birth of a stillborn infant. Syphilis, parvovirus, rubella, toxoplasmosis, malaria, Lyme borreliosis, listeriosis, and group B streptococcus are proven causes of stillbirth (Donders et al., 1993; Fletcher & Gordon, 1990; Minkoff et al., 1984).

Intrauterine growth restriction

Fetal growth restriction is generally defined as a birthweight less than the tenth percentile for gestational age. These data need to be cautiously interpreted as the standards used to define the 10th percentile birthweight for gestational age are highly variable and often do not apply to the population being evaluated (Goldenberg et al., 1989). Growth retardation can be caused by low maternal height, low maternal weight, smoking, preeclampsia, congenital anomalies, and intrauterine infection. With changes in obstetric recommendations regarding maternal weight gain over the last decades, the rate of growth retardation appears to be decreasing.

Many infections of the mother and fetus have been associated with growth retardation. Classically, infections such as rubella, toxoplasmosis, cytomegalovirus, varicella, listeriosis, and syphilis, which infect the fetus early in gestation, often result in congenital infection and subsequent growth restriction. For other pathogens, however, there is less evidence on whether an association with growth restriction exists. In developed countries, the majority of cases of growth restriction appear to result from below average maternal size, poor nutritional status, adverse health behaviours, and hypertension, rather than from an infectious source. Growth retardation has been associated in many, but not all, studies with an increased risk of neonatal death and neurological disability (Chard et al., 1993; Low et al., 1982).

Preterm birth

Preterm birth (defined as delivery < 37 weeks' gestation) complicates approximately 10% of all births in the USA. In spite of advances in obstetric care, the rate of prematurity has not changed and may actually have increased slightly in recent decades (Creasy, 1993). As the risk of neonatal mortality and morbidity near term is low, attention has focused on early preterm birth (23–32 weeks' gestation) (Allen et al., 1993). Although preterm birth rates in this gestational age group represent less than 1–2% of all deliveries, this group contributes to nearly 50% of long-term neurological morbidity and to about 60% of perinatal mortality. Spontaneous preterm labour accounts for 40–50% of all preterm births, with the remainder resulting from preterm premature rupture of membranes (25–40%) and obstetrically indicated preterm delivery (20–25%) (Tucker et al., 1991).

Survival of preterm babies is highly dependent on the gestational age at the time of birth (Gilstrap et al., 1985). Neonatal mortality rates also vary greatly based on the availability of neonatal intensive care. In the USA, survival rates of 20–30% have been noted in neonates delivered at 22–23 weeks' gestation. Many of the survivors, however, are often left with long-term neurological impairment (Hack & Fanaroff, 1989; McCormick, 1985). Neonatal survival dramatically improves as gestational age progresses, with over 50% surviving at 25 weeks' gestation, and over 90% by 28–29 weeks gestation (Copper et al., 1993).

There is a growing body of evidence that spontaneous preterm birth, especially ≤ 28 weeks' gestation, is associated with upper genital tract infection (Andrews et al., 1995; Gibbs et al., 1992). Infections of the decidua, fetal membranes, and amniotic fluid have been associated with preterm delivery (Krohn et al., 1991). Chorioamnionitis has been strongly associated with prematurity and extremely low birthweight (≤ 1000 grams) (Guzik & Winn, 1985; Hillier et al., 1988; Mueller-Heubach et al., 1990). Additionally, Hillier et al. (1991), Watts et al. (1992), Cassell et al. (1993), and others have provided evidence that specific organisms, such as *Ureaplasma*, *Mycoplasma*, *Gardnerella*, *Bacteroides*, and *Mobiluncus* species, are associated with histological chorioamnionitis. Further support for this hypothesis is derived from data linking the presence of pathogenic organisms in both the amniotic fluid and chorioamnion with spontaneous labour in otherwise asymptomatic women with intact membranes (Krohn et al., 1991). Women with spontaneous preterm labour are twice as likely to have microbial colonization of the chorioamnion compared to the amniotic fluid (Andrews et al., 1995). Importantly, there is an inverse relationship between a positive chorioamnion or amniotic fluid culture and lower gestational age at delivery in women with spontaneous preterm labour (Cassell et al., 1993). Chorioamnion colonization may account for up to 80% of very early spontaneous preterm births. In contrast, microbial colonization of the upper genital tract appears to play a much less important role in the initiation of parturition at or near term. As previously discussed, bacterial vaginosis is associated with a twofold increase in the rate of preterm delivery. Interestingly, many of the pathogens identified with occult upper genital tract infection are associated with bacterial vaginosis. Thus bacterial vaginosis may be a marker for occult upper genital tract infection.

Many other maternal infections/colonizations have been reported to be associated with preterm birth (Elliot et al., 1990; Berman et al., 1987; Gravett et al., 1986; Hay et al., 1994; Lamont et al., 1986, 1987; Martin et al., 1982; Martius et al., 1988). Nearly all of the organisms identified in Table 3.2 have been associated with preterm birth. One of the difficult questions to answer is whether these relationships are causal or merely associations. Gonorrhoea, chlamydia, *Trichomonas*, syphilis and other genital pathogens are more frequently found in women who have a spontaneous preterm birth. However, the population of women affected by these infections often have other risk factors for preterm birth (low socioeconomic status, malnutrition, smoking, substance abuse, bacterial vaginosis, etc). For example, initial analysis of data from the NICHD/MFM Network Prematurity Prediction Study conducted in the USA, revealed that the presence of chlamydia at 24 weeks' gestation was associated with a twofold increased risk for preterm birth (Andrews et al., 1997). However, after adjusting for other risk factors, this association was no longer significant. These confounding variables make it difficult to establish causality since most studies have not controlled for these variables. Conflicting data exist regarding the relative risk of many of the pathogens noted in Table 3.2. In general, gonorrhoea and chlamydia have been associated with a twofold increased risk for preterm delivery (Sweet et al., 1987, Polk et al., 1989). Similarly, trichomoniasis appears to be associated with a 1.3-fold increased risk for preterm delivery (Cotch et al., 1997; Ross & Van Middelkoop, 1983). Group B streptococcus has been associated with prematurity in some studies, however, the majority of studies demonstrate no association (Hastings et al., 1986; Moller et al., 1984; Regan et al., 1981; Thomsen et al., 1987; White et al., 1984). Many of the other sexually transmitted diseases, such as HIV, hepatitis B, and genital herpes simplex virus, have been associated with an increased risk for spontaneous preterm birth in some, but not most, studies. Syphilis is widely reported to be associated with a twofold increased risk of preterm birth, and this relationship is relatively consistent among most studies.

Neonatal death

Neonatal deaths are defined as deaths occurring within the first 28 days of life. In most western countries, neonatal death occurs at a rate of between 4 and 8 per 1000 live births. Seventy per cent of these deaths are associated with a preterm birth, 25% associated with a major congenital anomaly, with the remainder due to asphyxia, sepsis, meconium aspiration, birth trauma, and rarer conditions such as immune or non-immune hydrops. Infection-related neonatal deaths are a frequent complication of preterm birth. Often infection occurs in the setting of other morbidities associated with prematurity, including respiratory distress syndrome, intraventricular haemorrhage and necrotizing enterocolitis. Group B streptococcus and *E. coli* are common causes of neonatal sepsis (Schuchat et al., 1990; Rouse et al., 1994). However, many other organisms, including those that normally colonize the vagina and those that are acquired in the nursery, have been implicated in sepsis-related neonatal deaths. In addition, infections such as CMV, HSV, rubella, varicella, echovirus, measles, listeriosis, tuberculosis, and syphilis, may result in neonatal or postnatal death, even in the term neonate.

Postneonatal deaths

Postneonatal deaths (defined as deaths occurring after the 27th day of life and before 1 year of age) occur in approximately 3 to 4 infants per 1000 live births in the USA. Sudden infant death syndrome is the most common aetiology. Congenital anomalies, accidents, and infection account for most of the remainder. Infection-related causes of post neonatal mortality include meningitis, pneumonia, and diarrhoea. Although deaths from these causes are rare in middle-class women in western countries, they are more frequently seen in rural areas and among the poor. In less-developed countries, infection may cause up to several hundred deaths per thousand live births. Table 3.2 lists the pathogens which have been associated with postnatal death. Hepatitis B and C virus infections result in an indolent chronic infection that may cause morbidity and mortality well beyond the postnatal period. Similarly, neonatal HIV infection may be asymptomatic during the neonatal and postnatal period, only later developing into AIDS.

Long-term disability

There is a wide range of permanent structural and neurological morbidities that have been associated with maternally transmitted infectious diseases. These include (i) structural congenital anomalies with a defect in one or more organs, (ii) structural or functional damage to the brain resulting in decreased cognitive ability, mental retardation, or both, and (iii) a motor disorder such as a diminution of fine or gross motor skills or an increase in spasticity or athetosis such as that associated with cerebral palsy. These morbidities, in addition to blindness, deafness, and hydrocephalus, have all been associated with infectious diseases (Alberman & Stanley, 1984).

Relating long-term neurologic outcomes to specific birth-related diagnoses is much more difficult than assessment of mortality. These difficulties stem from the lack of sufficient long-term data on these outcomes and the variable definitions in use. Cerebral palsy, defined as a non-progressive motor dysfunction with origin around the time of birth, complicates approximately 2 per 1000 live births. The majority of cases of cerebral palsy do not have a specific identifiable aetiology. Some cases are associated with neonatal infections, such as group B streptococcus, HSV, and CMV. While the majority of cases of cerebral palsy occur in term infants, the relative risk for an early preterm infant developing cerebral palsy is nearly 40 times that of term infants. Approximately 10% percent of surviving newborns born weighing less than 1000 grams will develop cerebral palsy (Alberman & Stanley, 1984).

Intraventricular haemorrhage and periventricular leukomalacia are useful predictors of cerebral palsy in the newborn period (Leviton & Paneth, 1990, Dammann & Leviton, 1997; Roth et al., 1993). The association between intrauterine infection and subsequent development of periventricular leukomalacia, intraventricular haemorrhage, and cerebral palsy is well established (Dammann & Leviton, 1996; Nelson & Ellenberg, 1986; Torfs et al., 1990). Additionally, a clear relationship between both clinical chorioamnionitis and histologic chorioamnionitis with cerebral palsy has been established (Ellenberg & Nelson, 1979). Subsequent studies have confirmed this relationship in both term and preterm infants. The reason for this relationship is not entirely clear, but in preterm infants, towards the end of the second trimester, myelinization of the periventricular pyramidal motor tracks is beginning, making these neurons particularly vulnerable. Intrauterine infection and the various inflammatory cytokines appear to substantially increase the risk of

cell death resulting in 'leukomalacia' and periventricular hemorrhage, and ultimately in cerebral palsy (Yoon et al., 1996; Leviton & Paneth, 1990). Infants born
at the same gestational age, but without evidence of infection, appear to have a
substantially lower risk for periventricular damage and cerebral palsy.

Mental retardation is another outcome measure of great importance, but one
whose prevalence in the population is difficult to determine with certainty.
Difficulties occur due to inconsistencies in definitions, variations in the timing of
testing, and many other factors. Premature neonates, as well as those born with
low birthweight following intrauterine growth restriction, are all at risk for the
development of mental retardation regardless of the definition used. Most
preterm and growth-restricted neonates, however, will eventually have normal IQs
although mean population scores are lower. Perinatal infections such as group B
streptococcus, rubella, varicella, listeriosis, HSV, CMV, syphilis, and toxoplasmosis all are demonstrated causes of mental retardation.

Prevention

Prompt identification and treatment of maternal infection is often essential to
reduce risk for maternal and/or neonatal morbidity and mortality. Access to
medical care and appropriate therapy is essential to achieve this goal. Effective
antimicrobial, antiviral, and antiprotozoal agents are available for many human
pathogens. Prompt treatment of syphilis has been shown to significantly lower risk
for long-term maternal sequelae and for congenital infection (Alexander et al.,
1999). Use of antimalarial agents has also resulted in improved maternal and
neonatal outcomes. Treatment of bacterial vaginosis in patients at high risk has
been shown to effectively reduce risk for preterm delivery (Hauth et al., 1995;
Morales et al., 1994). Routine use of prophylactic antibiotics or silver nitrate in the
infant's eyes following delivery has dramatically reduced long-term ophthalmologic sequelae resulting from chlamydia and gonorrhoea acquired at birth.
Adoption of the 1997 Centers for Disease Control guidelines for screening and
intrapartum treatment of maternal group B streptococcal colonization appears to
have resulted in a decrease in neonatal morbidity and mortality resulting from
neonatal group B streptococcal sepsis and meningitis (Centers for Disease Control
and Prevention, 1996). Similarly, use of antepartum, intrapartum and postpartum
zidovudine (AZT) prophylaxis has been shown to significantly reduce vertical
transmission of HIV (Connor et al., 1994; Rouse et al., 1995).

For some of the infections discussed, no effective treatments are available,
however, active or passive immunization strategies have been shown to be effective. Aggressive public health vaccination efforts have dramatically reduced maternal and neonatal sequelae resulting from rubella and measles. As a result,

congenital rubella, once an important cause of congenital heart disease and deafness, is now rare in developed countries. The recent introduction of the hepatitis B vaccine and varicella vaccine likely will result in similar positive effects on maternal and neonatal health (Centers for Disease Control and Prevention, 1990, 1991). Use of passive immunization, with hepatitis B immunoglobulin (HBIG) and varicella zoster immunoglobulin (VZIG), in the setting of active hepatitis B and a varicella infection, respectively, has been shown to markedly reduce intrapartum transmission. Effective intervention strategies, however, are not available for all potential human pathogens.

Lastly, premature birth resulting from genital tract infection represents a major target for prevention strategies. Since the costs and morbidities associated with preterm birth are high, strategies which identify and eradicate these infections have the potential to achieve a significant reduction in preterm birth and may significantly improve neonatal outcomes and health care expenditures. In a previous publication, we estimated the likely numbers of fetuses or infants born each year in the USA, who die or suffer long-term neurologic damage as a result of direct infection by many of the organisms discussed (Goldenberg et al., 1997, 1999). The range of these postulated direct effects (perinatal mortality and long-term neurologic sequelae) are relatively small, ranging from 800 infants infected with HSV to 1600 infants with group B streptococcus to over 2000 infants annually for syphilis and CMV infection. In contrast, maternal infection with bacterial vaginosis, chlamydia, gonorrhoea, syphilis, and trichomoniasis may result in an excess of 100 000 preterm births. Associated with this excess rate of premature birth, it is likely that more than 5000 infants will die in the perinatal period, with an additional 5000 infants suffering long-term neurologic morbidity. Virtually any strategy which achieves a significant decrease in the preterm birth rate or residual major neurologic handicap will be highly cost effective.

Summary

We have reviewed many of the major human pathogens which have been reported to complicate pregnancy. In addition to addressing specific issues related to common maternal infections, we have also explored the specific types of fetal/neonatal transmission, the various factors which affect such transmission, and the array of adverse pregnancy outcomes attributable to maternal, fetal, and neonatal infection. The reported estimates of disease prevalence, transmission rates, and outcomes demonstrate the scope of the problem related to maternal infection. Although the adverse perinatal outcomes resulting from classic perinatal infections such as syphilis and rubella are important, preterm birth, likely associated with bacterial vaginosis and occult intrauterine infection, probably contributes more to the overall burden of adverse pregnancy outcomes. Finally, we provided a brief discussion of several successful treatment and prevention strategies which have reduced sequelae related to maternal infection during pregnancy.

Acknowledgement

Supported in part by the Agency for Health Care Policy Research Contract No. DHHS 290-92-0055.

REFERENCES

Alberman, E. & Stanley, F. (1984). Guidelines to the epidemiological approach. In *Clinics in Developmental Medicine No. 87, The Epidemiology of the Cerebral Palsies*, ed. F. Stanley & E. Alberman, pp. 27–31. Lavenham, Suffolk: Spastics International Medical.

Alexander, E. R. (1984). Maternal and infant sexually transmitted diseases. *Urol. Clin. North Am.*, 11, 131–9.

Alexander, E. R. & Harrison, H. R. (1983). Role of *Chlamydia trachomatis* in perinatal infection. *Rev. Infect Dis.*, **5**, 713–19.

Alexander, J. M., Sheffield, J. S., Sanchez, P. J., Mayfield, J. & Wendel, G. D. Jr (1999). Efficacy of treatment for syphilis in pregnancy. *Obstet. Gynecol.*, **93**, 5–8.

Alger, L. S., Lovchik, J. C., Hebel, J. R., Blackmon, L. R. & Crenshaw, M. C. (1988). The association of *Chlamydia trachomatis, Neisseria gonorrhoeae*, and group B streptococci with preterm rupture of the membranes and pregnancy outcome. *Am. J. Obstet. Gynecol.*, **159**, 397–404.

Allen, M. C. (1984). Developmental outcome and followup of the small for gestational age infant. *Semin. Perinatol.*, **8**, 123–56.

Allen, M. C., Donohue, P. K. & Dusman, A. E. (1993). The limit of viability – neonatal outcome of infants born at 22 to 25 weeks' gestation. *N. Engl. J. Med.*, **329**, 1597–601.

American College of Obstetricians and Gynecologists. (1992). *Group B streptococcal infections in pregnancy. ACOG Technical Bulletin 170.* Washington, DC: American College of Obstetricians and Gynecologists.

American College of Obstetricians and Gynecologists. (1994). *Gonorrhoea and chlamydial infections. ACOG Technical Bulletin 190.* Washington, DC: American College of Obstetricians and Gynecologists.

Andrews, W. W., Goldenberg, R. L. & Hauth, J. C. (1995). Preterm labor: emerging role of genital tract infections. *Infect. Agents & Dis.*, **4**, 196–211.

Andrews, W. W., NICHD MFMU Network. (1997). The preterm prediction study: association of mid-trimester genital chlamydia infection and subsequent spontaneous preterm birth. *Am. J. Obstet. Gynecol.*, **176**, S55 (Abstract 151).

Armer, T. L. & Duff, P. (1991). Intraamniotic infection in patients with intact membranes and preterm labor. *Obstet. Gynecol. Surv.*, **46**, 589.

Benedetti, T. J., Valle, R. & Ledger, W. J. (1982). Antepartum pneumonia in pregnancy. *Am. J. Obstet. Gynecol.*, **144**, 413–17.

Berman, S. M., Harrison, H. R., Boyce, W. T., Haffner, W. J. J., Lewis, M. & Arthur, J. B. (1987). Low birth weight, prematurity and postpartum endometritis: association with prenatal cervical *Mycoplasma hominis* and *Chlamydia trachomatis* infections. *J.A.M.A.*, **257**, 1189–94.

Cassell, G., Hauth, J., Andrews, W., Cutter, G. & Goldenberg, R. (1993). Chorioamnion colonization: correlation with gestational age in women delivered following spontaneous labor versus indicated delivery. *Am. J. Obstet. Gynecol.*, **168**, 425.

Centers for Disease Control and Prevention. (1990). Protection against viral hepatitis. Recommendations of the Immunization Practices Advisory Committee (ACIP). *M.M.W.R.* **39**, 1–26.

Centers for Disease Control and Prevention. (1991). Hepatitis B virus: a comprehensive strategy for eliminating transmission in the United States through universal vaccination: Recommendations of the Immunization Practices Advisory Committee (ACIP). *M.M.W.R.*, **40**,1–25.

Centers for Disease Control and Prevention. (1996). Prevention of perinatal group B streptococcal disease: a public health perspective. *M.M.W.R.*, **45** (RR-7),1–24.

Chapman, S. & Duff, P. (1993). Varicella in pregnancy. *Semin. Perinatol.*, **17**, 403.

Chard, T., Yoong, A. & Macintosh, M. (1993). The myth of fetal growth retardation at term. *Br, J, Obstet, Gynaecol.*, 100, 1076–81.

Cohen, I., Veille, J. C. & Calkins, B. M. (1990). Improved pregnancy outcome following successful treatment of chlamydial infection. *J.A.M.A.*, **263**, 3160–3.

Connor, E. M., Sperling, R. S., Gelber, R., Kiseles, P., Scott, G., O'Sullivan, M. J., Van Dyke, R., Bey, M., Shearer, W., Jacobson, R. L. et al.(1994). Reduction of maternal-fetal transmission of human immunodeficiency virus type I with zidovudine treatment. *N. Engl. J. Med.*, **331**, 1173–80.

Copper, R. L., Goldenberg, R. L., Creasy, R. K., DuBard, M. B., Davis, R. O., Entman, S. S., Iams, J. D. & Cliver, S. P. (1993). A multicenter study of preterm birth weight and gestational age specific neonatal mortality. *Am. J. Obstet. Gynecol.*, **168**, 78–84

Copper, R. L., Goldenberg, R. L., DuBard, M. B., Davis, R. O. & Collaborative Group on Preterm Birth Prevention (1994). Risk factors for fetal death in white, black and hispanic women. *Obstet. Gynecol.*, **84**, 490–5.

Cotch, M. F., Pastorek, J. G., Nuget, R. P., Hillier, S. L., Gibbs, R. S., Martin, D. H., Eschenbach, D. A., Edelman, R., Carey, J. C., Regan, J. A., Krohn, M. A., Klebanoff, M. A., Rao, A. V. & Rhoads, G. G. (1997). *Trichomonas vaginalis* associated with low birth weight and preterm delivery. *Sex. Transm. Dis.*, **24**, 353–60

Covell, G. (1950). Congenital malaria. *Trop. Dis. Bull.*, **47**, 1147.

Creasy, R. K. (1993). Preterm birth prevention: where are we? *Am. J. Obstet. Gynecol.*, **168**, 1223–30

Cunningham, F. G., Morris, G. B. & Mickal, A. (1973). Acute pyelonephritis of pregnancy: a clinical review. *Obstet. Gynecol.*, **43**, 112.

Dammann, O. & Leviton, A. (1996). Maternal intrauterine infection, cytokines, and brain damage in the preterm newborn. *Pediatr. Res.*, **42**, 1–8.

Dammann, O. & Leviton, A. (1997). The role of perinatal brain damage in developmental disabilities: an epidemiologic perspective. *Ment. Ret. Dev. Dis. Res. Rev.*, **3**, 13–21.

Davis, S. F., Byers, R. H., Lindegren, L. M., Caldwell, M. B., Karon, H. M. & Gwinn, M. (1995). Prevalence and incidence of vertically acquired HIV infection in the United States. *J.A.M.A.*, **274**, 952–5.

De Rossi, A., Ometto, L., Mammano, F., Zanotto, C., Giaquinto, C. & Chieco-Bianehi, L. (1992). Vertical transmission of HIV-1: lack of detectable virus in peripheral blood cells of infected children at birth. *AIDS*, **6**, 1117–20.

Dildy, G. A., Martens, M. G., Faro, S. & Lee, W. (1990). Typhoid fever in pregnancy: a case report. *J. Reprod. Med.*, **35**, 273.

Donders, G. G., Desmyter, J., De Wet, D. H. & Van Assche, F. A. (1993). The association of gonorrhoea and syphilis with premature birth and low birthweight. *Genitourin. Med.*, **69**, 98–101.

Duff, P. (1984). Pyelonephritis in pregnancy. *Clin. Obstet. Gynecol.*, **27**, 17.

Edwards, L. E., Barrada, M. I., Hamann, A. A. & Hakanson, E. Y. (1978). Gonorrhoea in pregnancy. *Am. J. Obstet. Gynecol.*, **132**, 637–41.

Ellenberg, J. & Nelson, K. (1979). Birth weight and gestational age in children with cerebral palsy or seizure disorders. *Am. J. Dis. Child.*, **133**, 1044–8.

Elliott, B., Brunham, R. C., Laga, M., Piot, P., Ndinya-Achola, J. O., Maitha, G., Cheang, M. & Plummer, F. A. (1990). Maternal gonococcal infection as a preventable factor for low birth weight. *J. Infect. Dis.*, **161**, 531–6.

Eschenbach, D. A. (1993). History and review of bacterial vaginosis. *Am. J. Obstet. Gynecol.*, **169**, 441–5.

Eschenbach, D. A., Gravett, M. G., Chen, K. C., Hoyme, U. B. & Holmes, K. K. (1984). Bacterial vaginosis during pregnancy. An association with prematurity and postpartum complications. *Scand. J. Urol. Nephrol.* Suppl. **86**, 213–22.

European Collaborative Study. (1992). Risk factors for mother-to-child transmission of HIV-1. *Lancet*, **339**, 1007–12.

Fiscella, K. (1996a). Race, perinatal outcome, and amniotic infection. *Obstet. Gynecol. Surv.*, **51**, 60–6.

Fiscella, K. (1996b). Racial disparities in preterm births: the role of urogenital infections. *Public Health Rep.*, **111**, 104–13.

Fiumara, N. J., Fleming, W. L., Downing, J. G. & Good, F. L. (1952). The incidence of prenatal syphilis at the Boston City Hospital. *N. Engl. J. Med.*, **247**, 48–52.

Fletcher, J. L. & Gordon, R. C. (1990). Perinatal transmission of bacterial sexually transmitted diseases. Part I: syphilis and gonorrhoea. *J. Fam. Pract.*, **30**, 448–56.

Foulon, W., Villena, I., Stray-Pedersen, B., Decoster, A., Lappalainen, M., Pinon, J. M., Jenum, P. A., Hedman, K. & Naessens, A. (1999). Treatment of toxoplasmosis during pregnancy: a multicenter study of impact on fetal transmission and children's sequelae at age 1 year. *Am. J. Obstet. Gynecol.*, **180**, 410–15.

Fowler, K. B., Stagno, S., Pass, R. F., Britt, W. J., Boll, T. J. & Alford, C. A. (1992). The outcome of congenital cytomegalovirus infection in relation to maternal antibody status. *N. Engl. J. Med.*, **326**, 663–7.

Gibbs, R. S. & Duff, P. (1991). Progress in pathogenesis and management of clinical intraamniotic infection. *Am. J. Obstet. Gynecol.*, **164**, 1317.

Gibbs, R. S., Romero, M. D., Hillier, S. L., Eschenbach, D. A. & Sweet, R. L. (1992). A review of premature birth and subclinical infection. *Am. J. Obstet. Gynecol.*, **166**, 1515–28.

Gilstrap, L. C., III, Hauth, J. C., Bell, R. E., Ackerman, N. B., Yoder, B. A. & Delemos, R. (1985). Survival and short-term morbidity of the premature neonate. *Obstet. Gynecol.*, **65**, 37–41.

Goldenberg, R. L., Cutter, G. R., Hoffman, H., Foster, J. M., Nelson, K. G. & Hauth, J. C. (1989). Intrauterine growth retardation, standards for diagnosis. *Am. J. Obstet. Gynecol.*, **161**, 271–7.

Goldenberg, R. L., Klebanoff, M. A., Nugent, R., Krohn, M. A., Hillier, S. & Andrews, W. W. (1996). Bacterial colonization of the vagina during pregnancy. *Am. J. Obstet. Gynecol.*, **174**, 1618–21.

Goldenberg, R. L., Andrews, W. W., Yuan, A. C., MacKay, H. T. & St. Louis, M. E. (1997). Sexually transmitted diseases and adverse outcomes of pregnancy. *Clin. Perinatol.*, **24**, 23–41.

Goldenberg, R. L., Vermund, S. H., Goepfert, A. R. & Andrews, W. W. (1998). Choriodecidual inflammation, a potentially preventable cause of perinatal HIV-1 transmission. *Lancet*, **352**, 1927–30.

Goldenberg, R. L., Andrews, W. W., Yuan, A., MacKay, T. & St. Louis, M. (1999). Pregnancy outcome related to sexually transmitted diseases. In *Sexually Transmitted Diseases and Adverse Outcomes of Pregnancy*, ed. P. J. Hitchcock, H. T. MacKay, J. N. Wasserheit & R. Binder, pp. 1–24. Washington, DC: ASM Press.

Good, J. T., Iseman, M. D., Davidson, P. T., Lakshminarayan, S. & Sahn SA (1981). Tuberculosis in association with pregnancy. *Am. J. Obstet. Gynecol.*, **140**, 492–8.

Gravett, M. G., Nelson, H. P., DeRouen, T., Crirchlow, C., Eschenbach, D. A. & Holmes, K. K. (1986). Independent associations of bacterial vaginosis and *Chlamydia trachomatis* infection with adverse pregnancy outcome. *J.A.M.A.*, **256**, 1899–903.

Gray, D. J., Robinson, H. B., Malone, J. & Thomson, R. B. Jr. (1992). Adverse outcome in pregnancy following amniotic fluid isolation of *Ureaplasma urealyticum*. *Prenat. Diagn.*, **12**, 111–17.

Guzik, D. S. & Winn, K. (1985). The association of chorioamnionitis with preterm delivery. *Obstet. Gynecol.*, **65**, 11–15.

Gwinn, M., Pappaioanou, M., George, J. R., Hannon, W. H., Wasser, S. C., Redus, M. A., Hoff, R., Grady, G. F., Willoughby, A., Novello, A. C., Petersen, L. R., Dondero, T. J. & Curran, J. W. (1991). Prevalence of HIV infection in childbearing women in the United States. *J.A.M.A.*, **265**, 1704–8.

Hack, M. & Fanaroff, A. A. (1989). Outcomes of extremely-low-birth-weight infants between 1982 and 1988. *N. Engl. J. Med.*, **321**, 1642–7.

Hack, M. & Fanaroff, A. A. (1993). Outcomes of extremely immature infants – a perinatal Dilemma. *N. Engl. J. Med.*, **329**, 1649–50.

Hagay, Z. J., Biran, G., Ornoy, A. & Reece, E. A. (1996). Congenital cytomegalovirus infection, a long-standing problem still seeking a solution. *Am. J. Obstet. Gynecol.*, **174**, 241–5.

Hammed, C., Tejani, N., Verma, U. L. & Archbald, F. (1984). Silent chorioamnionitis as a cause of preterm labor refractory to tocolytic therapy. *Am. J. Obstet. Gynecol.*, **149**, 726–30.

Hanshaw, J.B. (1994). Congenital cytomegalovirus infection. *Pediatr. Ann.*, **23**, 124–8.

Hardy, P. H., Hardy, J. B., Nell, E. E., Graham, D. A., Spence, M. R. & Rosenbaum, R. C. (1984).

Prevalence of six sexually transmitted disease agents among pregnant inner-city adolescents and pregnancy outcome. *Lancet*, **ii**, 333–7.

Harris, J. W. (1919). Influenza occurring in pregnant women. *J.A.M.A.*, **72**, 978–80.

Harrison, H. R., Alexander, E. R., Weinstein, L., Lewis, M., Nash, M. & Sim, D. A. (1983). Cervical *Chlamydia trachomatis* and mycoplasmal infections in pregnancy, epidemiology and outcomes. *J.A.M.A.*, **250**, 1721–7.

Harter, C. A. & Benirschke, K. (1976). Fetal syphilis in the first trimester. *Am. J. Obstet. Gynecol.*, **124**, 705–11.

Hastings, M. J., Easmon, C. S., Neill, J., Bloxham, B. & Rivers, R. P. (1986). Group B streptococcal colonization and the outcome of pregnancy. *J. Infect.*, **12**, 23–9.

Hauth, J. C., Goldenberg, R. L., Andrews, W. W., DuBard, M. B. & Copper, R. L. (1995). Reduced incidence of preterm delivery with metronidazole and erythromycin in women with bacterial vaginosis. *N. Engl. J. Med.*, **333**, 1732–36.

Hay, P. E., Lamont, R. F., Taylor-Robinson, D., Morgan, D. J., Ison, C. & Pearson, J. (1994). Abnormal bacterial colonization of the genital tract and subsequent preterm delivery and late miscarriage. *Br. Med. J.*, **308**, 295–8.

Hill, G. B. (1993). The microbiology of bacterial vaginosis. *Am. J. Obstet. Gynecol.*, **169**, 450–4.

Hill, G. B. (1998). Preterm birth, associations with genital and possibly oral microflora. *Ann. Periodontol.*, **3**, 222–32.

Hillier, S. L., Martius, J., Krohn, M., Kiviat, N., Holmes, K. K. & Eschenbach, D. A. (1988). A case-control study of chorioamnionic infection and histologic chorioamnionitis in prematurity. *N. Engl. J. Med.*, **319**, 972–8.

Hillier, S. L., Krohn, M. A., Kiviat, N. B., Watts, D. H. & Eschenbach, D. A. (1991). Microbiologic causes and neonatal outcomes associated with chorioamnion infection. *Am. J. Obstet. Gynecol.*, **165**, 955–61.

Hillier, S. L. (1993). Diagnostic microbiology of bacterial vaginosis. *Am. J. Obstet. Gynecol.*, **169**, 455–9.

Hopwood, H. G. (1965). Pneumonia in pregnancy. *Obstet. Gynecol.*, **25**, 875–9.

Hulbert, T. V. (1992). Congenital malaria in the United States, report of a case and review. *Clin. Infect. Dis.*, **14**, 922.

Hutto, C., Arvin, A., Jacobs, R., Steele, R., Stagno, S., Lyrene, R., Willett, L., Powell, D., Andersen, R., Werthammer, J., Ratcliff, G., Nahmias, A., Christy, C. & Whitley, R. (1987). Intrauterine herpes simplex virus infections. *J. Pediatr.*, **110**, 97–101.

Judson, F. N. (1985). Assessing the number of genital chlamydial infections in the United States. *J. Reprod. Med.*, **30**, 269–72.

Klebanoff, M., Carey, J. C. & NICHD MFMU Network (1999). Metronidazole did not prevent preterm birth in asymptomatic women with bacterial vaginosis. *Am. J. Obstet. Gynecol.*, **180**, S2 (Abstract 1).

Korn, A. P., Bolan, G., Padian, N., Ohm-Smith, M., Schachter, J. & Landers, D. V. (1995). Plasma cell endometritis in women with symptomatic bacterial vaginosis. *Obstet. Gynecol.*, **85**, 387–90.

Kort, B. A., Cefalo, R. C. & Baker, V. V. (1986). Fatal influenza A pneumonia in pregnancy. *Am. J. Perinatol.*, **3**, 179–82.

Krohn, M. A., Hillier, S. L., Lee, M. L., Rabe, L. K. & Eschenbach, D. A. (1991). Vaginal bacteroides species are associated with an increased rate of preterm delivery among women in preterm labor. *J. Infect. Dis.*, **164**, 88–93.

Krohn, M. A., Hillier, S. L., Nugent, R. P., Cotch, M. F., Carey, J. C., Gibbs, R. S. & Eschenbach, D. A. for the Vaginal Infection and Prematurity Study Group (1995). The genital flora of women with intraamniotic infection. *J. Infect. Dis.*, **171**, 1475–8.

Kurki, T., Sivonen, A., Renkonen, O. V., Savia, E. & Ylikorkala, O. (1992). Bacterial vaginosis in early pregnancy and pregnancy outcome. *Obstet. Gynecol.*, **80**, 173–7.

Lamont, R. F., Taylor-Robinson, D., Newman, M., Wigglesworth, J. & Elder, M. G. (1986). Spontaneous early preterm labour associated with abnormal genital bacterial colonization. *Br. J. Obstet. Gynaecol.*, **93**, 804–10.

Lamont, R. F., Taylor-Robinson, D., Wigglesworth, J., Furr, P. M., Evans, R. T. & Elder, M. G. (1987). The role of mycoplasmas, ureaplasmas and chlamydiae in the genital tract of women presenting in spontaneous early preterm labour. *J. Med. Microbiol.*, **24**, 253–7.

Lawson, H. W., Atrash, H. K., Saftlas, A. F., Franks, A. L., Finch, E. L. & Hughes, J. M. (1988). Ectopic pregnancy surveillance, United States, 1970–1978. *M.M.W.R.*, **39**(SS-4), 9–17.

Leviton, A. & Paneth, N. (1990). White matter damage in preterm newborns – an epidemiologic perspective. *Early Hum. Dev.*, **24**, 1–22.

Lewin, E. B. & Amstey, M. S. (1981). Natural history of group B streptococcus colonization and its therapy during pregnancy. *Am. J. Obstet. Gynecol.*, **139**, 512–15.

Low, J., Galbraith, R., Muir, D., Killen, H., Pater, B. & Karchmar, J. (1982). Intrauterine growth retardation, a study of long-term morbidity. *Am. J. Obstet. Gynecol.*, **142**, 670–7.

Luby, J. P. (1987). Pneumonia in adults due to *Mycoplasma, Chlamydia* and viruses. *Am. J. Med. Sci.*, **294**, 45–64.

Luzuriaga, K. & Sullivan, J. L. (1994). Pathogenesis of vertical HIV-1 infection, implications for intervention and management. *Pediatr. Ann.*, **23**, 159–66.

McCormick, M. C. (1985). The contribution of low birth weight to infant mortality and childhood morbidity. *N. Engl. J. Med.*, **312**, 82–90.

McDonald, H. M., O'Loughlin, J. A., Jolly, P., Vigneswaran, R. & McDonald, P. J. (1991). Vaginal infection and preterm labour. *Br. J. Obstet. Gynecol.*, **98**, 427–35.

McDonald, H. M., O'Loughlin, J. A., Jolly, P., Vigneswaran, R. & McDonald, P. J. (1992). Prenatal microbiological risk factors associated with preterm birth. *Br. J. Obstet. Gynecol.*, **99**, 190–6.

McDonald, H. M., O'Loughlin, J. A., Vigneswaran, R., Jolley, P. T., Harvey, J. A., Bof, A. & McDonald, P. J. (1997). Impact of metronidazole therapy on preterm birth in women with bacterial vaginosis flora (*Gardnerella vaginalis*), a randomised, placebo controlled trial. *Br. J. Obstet. Gynaecol.*, **104**, 1391–7.

McGregor, J. A. & French, J. I. (1991). *Chlamydia trachomatis* infection during pregnancy. *Am. J. Obstet. Gynecol.*, **164**, 1782–88.

Mandelbrot, L., Mayaux, M-J., Bongain, A., Berrebi, A., Moudoub-Jeanpetit, Y., Benifla, J. L., Ciraru-Vigneron, N., Le Chenadec, J., Blanche, S. & Delfraissy, J. F. (1996). Obstetric factors and mother-to-child transmission of human immunodeficiency virus type 1, The French perinatal cohorts. *Am. J. Obstet. Gynecol.*, **175**, 661–7.

Martin, D. H., Koutsky, L., Eschenbach, D. A., Daling, J. R., Alexander, E. R., Benedetti, J. K. & Holmes, K. K. (1982). Prematurity and perinatal mortality in pregnancies complicated by maternal *Chlamydia trachomatis* infections. *J.A.M.A.*, **247**, 1585–8.

Martius, J., Krohn, M. A., Hillier, S. L., Stamm, W. E., Holmes, K. K. & Eschenbach, D. A. (1988). Relationships of vaginal lactobacillus species, cervical *Chlamydia trachomatis*, and bacterial vaginosis to preterm birth. *Obstet. Gynecol.*, **71**, 89–95.

Mason, P. R. & Brown, I. M. (1980). *Trichomonas* in pregnancy. *Lancet*, **ii**, 1025–6.

Mayaux, M. J., Blanche, S., Rouzioux, C., Le Chenadec, J., Chambrin, V., Firtion, G., Allemon, M. C., Vilmer, E., Vigneron, N. C., Tricoire, J., *et al.* (1995). Maternal factors associated with perinatal HIV-1 transmission, The French cohort study – 7 years of follow-up observation. *J. Acquir. Immune Defic. Syndr. Hum. Retrovirol.*, **8**, 188–94.

Meis, P., Goldenberg, R., Iams, J., Mercer, B., Moawad, A., McNellis, D., Roberts, J., Das, A., Copper, R., Thom, E., Johnson, F., Andrews, W. & NICHD MFMU Network (1995). Vaginal infections and spontaneous preterm birth. *Am. J. Obstet. Gynecol.*, **172**, 548.

Minkoff, H., Grunebaum, A. N., Schwarz, R. H., Feldman, J., Cummings, M., Crombleholme, W., Clark, L., Pringle, G. & McCormack, W. M. (1984). Risk factors for prematurity and premature rupture of membranes, a prospective study of the vaginal flora in pregnancy. *Am. J. Obstet. Gynecol.*, **150**, 965–72.

Minkoff, H., Burns, D. N., Landesman, S., Youchah, J., Goedert, J. J., Nugent, R. P., Muenz, L. R. & Willoughby, A. D. (1995). The relationship of the duration of ruptured membranes to vertical transmission of human immunodeficiency virus. *Am. J. Obstet. Gynecol.*, **173**, 585–9.

Moller, M., Thomsen, A. C., Borch, K., Dinesen, K. & Zdravkovic, M. (1984). Rupture of fetal membranes and premature delivery associated with group B streptococci in urine of pregnant women. *Lancet*, **ii(8394)**, 69–70.

Morales, W. J., Schorr, S. & Albritton, J. (1994). Effect of metronidazole in patients with preterm birth in preceding pregnancy and bacterial vaginosis, a placebo-controlled, double-blind study. *Am. J. Obstet. Gynecol.*, **171**, 345–9.

Mueller-Heubach, E., Rubinstein, D. N. & Schwarz, S. S. (1990). Histologic chorioamnionitis and preterm delivery in different patient populations. *Obstet. Gynecol.*, **75**, 622–6.

Mullooly, J. P., Barker, W. H., Nolan, T. F. Jr (1986). Risk of acute respiratory disease among pregnant women during influenza A epidemics. *Public Health Rep.*, **101**, 205–11.

Nadel, D., Hunziker, U. A., Bucher, H. V., Hitzig, W. H. & Duc, G. (1989). Infants born to mothers with antibodies against *Borrellia burgdorferi* at delivery. *Eur. J. Pediatr.*, **148**, 426–7.

Nelson, K. B. & Ellenberg, J. H. (1986). Antecedents of cerebral palsy. Multivariate analysis of risk. *N. Engl. J. Med.*, **315**, 81–6.

Nemir, R. & O'Hare, D. (1985). Congenital tuberculosis, review and diagnostic guidelines. *Am. J. Dis. Child.*, **139**, 284–7.

Newell, M. L. & European Collaborative Study Group (1994). Perinatal findings in children born to HIV-infected mothers. *Br. J. Obstet. Gynaecol.*, **101**, 136–41.

Offenbacher, S., Katz, V., Fertik, G., Collins, J., Boyd, D., Maynor, G., McKaig, R. & Beck, J. (1996). Periodontal infection as a possible risk factor for preterm low birth weight. *J. Periodontol.*, **67**, 1103–13.

Overall, J. C. (1994). Herpes simplex virus infection of the fetus and newborn. *Pediatr. Ann.*, **23**, 131–36.

Oxorn, H. (1955). The changing aspects of pneumonia complicating pregnancy. *Am. J. Obstet. Gynecol.*, **70**, 1057–63.

Polk, B. F., Berlin, L., Kanchanaraksa, S., Munoz, A., Kramer, F., Spence, M., Quinn, T., Hoffman, G., Winn, K., Repke, J., Jones, M. D. Jr, Bartlett, J., Laughon, B., Bobo, L., Hern, J., Kappus, B., Mattern, C. F. T., Brockman, M., Donohue, P., Lievers, V., Wheeler, J., Nugent, R. & Rhoads, G. (1989). Association of *Chlamydia trachomatis* and *Mycoplasma hominis* with intrauterine growth retardation and preterm delivery. *Am. J. Epidemiol,* **129**, 1247–57.

Prober, C. G., Sullender, W. M., Yasukawa, L. L., Au, D. S., Yeager, A. S. & Arvin, A. M. (1987). Low risk of herpes simplex virus infections in neonates exposed to the virus at the time of vaginal delivery to mothers with recurrent genital herpes simplex virus infections. *N. Engl. J. Med.*, **316**, 240–4.

Ray, J. G. (1995) Lues-lues, maternal and fetal considerations of syphilis. *Obstet. Gynecol. Surv.* **50**, 845–9.

Regan, J. A., Chao, S. & James, L. S. (1981). Premature rupture of membranes, preterm delivery, and group B streptococcal colonization of mothers. *Am. J. Obstet. Gynecol.*, **141**, 184–6.

Regan, J. A., Klebanoff, M. A. & Nugent, R. P. (1991). The epidemiology of group B streptococcal colonization in pregnancy. *Obstet. Gynecol.*, **77**, 604–10.

Remington, J. S. & Klein, J. O. (1995). *Infectious Diseases of the Fetus and Newborn Infant*, 4th edn. Philadelphia: W. B. Saunders.

Reyes, M. P., Hunt, N., Ostrea, E. M. Jr & George, D. (1993). Maternal/congenital syphilis in a large tertiary-care urban hospital. *Clin. Infect. Dis.*, **17**, 1041–6.

Reynolds, D. W., Stagno, S., Hosty, T. S., Tiller, M. & Alford, C. A. Jr (1973). Maternal cytomegalovirus excretion and perinatal infection. *N. Engl. J. Med.*, **289**, 1–5.

Ricci, J. M., Fojaco, R. M. & O'Sullivan, M. J. (1989). Congenital syphilis, The University of Miami/Jackson Memorial Medical Center experience, 1986–1988. *Obstet. Gynecol.*, **74**, 687–93.

Riduan, J. M., Hillier, S. L., Utomo, B., Wiknjosastro, G., Linnan, M. & Kandun, N. (1993). Bacterial vaginosis and prematurity in Indonesia, association in early and late pregnancy. *Am. J. Obstet. Gynecol.*, **169**, 175–8.

Romero, R., Sirtori, M., Oyarzun, E., Avila, C., Mazor, M., Callahan, R., Sabo, V., Athanassiadis, A. P. & Hobbins, J. C. (1989). Infection and labor. V. Prevalence, microbiology, and clinical significance of intra-amniotic infection in women with preterm labor and intact membranes. *Am. J. Obstet. Gynecol.*, **161**, 817–24.

Ross, S. M. & van Middelkoop, A. (1983). *Trichomonas* infection in pregnancy – does it affect perinatal outcome? *S. Afr. Med. J.*, **63**, 566–7.

Roth, S. C., Baudin, J., McCormick, D. C., Edwards, A. D., Townsend, J., Stewart, A. L. & Reynolds, E. O. R. (1993). Relation between ultrasound appearance of the brain of very preterm infants and neurodevelopmental impairment at eight years. *Dev. Med. Child. Neurol.*, **35**, 755–68.

Rouse, D. J., Goldenberg, R. L., Cliver, S. P., Cutter, G. R., Mennemeyer, S. T. & Fargason, C. A. Jr (1994). Strategies for the prevention of early-onset neonatal group B streptococcal sepsis, a decision analysis. *Obstet. Gynecol.*, **83**, 483–94.

Rouse, D. J., Owen, J., Goldenberg, R. L. & Vermund, S. H. (1995). Zidovudine for the prevention of vertical HIV transmission, a decision analytic approach. *J. Acquir. Immun. Def. Syndr. Hum. Retrovirol.*, **9**, 401–7.

Rouzioux, C., Costagliola, D., Burgard, M., Blanche, S., Mayaux, M. J., Griscelli, C. & Valleron, A. J. (1995). Estimated timing of mother-to-child human immunodeficiency virus type I (HIV-1) transmission by use of a Markov model. *Am. J. Epidemiol.*, **142**, 1330–7.

Schachter, J., Grossman, M., Sweet, R. L., Holt, J., Jordan, C. & Bishop, E. (1986). Prospective study of perinatal transmission of *Chlamydia trachomatis*. *J.A.M.A.*, **255**, 3374–7.

Schlesinger, P. A., Duray, P. H., Burke, B. A., Steere, A. C. & Stillman, M. T. (1985). Maternal–fetal transmission of the Lyme disease spirochete, *Borrelia burgdorferi*. *Ann. Intern. Med.*, **103**, 67–8.

Schuchat, A., Oxtoby, M., Cochi, S., Sikes, R. K., Hightower, A., Plikaytis, B. & Broome, C. V. (1990). Population-based risk factors for neonatal group B streptococcal disease. Results of a cohort study in metropolitan Atlanta. *J. Infect. Dis.*, **162**, 672–7.

Sehgal, V. M., Siddiqui, W. A. & Alpers, M. P. (1989). A seroepidemiological study to evaluate the role of passive immunity to malaria in infants. *Trans. R. Soc. Trop. Med. Hyg.*, **83**, 105.

Sever, J. L., Larsen, J. W. Jr & Grossman, J. H. (1989). *Handbook of Perinatal Infections*, 2nd edn, Boston: Little, Brown and Company, Inc.

Silverstein, A. M. (1962). Congenital syphilis and the timing of immunogenesis in the human fetus. *Nature*, **194**, 196–7.

Smego, R. & Asperilla, M. O. (1991). Use of acyclovir for varicella pneumonia during pregnancy. *Obstet. Gynecol.*, **78**, 1112.

Snydman, D. R. (1985). Hepatitis in pregnancy. *N. Engl. J. Med.*, **313**, 1398–401.

St Louis, M. E., Kamenga, M., Brown, C., Nelson, A. M., Manzila, T., Batter, V., Behets, F., Kabagabo, U., Ryder, R. W., Oxtoby, M., et al. (1993). Risk for perinatal HIV-1 transmission according to maternal, immunologic, virologic and placental factors. *J.A.M.A.*, **269**, 2853–9.

Stagno, S., Pass, R. F., Cloud, G., Britt, W. J., Henderson, R. E., Walton, P. D., Veren, D. A., Page, F. & Alford, C. A. (1986). Primary cytomegalovirus infection in pregnancy. Incidence, transmission to fetus, and clinical outcome. *J.A.M.A.*, **256**, 1904–08.

Stone, K. M., Brooks, C. A., Guinan, M. E. & Alexander, E. R. (1989). National surveillance for neonatal herpes simplex virus infection. *Sex Transm. Dis.*, **16**, 152–6.

Strobino, B. A., Williams, C. L., Adib, S., Chalson, R. & Spierling, P. (1993). Lyme disease and pregnancy outcome, a prospective study of 2000 prenatal patients. *Am. J. Obstet. Gynecol.*, **169**, 367–74.

Sweet, R. L. (1990). Hepatitis B infection in pregnancy. *Obstet. Gynecol. Rep.*, **2**, 128-39.

Sweet, R. L., Landers, D. V., Walker, C. & Schachter, J. (1987). *Chlamydia trachomatis* infection and pregnancy outcome. *Am. J. Obstet. Gynecol.*, **156**, 824–33.

Thomsen, A. C., Morup, L. & Hansen, K. B. (1987). Antibiotic elimination of group-B streptococci in urine in prevention of preterm labour. *Lancet*, **i(8533)**, 591–3.

Torfs, C. P., van den Berg, B., Oechsli, F. W. & Cummins, S. (1990). Prenatal and perinatal factors in the etiology of cerebral palsy. *J. Pediatr.*, **116**, 615-19.

Tucker, J. M., Goldenberg, R. L., Davis, R. O., Baker, R. C., Winkler, C. L., Hauth, J. C. & Owen, J. (1991). Etiologies of preterm birth in an indigent population. Is prevention a logical expectation? *Obstet. Gynecol.*, **77**, 343-7.

Valeur-Jensen, A. K., Pedersen, C. B., Westergaard, T., Jensen, I. P., Lebech, M., Andersen, P. K., Aaby, P., Pedersen, B. N. & Melbye, M. (1999). Risk factors for parvovirus B19 infection in pregnancy. *J.A.M.A.*, **281**, 1099-105.

Vaules, M. B., Ramin, K. D. & Ramsey, P. S. (2000). Syphilis in pregnancy, a review. *Primary Care Update* for *Obstet. Gynecol.*, **7**, 26–30.

Watts, D. H., Krohn, M. A., Hillier, S. L. & Eschenbach, D. A. (1992). The association of occult amniotic fluid infection with gestational age and neonatal outcome among women in preterm labor. *Obstet. Gynecol.*, **79**, 351-7.

Watts, D. H., Koutsky, L. A., Holmes, K. K., Goldman, D., Kuypers, J., Kiviat, N. B. & Galloway, D. A. (1998). Low risk of perinatal transmission of human papillomavirus, results from a prospective cohort study. *Am. J. Obstet. Gynecol.*, **178**, 365-73.

Wendel, G. D. (1988). Gestational and congenital syphilis. *Clin. Perinatol.*, **15**, 287-303.

Wendel, P. J. & Wendel, G. D. Jr, (1993). Sexually transmitted diseases in pregnancy. *Semin. Perinatol.*, **17**, 443-51.

Westrom, L. (1980). Incidence, prevalence, and trends of acute pelvic inflammatory disease and its consequences in industrialized countries. *Am. J. Obstet. Gynecol.*, **138**, 880.

White, C. P., Wilkins, E. G. L., Roberts, C. & Davidson, D. C. (1984). Premature delivery and group B streptococcal bacteriuria. *Lancet*, **ii(8402)**, 586.

Whitley, R. J. & Hutto, C. (1985). Neonatal herpes simplex virus infections. *Pediatr. Rev.*, **7**, 119.

Whitley, R., Arvin, A., Prober, C., Corey, L., Burchett, S., Plotkin, S., Starr, S., Jacobs, R., Powell, D., Nahmias, A. et al.(1991). Predictors of morbidity and mortality in neonates with herpes simplex virus infections. *N. Engl. J. Med.*, **324**, 450-4.

Yoon, B. H., Romero, R., Kim, C. J., Park, K. H., Hong, S. A., Jun, J. K., Ghezzi, F. & Syn, H. C. (1996). High expression of interleukin-6, interleukin-1β, and tumor necrosis factor-α in periventricular leukomalacia. *Am. J. Obstet. Gynecol.*, **174**, 399.

4

Assessing the scientific value of screening for antenatal infections

Edgardo J. Abalos, A. Metin Gülmezoglu and Guillermo Carroli

Introduction

One of the major, possibly preventable, causes of perinatal mortality and morbidity is infection. Infection during pregnancy is a relatively common occurrence. Although most infections do not have serious consequences on obstetric or perinatal outcomes, some are important causes of fetal and neonatal mortality and morbidity. Adverse consequences on the infant can be either directly due to fetal infection, such as toxoplasmosis, syphilis, rubella or herpes (Charles, 1994; Arias, 1993) or indirectly through another pathology caused by the maternal infection, such as preterm birth (Hillier et al., 1995; Romero et al., 1989; Meis et al., 1995; Smaill. 1998; McGregor et al., 1995). Infections may also cause significant maternal complications (Charles, 1994).

The implementation of any intervention for promoting health care begins with knowledge about the presence or absence of pathological or abnormal conditions that could be prevented through intervention, and detection of these conditions depends on the ability of the method used for that purpose. Thus, diagnosis is a very important component of medical care, and much medical research is carried out to try new methods of diagnosis. When a preventable, treatable, or curable condition is identified a cascade of medical and non-medical interventions is initiated, but not always in a cost-effective way. Cost-effectiveness is a trade-off between cost and medical benefit (Doubilet et al., 1986). Rapid developments in medical technology along with an increasing pressure for cost reduction within the health care system have led to a growing interest in cost-effectiveness analysis in medical literature. Unfortunately, published economic analyses in the obstetrics and gynaecology literature seldom adhere to the recommended standards for methodological assessment (Smith & Blackmore, 1998).

While striving to restrain health care costs, clinicians must focus on the primary goal of providing quality care for women. All analyses of cost containment proposals should begin by asking the following questions: what impact will this have on the quality of women's health care; will this be effective in appropriately containing health care costs and will this simply shift costs to another group or individual? (Committee on Practice Management, 1996). Technology increases in an exponential way, and thousands of new methods for diagnostic or screening proposals are reported in the medical literature each year. Clinicians must decide whether to incorporate these new developments into practice or to regard them as purely of 'academic' interest. A substantial number of diagnostic or screening tests have been accepted in clinical practice before their effectiveness has been demonstrated, whereas in other topics, despite the presence of solid evidence of the benefit of screening and treating patients (Romero et al., 1989; Meis et al., 1995), these findings have not been transferred to clinical practice (Lelekis et al., 1994).

Before introducing a screening test, which will be applied to large numbers of asymptomatic women, firm evidence is required to support the premise that early diagnosis and subsequent therapy or prophylaxis will do more good than harm. A false negative test could miss the opportunity of a prompt treatment, and the chance of the individual to be cured. On the other hand, diagnosis can be wrong, and large numbers of women could be exposed to treatments or other unnecessary procedures, with health, economic and behavioural consequences. Several studies have shown clear links between the intensity of diagnostic testing and subsequent therapy (Wennberg et al., 1996; Verrilli & Welch., 1996). It is worth noting that a policy of screening has to be followed by an intervention (preventive, therapeutic or corrective) of proven efficacy, because the screening itself may have harmful effects (Bastian et al., 1998). For this reason, sound evidence based on systematic reviews of randomized trials showing that early diagnosis and subsequent specific forms of care do more good than harm is required before these tests are introduced in practice (Sackett et al., 1991).

To interpret the validity of diagnostic or screening tests, clinicians must have a basic understanding of the assessment of diagnostic accuracy of the method, on one hand, and the characteristics of the population tested on the other. In this chapter we will focus on the assessment of screening tests before their introduction in clinical practice.

Screening

A screening test is defined as the systematic application of a test or inquiry to identify individuals at sufficient risk of a specific disorder to warrant further investigation or direct preventive action, amongst persons who have not sought medical attention on account of symptoms of that disorder (Gray, 1998). Many of the laboratory tests ordered in outpatient management, and many (if not most) of the tests ordered when patients are admitted to the hospitals are performed as acts of screening (Feinstein, 1985).

The goal of a screening test is to reduce morbidity or mortality from the disease among the people screened; this goal is attained by early treatment of the cases identified. Thus, the objective of screening is the examination of asymptomatic people in order to classify them as likely or unlikely to have the disease. People who appear likely to have the disease are further investigated to arrive at a final diagnosis. Those people who are then found to have the disease are treated (Morrison, 1998). However, the natural history of the disease, and the 'critical point' before which intervention is either more effective or easier to apply as compared to later when the disease is symptomatic, is critical for the evaluation of a screening strategy. To be suitable for control by a programme of early detection, confirmation, and treatment, a disease not only has to be detectable, but early treatment must offer some advantage over later treatment (Sackett et al., 1991).

Cadman et al. (1984) propose some questions as a guide that may help clinicians to decide when, and on which patients they should attempt the early diagnosis of presymptomatic disease:

 (i) Does early diagnosis really lead to improved clinical outcomes? Beneficial effects of the intervention in survival, function, quality of life or all three have to be demonstrated to justify the introduction of any screening strategy. For example, screening for HIV infection during pregnancy leading clinicians to start interventions that reduce the risk of mother-to-child transmission (Thorne et al., 1998).

 (ii) Can you manage the additional clinical time and afford additional tests required to confirm the diagnosis and provide long-term care for those whose screening was positive? Following the previous example, if a patient's screening is positive, additional tests may be required to confirm the presence of the disease. Diagnosis of HIV status has to be followed by an intervention of proven efficacy in order to achieve a specific outcome (in this case a decrease in perinatal transmission) (Thorne et al., 1998; Olaitan et al., 1998). However, in this case interventions to reduce the risk of transmission should be in place for the screening to be beneficial.

 (iii) Will the patients in whom an early diagnosis is achieved comply with your subsequent recommendations and treatment regimens? No programme of early detection and intervention can be effective if patients cannot follow the instructions prescribed. Strategies to ensure that screening results can be followed with the appropriate intervention should be in place when a screening programme is initiated. For example: the feasibility of introducing a same-day screen-and-treat policy should be considered for syphilis screening in rural communities where adequate follow-up and full compliance with treatment is difficult. (Fitzgerald et al., 1998; Narducci et al., 1998).

 (iv) Has the effectiveness of individual components of a periodic health examination or multiphasic-screening programme been demonstrated prior to their combination? A screening procedure usually initiates the series of actions that leads clinicians to reach the final diagnosis. The widespread implementation of untested methods of screening renders their subsequent rigorous evaluation much more difficult, because practitioners and users may have incorporated them into practice. For that reason, each component of this cascade has to be scientifically validated before inclusion as a part of the decision tree.

(v) Does the burden of disability from the target disease warrant action? The disease that is the objective of screening has to be related directly or indirectly with a deleterious perinatal outcome to warrant all the work and expenses of detecting it in a pre-symptomatic stage. For example: one of the risk factors for preterm labour and delivery is urinary tract infection (Romero et al., 1989; Meis et al., 1995), and screening and treatment of asymptomatic bacteriuria (a presymptomatic stage of urinary tract infection) has been demonstrated to be effective in preventing preterm birth (Smaill, 1998). Thus, interventions aimed to detect asymptomatic bacteriuria during pregnancy followed by treatment of positive cases are justified on the basis of this evidence.

(vi) Are the cost, accuracy and acceptability of the screening test adequate for your purpose? Clinicians and policy-makers have to consider this issue before the implementation of any practice, no matter how attractive it may seem. A systematic evaluation of the diagnostic accuracy of the test, with an appropriate assessment of the validity of the studies that report them should be done for each intervention proposed prior to its implementation. Moreover, a cost-effectiveness analysis, and an assessment of satisfaction of users and practitioners are also desirable for the evaluation of the screening strategy.

Critical evaluation of diagnostic or screening tests

Methodological standards have been proposed to evaluate the reports of diagnostic or screening tests (Sackett et al., 1991; Greenhalgh, 1997; Reid et al., 1995). Unfortunately, a substantial amount of published literature indicates that diagnostic tests are still inadequately appraised (Reid et al., 1995). Systematic evaluation of screening or diagnostic tests is the first step in eliminating ineffective tests before widespread application, and the introduction of those that have demonstrated their effectiveness. The following factors should be considered to appraise a screening test and to decide whether to implement it or not:

Usefulness of the test

To be suitable for general use, a programme of early detection and treatment should meet several criteria in addition to reducing morbidity and mortality. Even if diagnostic accuracy of the test or screening procedure was excellent, would it identify a treatable disorder, or any preventable consequence of the disease? If so, would clinicians use it in preference to the currently used test? Is it affordable? Would the individuals consent to it? Would it change the treatment plan or policies of health care (Sackett et al., 1991)? The screening procedures must be convenient and virtually free of discomfort or risk. People must be screened efficiently and economically, positive screens must have appropriate diagnostic studies, and confirmed cases must be treated. The screening programme should lead to a high number of case detections and a reasonably low number of false-positive test results. For example, antenatal screening for hepatitis B allows clinicians to detect infected mothers enabling paediatricians to initiate prompt treatment of newborns with the specific immunoglobulin and hepatitis B vaccine, interventions of proven efficacy (Cunningham et al., 1998; Jordan & Law, 1997).

Reference standard

The best way of determining the diagnostic accuracy of a test is by comparing it with the 'truth'. For all patients in which the test was performed, an appropriate reference standard (gold standard) should be applied to confirm or reject the presence of the disease. A gold standard can be defined as the method, procedure or measurement that is widely accepted as being the best available against which new interventions should be compared (Last, 1988). The biggest problem in selecting a definitive standard, however, occurs when conclusive evidence cannot be obtained. This problem could be resolved by applying a different type of procedure (such as an expert consensus), or letting the diagnosis be confirmed or refuted by the subsequent clinical course. For example, quantitative cultures have been defined as the reference standard for detecting the presence of bacteria in urine samples (Millar & Cox, 1997; Patterson & Andriole, 1997; Andrews et al., 1990). However, urine culture cannot be viewed as a precise quantitative assay in diagnosing urinary tract infections, since many clinical, microbiologic and technical conditions may result in a relatively low quantitative yield of pathogenic microorganisms. It is only one of the factors in making that diagnosis (Kellogg et al., 1987; Pollock, 1983).

Spectrum composition

If the spectrum of tested individuals is not specified, the reported indices of accuracy (sensitivity, specificity or likelihood ratios) may have limited clinical applicability. For example: diagnostic test studies sometimes enrol diseased patients who are symptomatic or have severe disease, some of which are on treatment, and some are not. These tests are often offered as mass screening tests, and when later applied to general population, they can be misleading. If the test is to be used as a screening procedure for discovering disease in asymptomatic individuals, it is not possible to rely on indices of sensitivity, specificity, or likelihood ratios calculated from results found in symptomatic hospitalized patients. In other words, a single test may have different diagnostic accuracy depending on the degree of the illness in which the test was performed (Lachs et al., 1992).

Analysis of pertinent subgroups

Even if the spectrum of evaluated individuals has been adequately described, the indices of accuracy represent average values for the entire group. These indices may vary in different subgroups (determined by their own characteristics such as age or some other particular criteria), and the test may do well in certain groups and poorly in others. One good example is the different ability of a dipstick test for detecting urinary tract infection when it is performed on asymptomatic or symptomatic individuals (Lachs et al., 1992).

Avoidance of work-up bias

When individuals are referred to receive the gold standard procedure only depending on the test result that is being studied, work-up or verification bias occurs. If the test is positive, the clinician may look intensely for the disease, thereby ordering the definitive diagnostic procedure, which is rarely ordered if the test is negative. These selective decisions in ordering definitive procedures are more common if the test to be ordered is non-invasive, cheap, or easy to perform.

Avoidance of review bias

Review bias can be introduced if either the screening test or the gold standard procedure is appraised without precautions to achieve objectivity in their sequential interpretation. If the screening test is done first, knowledge of its result may have a falsely high rate of agreement when the gold standard procedure is subsequently interpreted. In either direction, review bias can lead to falsely higher indices of accuracy, but can be avoided if persons unaware of the results of the other test interpret the diagnostic test and the gold standard procedure separately and objectively. For example, those indeterminate or equivocal results could be falsely interpreted as positive if the person in charge of their reading knows that the test performed was positive. This is one of the reasons why some tests reported as highly effective in medical literature show very low diagnostic accuracy when applied in clinical practice.

Test result	Target condition	
	Present	Absent
Positive	a	b
Negative	c	d

Sensitivity = a/a+c
Specificity = d/b+d
Prevalence = (a+c)/(a+b+c+d)
Positive predictive value = a/a+b
Negative predictive value = d/c+d
Positive likelihood ratio (LR+) = sensitivity / 1-specificity
Negative likelihood ratio (LR−) = 1-sensitivity/specificity

Figure 4.1   Determining diagnostic accuracy.

Determine diagnostic accuracy of the test

Clinical usefulness of a diagnostic test is mainly determined by its precision in identifying the target disease. Traditionally, diagnostic accuracy of a test has been reported using measures such as sensitivity (defined as the probability of a positive test result in diseased patients), specificity (the probability of a negative test result in healthy individuals), positive predictive value (the probability of disease in a patient with a positive test result), or negative predictive value (the probability of no disease in an individual with a negative test result). (See Fig. 4.1.)

Sensitivity and specificity have some limitations. In clinical practice the test result is all that is known, and the interest of clinicians is to know what proportion of patients with abnormal test results are truly abnormal. These measures do not give this information. The probability of the test in giving the correct diagnosis (whether is it positive or negative) is reflected in the predictive values, but these measures are strongly affected by prevalence.

An alternative to describe test performance is to specify the likelihood ratios of a positive and a negative test result. The likelihood ratio is defined as the odds that a given finding would occur in an individual with, as opposed to without, the target disorder or condition. The likelihood ratio of a positive test result (LR+) is the probability of a positive test in a patient with the disease divided by the probability of a positive test in a patient without the disease. The likelihood ratio of a negative test result (LR−) is the probability of a negative test in a patient with the disease divided by the probability of a negative test in a patient without the disease (Sackett et al., 1991; Mulley & Silverstein 1988; Jaeschke et al., 1994; Altman, 1991). It can easily be calculated from the sensitivity and specificity of a diagnostic test (LR+ = sensitivity/[1-specificity], and LR− = [1-sensitivity] / specificity) (Sackett et al., 1997).

For example, a diagnostic method is applied to a patient with a suspected disease (the pretest probability) and the likelihood ratios estimated for that test are known. The application of the likelihood ratio to that probability leads the clinician to rank the patient in another category. Depending on the test result being positive or negative, the possibility of having the disease would be higher or lower, respectively (the post-test probability). If the probability of having the disease remains unchanged after its application, the test is not helpful in reaching the diagnosis. The use of likelihood ratios offers several distinct advantages. First, it is not affected by the prevalence of disease. Secondly, different likelihood ratios can be calculated for different test result intervals with lower and higher ratios for milder and more severe degrees of test abnormality. Thirdly and lastly, it is easy in revising probabilities that can be performed sequentially, so the post-test probability from one diagnostic test becomes the pre-test probability for the next, and combine clinical judgement with laboratory science (Mulley & Silverstein 1988; Moore, 1998).

Precision of results of test accuracy

The indices of accuracy expressed as sensitivity, specificity, or likelihood ratios can be unreliable if too few patients have been evaluated. Quantitative uncertainty can be appraised from confidence intervals, which progressively narrow as sample size increases. Confidence intervals can be defined as the range within which the 'true' value is expected to lie with a given degree of certainty (Last, 1988). Confidence intervals are important in providing the level of uncertainty from clinical investigations, especially when comparing data from different populations or sites. As with other epidemiological studies, the calculation of an appropriate sample size is critical for achieving meaningful results in research studies designed to evaluate diagnostic or screening tests. Recommendations for determining appropriate sample sizes for screening tests have been published (Arkin & Wachtel, 1990; Simel et al., 1991; Buderer 1996).

Presentation of indeterminate test results

The frequency of unclear results (indeterminate, equivocal or non-diagnostic) in a new diagnostic test is very important, if the test is to be clinically useful. Cost-effectiveness is reduced if additional diagnostic evaluations are needed frequently. The indices of accuracy are compromised or distorted if the results are presented only in terms of a dichotomous, unequivocally positive or negative diagnostic or gold standard test. The frequency of indeterminate results and the way these results are used in the calculation of the test performance represent critical, important information for assessing the clinical effectiveness of the test.

Test reproducibility

Because of the variation in laboratory procedures or observers' judgement, the test may not consistently yield the same result when repeated. If the test requires observer interpretation, reproducibility is particularly important. Authors have to specify if the test has inter- or intraobserver variability, and how they tried to resolve that. Every aspect of the test that can influence its performance should be described in detail, including references to laboratories, measures, dilutions, proportions, timing, etc.

Systematic reviews of screening or diagnostic tests

Because of the exponentially increasing amount of existing information in health care, it is hard, and sometimes impossible, for clinicians to read and appraise all reports relating to a single clinical question. Thus clinicians, researchers and policy-makers need an efficient method that allows them to integrate the available information for a rational decision-making. A systematic review is a thorough review of the literature about a clearly defined question, performed by using a systematic and explicit method to identify, select and critically assess relevant studies. Statistical methods (meta-analysis) may or may not be used to analyse or summarize the data coming from primary studies.

Although systematic reviews of randomised controlled trials are widely used to summarize the effectiveness of interventions, the methodology can be applied to all types of epidemiological studies. In preparing a systematic review, it is useful to start with a protocol as in any other research project. The protocol for a systematic review states the objectives, the participants, the outcomes of the review, and the methods of searching, appraising and including the primary studies. In doing so, the reviewer avoids bias that may creep in by looking at the results of the primary studies.

Systematic reviews are potentially useful for the assessment of the diagnostic accuracy of a screening or diagnostic test as well as evaluating effectiveness of interventions. By the use of systematic reviews, it becomes possible to provide an overall summary of diagnostic accuracy; to determine whether estimates of diagnostic accuracy depend on the study design characteristics (study validity) of the primary studies and whether diagnostic accuracy differs in subgroups defined by the characteristics of the patients and tests; and to identify areas for further research (Irwig et al., 1994). Guidelines to help readers appraise systematic reviews of diagnostic or screening tests have been published (Irwig et al., 1994).

The methods of systematic reviews of diagnostic or screening tests are similar to those of randomized controlled trials but some modifications are needed.

Determine the objectives and scope of the systematic review

The objectives of the review should be clearly presented. It is important to clarify if the aim of the review is to assess the diagnostic accuracy of a test used for mass screening, or as a confirmatory test. Once the objective of the systematic review is clearly stated, then the participants of the studies, the characteristics of the test(s) to be studied and the outcome of interest for the systematic review should be established. Characteristics of the participants of primary studies are essential because the usefulness of the test would be different if it was performed in the general population from outpatient clinics, or if its efficacy was assessed in a sample of patients with some particular conditions. The test of interest has to be defined, and its results have to be compared with those obtained using an appropriate and defined reference standard. An example of how to structure a systematic review of a screening test is given in Table 4.1 using asymptomatic bacteriuria screening during pregnancy as an example.

Retrieve relevant literature

In order to find the relevant publications a comprehensive search should be conducted. The search strategy should be explicit so that the readers of the review can see both the search terms used and the databases searched. Search strategies usually include computerized bibliographic systems (such as Medline, Embase, Lilacs, the Cochrane Controlled Trials Register), hand-searching of appropriate journals, identification of studies using the reference lists of studies already obtained, and personal contact with authors or experts in the field (Sackett et al., 1991, 1997). Assistance from a librarian can be useful to develop the search terms. A comprehensive search strategy is common to all systematic reviews, but some specific rules related to diagnostic tests, screening and prognosis to be taken into account have been reported (McKibbon & Walker-Dilks, 1994). Efforts should be made to look for unpublished studies and search the grey literature to avoid publication bias (Egger & Smith, 1998). Inclusion and exclusion criteria for eligible articles have to be formally reported, to make it replicable, and reporting the reason for exclusion of potentially eligible papers helps readers understand how the criteria were applied.

Extract and present the data

The methodological quality of papers identified in a systematic review is assessed and reported systematically. Usually, two or more reviewers extract this information independently from each article, and disagreements between them are resolved in a prespecified way. Characteristics of each primary study (included or not) are reported to allow other readers or researchers to decide if they agree with the judgements made or not. Table 4.2 summarizes the characteristics of studies identified in the review of reagent strips.

Table 4.1. A systematic review of the diagnostic accuracy of rapid reagent strips for diagnosing asymptomatic bacteriuria during pregnancy: the review protocol

Objective	To evaluate the diagnostic accuracy of rapid reagent strips for diagnosing asymptomatic bacteriuria during pregnancy
Types of studies	Prospective case series
Participants	Asymptomatic pregnant women
Interventions	Nitrite and leukocyte esterase reagent strips
	Gold standard: quantitative urine culture
Outcome	Indicators of the presence of bacteriuria in strips

From Abalos, 1998.

Estimate diagnostic accuracy

In general terms, when estimating separately the mean sensitivity and specificity of a diagnostic or screening test, accuracy could be underestimated, even if they have been weighted in the same way for the sample size of each study. This is common because different studies are likely to use different explicit or implicit thresholds (cut-off point or positivity criterion) (Irwig et al., 1994). A likelihood ratio at each possible value of a multicategory or continuous test to get a result-specific likelihood ratio can be estimated thus avoiding the need to decide on a single cut-off value dichotomising a test as positive or negative (Sackett et al., 1991). Summary likelihood ratios or summary receiver operating characteristic curves can be estimated extracting the data from each primary study (Irwig et al., 1994).

Assess the effect of variation in study validity on estimates of diagnostic accuracy

The reliability of the overall assessment of diagnostic accuracy of a method depends on the quality of primary studies. If the quality of included studies is high, it may be possible to provide a bias-free overall estimate of accuracy. The most important sources of bias in assessing diagnostic accuracy are the lack of an appropriate reference standard, absence of independent observations, and verification bias. Obtaining diagnostic accuracy information from different primary studies could be particularly difficult in conducting systematic reviews. Integration of different types of evidence within a single review needs a careful judgement; differences in diagnostic accuracy may reflect differences in study characteristics that are unlikely to be adequately controlled by using statistical adjustments in the meta-analysis. Heterogeneity among studies may exist at one or more levels. Different outcome measures are used in different studies, and similar outcomes are sometimes measured or reported differently. Various study designs could be used, and heterogeneity of methodological features occurs within a given design (Murlow et al., 1997). Sometimes overall results can be adjusted by these sources

Table 4.2. A systematic review of the diagnostic accuracy of rapid reagent strips for diagnosing asymptomatic bacteriuria during pregnancy: description of studies

Number of potentially eligible studies	16
Excluded	10
Reasons for exclusion	Different inclusion criteria (symptomatic (4), puerperal (1), high-risk (1)), another gold standard (4), work-up bias (2)
Included	All were conducted in developed countries between 1984 and 1998, sample sizes ranged from 65 to 1047 patients (overall 3341)
Other relevant information	Prevalence of disease ranged from 2.3% to 9.3%
	Socio-economic status of women was low, middle and high (described in three studies). Gestational age ranged from 9 to 17 weeks (presented in other three)

From Abalos, 1998.

of bias, and sometimes heterogeneity is such that the combination of the studies selected for the review may be inappropriate.

By preparing a systematic review protocol *a priori*, which states the types of studies that will be included and minimum methodological quality criteria that a study should meet introduction of bias to the systematic review can be avoided. The standards for study validity were met only in a few studies included in the review given as examples (Table 4.3).

Assess the effect of variation in the characteristic of patients and test on estimates of diagnostic accuracy (generalizability)

Valid estimates of diagnostic accuracy of a test applied in a given sample of patients may not be applicable to another population, and this could be caused by particular characteristics of the patients, or of the test, or both. Baseline conditions of patients in each primary study and the technical details of the screening method used should be described clearly. The technical details of tests may vary from one setting to another and limit generalizability. Study participants are often drawn from various settings and have a wide spectrum of baseline risk, disease severity and socio-demographic and cultural characteristics. Heterogeneity may allow reviewers to examine consistency of findings across studies of various types and their applicability in a variety of patients and settings (that is, it would be analysed as a source of variation that may increase generalizability). However, it may induce ambiguity into the synthesis of evidence and could limit the strength of the conclusions of the review (Murlow et al., 1997). Sometimes defined characteristics

Table 4.3. A systematic review of the diagnostic accuracy of rapid reagent strips for diagnosing asymptomatic bacteriuria during pregnancy: Methodological quality of included studies

Gold standard	Quantitative urine culture. Described in all studies
Work-up bias	Avoided in all studies
Review bias	Avoided only in two studies
Sample size	Estimation of sample size was not described in any of the studies
Results	Presented in all studies as positive and negative test results
Test reproducibility	Technical details of the method was described in all studies

From Abalos (1998).

of patients are very important for the assessment of a test performance. The same test could be strongly recommended for some patients, and discouraged for others (Columbia Presbyterian Medical Center, 1997). The reagent strips used as screening method for bacteriuria during pregnancy have to be assessed in a population of asymptomatic pregnant women. The results obtained from the evaluation of the method in the general population (with its wide spectrum) cannot be extrapolated to this specific subgroup, because conclusions about the efficacy of the test can be misleading.

Key points

A screening test should meet scientific and ethical criteria before widespread use among healthy people. Medical screening aims to identify those people who may have a previously unrecognized disease, or who are at risk of developing it. Practitioners' attitudes to the disease vary in order to achieve specified screening targets: some screening policies would be voluntary, while other programmes would be mandatory. Some diseases carry greater social and psychological stigma than others, and implications related to prospects for treatment, lifestyle, and long-term outcomes detected after applying a screening policy could be different (Bastian et al., 1998). Furthermore, inappropriate screening strategies may also entail a serious waste of resources.

It can be argued that improving person-centred outcomes (survival, quality of life) is the ultimate purpose of using a test. Therefore, the effect of testing on outcomes can be reliably assessed by randomized-controlled trials. It seems appropriate to assess whether the use of tests to detect conditions for which there is evidence that intervention is effective leads to improved outcomes. Because randomized trials and double-blind procedures have seldom been used for evaluating the value of screening or diagnostic tools, the compared groups and the accuracy of compared data can often be distorted by biases that occur when the tests are obtained in ordinary clinical activities. The advantages of large randomized trials are well known. The most important is that potential confounding factors will tend to be distributed equally between the screened and control groups as a result of the random allocation of subjects, if enough subjects are enrolled and successfully retained. Therefore, a properly conducted randomised study with high follow-up can provide a valid estimate of the gains that can be achieved by screening (Morrison, 1998).

REFERENCES

Abalos, E. J. (1998). Review of two rapid screening tests for asymptomatic bacteriuria during pregnancy. *Eighth Post-Graduate Course for Training in Reproductive Medicine and Reproductive Biology*, Geneva, Switzerland. MatWeb home page: http://matweb.hcuge.ch/matweb/

Altman, D. G. (1991). *Practical Statistics for Medical Research*, 1st edn. London: Chapman & Hall.

Andrews, W., Cox, S. & Gilstrap, L. C. (1990). Urinary tract infections in pregnancy. *Int. Urogynecol. J.*, **1**, 155–63.

Arias, F. (1993). Congenital infections. In *Practical Guide to High-Risk Pregnancy and Delivery*. 2nd edn, ed. F. Arias, pp. 354–81. London: Mosby Year Book, Inc.

Arkin, C. F. & Wachtel, M. (1990). How many patients are necessary to assess test performance? *J.A.M.A.*, **263**, 275–8.

Bastian, H., Keirse, M. N. J. C., Middleton, P. & Searle, J. (1998). Influencing people's experiences of screening (Protocol for a Cochrane Review). In *The Cochrane Library*, Issue 4. Oxford: Update Software.

Buderer, N. M. (1996). Statistical methodology: I. Incorporating the prevalence of disease into the sample size calculation for sensitivity and specificity. *Acad. Emerg. Med.*, **3**, 895–900.

Cadman, D., Chambers, L., Feldman, W., & Sackett, D. (1984). Assessing the effectiveness of community screening programs. *J.A.M.A.*, **251**, 1580.

Charles, D. (1994). In *Obstetric and Perinatal Infections*, 1st edn., ed. J. P. Stanford, D. A. J. Tyrrell, T. H. Weller & S. M. Wolff. London: Mosby-Year Book.

Columbia Presbyterian Medical Center (1997). Clinical Preventive Services, 2nd edn. *Infectious Diseases. Screening for Asymptomatic Bacteriuria*. CPMC net: http://cpmcnet.columbia.edu/texts/gcps/gcps0041.html.

Committee on Practice Management (1996). Cost containment in medical care. Committee opinion. *A. C. O. G.*, **171**, 1–2.

Cunningham, R., Northwood, J. L., Kelly, C. D., Boxall, E. H. & Andrews, N. J. (1998). Routine antenatal screening for hepatitis B using pooled sera: validation and review of ten year experience. *J. Clin. Pathol.*, **51**, 392–5.

Doubilet, P., Weinstein, M. C. & McNeil, B. J. (1986). Use and misuse of the term 'cost-effective' in medicine. *N. Engl. J. Med.*, **314**, 253–6.

Egger, M. & Smith, G. D. (1998). Meta-analysis. Bias in location and selection of studies. *B.M.J.*, **316**, 61–6.

Feinstein, A. R. (1985). Diagnostic and spectral markers. *Clinical Epidemiology*, Chap. 25, pp. 597–631. Philadelphia: W. B. Saunders.

Fitzgerald, D. W., Behetsm F. M., Lucet, C. & Roberfroid, D. (1998). Prevalence, burden, and control of syphilis in Haiti's rural Artibonite region. *Int. J. Infect. Dis.*, **2**, 127–31.

Gray, J. A. M. (1998). Screening. *Evidence Based Health Policy Managem.*, **2**, 85–6.

Greenhalgh, T. (1997). Papers that report diagnostic or screening tests. *B. M. J.*, **315**, 540–3.

Hillier, S. L., Nugent, R. P., Eschenbach, D. A., Krohn, M. A., Gibbs, R. S., Martin, D. H., Cotch, M. F., Edelman, R., Pastorek, II J. G., Vijaya Rao, A., McNellis, D., Regan, J. A., Carey, J. C. & Klebanoff, M. A. (1995). Association between bacterial vaginosis and preterm delivery of a low-birth-weight infant. *N. Engl. J. Med.*, **333**, 1737–42.

Irwig, L., Tosteson, A., Gatsonis, C., Lau, J., Colditz, G., Chalmers, T. & Monsteller, F. (1994). Guidelines for meta-analyses evaluating diagnostic tests. *Ann. Intern. Med.*, **120**, 667–76.

Jaeschke, R., Guyatt, G. H. & Sackett, D. L. (1994). Users' Guides to the medical literature. II. How to use an article about a diagnostic test. B. What are the results and will they help me in caring for my patients? *J.A.M.A.*, **271**, 703–7.

Jordan, R. & Law, M. (1997). An appraisal of the efficacy and cost effectiveness of antenatal screening for hepatitis B. *J. Med. Screening*, **4**, 117–27.

Kellogg, J. A., Manzella, J. P., Shaffer, S. N. & Schwartz, B. B. (1987). Clinical relevance of culture versus screens for the detection of microbial pathogens in urine specimens. *Am. J. Med.*, **83**, 739–45.

Lachs, M. S., Nachamkin, I., Edelstein, P. H., Goldman, J., Feinstein, A. R. & Schwartz, J. S. (1992). Spectrum bias in the evaluation of diagnostic tests: lessons from the rapid Dipstick Test for urinary tract infection. *Ann. Int. Med.*, **117**, 135–40.

Last, J. M. (1988). *A Dictionary of Epidemiology*, 2nd edn. Oxford: Oxford University Press.

Lelekis, M., Economou, E., Adamis, G., Gargalianos, P. & Kosmidis, J. (1994). Asymptomatic bacteriuria of pregnancy: do obstetricians bother? *J. Chemother*, **6**, 58–60.

McGregor, J. A., French, J. I., Parker, R., Draper, D., Patterson, E., Jones, W., Thorsgard, K. & McFee, J. (1995). Prevention of premature birth by screening and treatment for common genital tract infections: results of a prospective controlled evaluation. *Am. J. Obstet. Gynecol.*, **173**, 157–67.

McKibbon, K. A. & Walker-Dilks, C. J. (1994). Beyond ACP journal club: how to harness MEDLINE for diagnostic problems. *ACP Journal Club*, Sep/Oct 94, A10–A12.

Meis, P., Michielutte, R., Peters, T., Wells, H. B., Sands, R. E., Coles, E. C. & Johns, K. A. (1995). Factors associated with preterm birth in Cardiff, Wales. II. Indicated and spontaneous preterm birth. *Am. J. Obstet. Gynecol.*, **173**, 597–602.

Millar, L. K. & Cox, S. M. (1997). Urinary tract infections complicating pregnancy. *Infect. Dis. Clin. N. Am.*, **11**, 13–26.

Moore, R. A. (1998). On the need for evidence-based clinical biochemistry. *Evidence Based Medicine*, Jan–Feb, 7–8.

Morrison, A. S. (1998). Screening. In *Modern Epidemiology, 2nd edn,* ed. K. J. Rothman & S. Greenland, pp. 499–518. Lippincott-Raven.

Mulley, A. G. Jr & Silverstein, M. (1988). Clinical decision analysis. In *Data Analysis for Clinical Medicine: The Quantitative Approach to Patient Care in Gastroenterology.* 1st edn. ed. T. Chalmers, pp. 49–64. Via Udine 32–40, 00161 Rome, Italy: International University Press.

Murlow, C., Langhorne, P. & Grimshaw, J. (1997). Integrating heterogeneous pieces of evidence in systematic reviews. *Ann. Intern. Med.,* **127**, 989–95.

Narducci, F., Switala, I., Rajabally, R., Decocq, J. & Delahousse, G. (1998). Syphilis maternelle et congenitale. *J. Gynecol. Obstet. Biol. Reprod. Paris,* **27**, 150–60.

Olaitan, A., Madge, S., Jones, M. & Johnson, M. (1998). Reducing the vertical transmission of HIV. Screening programme has not failed (letter). *B.M.J.,* **316**, 1900–1.

Patterson, T. F. & Andriole, V. T. (1997). Detection, significance and therapy of bacteriuria in pregnancy. *Infect. Dis. Clin. N. Am.,* **11**, 593–608.

Pollock, H. (1983) Laboratory techniques for detection of urinary tract infection and assessment of value. *Am. J. Med.,* **75**, 79–84.

Reid, M. C., Lachs, M. S. & Feinstein, A. R. (1995). Use of methodological standards in Diagnostic test research. Getting better but still no good. *J.A.M.A.,* **274**, 645–51.

Romero R., Oyarzún, E., Mazor, M., Sirtori, M., Hobbins, J. & Bracken, M. (1989). Meta-Analysis of the relationship between asymptomatic bacteriuria and preterm delivery/low birth weight. *Obstet. Gynecol.,* **73**, 576–82.

Sackett, D. L., Haynes, R. B., Guyatt, G. H. & Tugwell, P. (1991). *Clinical Epidemiology. A Basic Science for Clinical Medicine.* 2nd edn. Boston: Little Brown.

Sackett, D. L., Richardson, W. S., Rosenberg, W. & Haynes, R. B. (1997). *Evidence-based Medicine. How to Practise and Teach EBM.* 1st edn. London: Churchill Livingstone.

Simel, D. L., Samsa, G. & Matchar, D. B. (1991). Likelihood ratios with confidence: sample size estimation for diagnostic test studies. *J. Clin. Epidemiol.,* **44**, 763–70.

Smaill, F. (1998). Antibiotic versus no treatment for asymptomatic bacteriuria during pregnancy. *Pregnancy and Childbirth Module. The Cochrane Database of Systematic Reviews.* Updated 1997. Issue 4, 1998. Oxford: Update Software.

Smith, W. J. & Blackmore, C. C. (1998). Economic analyses in obstetrics and gynecology: a methodologic evaluation of the literature. *Obstet. Gynecol.,* **91**, 472–8.

Thorne, C. Newell, M. L., Bailey, A. & Peckham, C. S. (1998). The European Collaborative Study. Therapeutic and other interventions to reduce the risk of mother-to-child transmission of HIV-1 in Europe. *Br. J. Obstet. Gynaecol.,* **105**, 704–9.

Verrilli, D. & Welch, H. G. (1996). The impact of diagnostic testing on therapeutic interventions. *J.A.M.A.,* **275**, 1189–91.

Wennberg, D. E., Kellett, M. A., Dickens, J. D., Malenka, D. J., Keilson, L. M. & Keller, R. B. (1996). The association between local diagnostic testing intensity and invasive cardiac procedures. *J.A.M.A.,* **275**, 1161–4.

Part II

Specific infections

5

Rubella infection in pregnancy

Desmond Martin and Barry Schoub

Introduction

Rubella virus belongs to the rubivirus genus of the family Togaviridae, for which humans are apparently the only host. Rubella is an enveloped single-stranded RNA virus which is relatively fragile, multiplies in and is transmitted from the respiratory tract of infected individuals. The virus gains access to the bloodstream resulting in widespread dissemination throughout the body. In pregnant women, rubella can infect the placenta leading to fetal infection with varying degrees of fetal damage. Attention was first drawn to the association between rubella and fetal damage when Gregg, an Australian ophthalmologist noted an epidemic of congenital cataracts following a large outbreak of rubella (Gregg, 1941). Similar reports followed from Sweden, the US and the UK and the role of rubella in congenital cataracts was confirmed. The coincidence of heart disease and deafness was also noted (Plotkin & Mortimer, 1994). Rubella infection is often asymptomatic or causes only mild disease, and the importance is confined to infection during pregnancy and its possible effects on the fetus, referred to as the congenital rubella syndrome (CRS).

Rubella infection is readily prevented by a highly effective and safe live attenuated vaccine which when given to all infants and susceptible adults, as is the case in much of the developed world, has virtually eliminated cases of the congenital rubella syndrome. However, rubella can still be prevalent in immigrant populations from countries where vaccination is not common (Tookey & Peckham, 1999).

Clinical features of rubella

In children rubella infection is usually either asymptomatic or with mild constitutional symptoms accompanied by an evanescent rash, which is often missed. In adults, infection is generally accompanied by an illness although this is likely to be mild. A prodrome lasting 1 to 5 days consisting of a low-grade temperature, headache, malaise, mild coryza and conjunctivitis is usually present. A generalized lymphadenopathy, particularly noticeable in the postauricular, occipital and posterior cervical lymph nodes, precedes the rash by a few days. The rash is characteristically a diffuse, fine maculopapular eruption which commences in the head and neck area and then progresses downward, generally noted in the exposed parts of the body. The rash usually clears after 3 or 4 days, and itching is uncommon. Arthritis (or arthalgia), usually felt as stiffness in the joints, occurs in approximately 70% of adult women. This condition has also been noted in adult women receiving rubella vaccination. Complications are rare, but may include thrombocytopaenia and encephalitis, probably occurring in less than in 5 in 10 000 cases (Morgan-Capner, 1999).

The clinical diagnosis of rubella can be difficult as the clinical picture mimics other diseases. It is therefore recommended that a serological confirmation of the presumptive diagnosis be performed. The differential diagnosis of rubella includes non-infectious conditions such as allergic rashes and infections due to enteroviruses (particularly Echo and Coxsackie virus), parvovirus, arboviruses, and measles. Indeed, many cases diagnosed clinically as measles prove to be rubella on laboratory testing.

Epidemiology

Rubella occurs throughout the world. Before the widespread use of rubella vaccine, rubella was an endemic disease with a seasonal peak in late winter and early spring and with epidemics occurring at irregular intervals of 5–7 years. Infection is uncommon in preschool children. Outbreaks occur in older schoolchildren, adolescents and adults living in closed quarters. Women of childbearing age often become infected after exposure to children within a household or after occupational exposure in nurseries or schools. An infected individual is infectious from 7 days before and for two weeks after the appearance of the rash. Excretion of virus may however persist for a longer period of time, especially in the urine. Congenitally infected infants excrete virus in all secretions and are an important source of infection for a year or more after birth.

Since rubella is not a notifiable disease in most countries, seroepidemiological studies provide a means to assess epidemiological trends of rubella infections. This can be done by determining seroprevalence of rubella antibodies in various age-groups. In the pre-vaccination era, 80–85% of women of childbearing age were found to be immune as a result of childhood infection. In the developing world, infection tends to occur at an earlier age (Miller, 1991). In addition, studies in parts of the developing world have shown that there is a relatively high rate of susceptibility to rubella, but unfortunately comparatively few data exist on the incidence of congenital rubella syndrome.

Congenitally acquired infection

Pathogenesis

Following maternal viraemia, placental infection occurs. The placenta may also become infected through ascending infection via the uterine cervix. This results in necrotizing of areas of the chorion and damage to endothelial cells, which in turn leads to virus-infected emboli which lodge in various organs. Virus replication follows in the absence of an inflammatory response due to a lack of a functioning fetal immune system. In addition, cell division slows due to a suppression of the mitotic rate of cells leading to impaired development of many organs including the heart, lens of the eye and inner ear. Additional damage to organs such as liver and myocardium may result from haemorrhages arising from the damaged endothelial cells in these sites. Persistence of the viral infection commonly occurs due to the impaired immune response.

Risk to the fetus (Table 5.1)

The risk of vertical transmission of the virus to the fetus depends on the timing of infection in the mother during pregnancy. If the mother is infected in the first 12 weeks of pregnancy, 80% of babies become infected, the rate is 67% during weeks 13 and 14 and declines steadily to 25% at the end of 26 weeks (Miller et al., 1982). In infected babies, rubella-associated defects occur in 100% if infection occurred in the first 11 weeks, 50% of those who were infected at 11 or 12 weeks and 35% of those who were infected between 13 and 16 weeks. If maternal rubella occurs after the 16th week, the risk to the fetus is negligible, with only rare cases of deafness being attributable to rubella (Morgan-Capner, 1999). The most common permanent defects are deafness, learning difficulties, cataracts, heart defects, sight problems and cerebral palsy. Diabetes in early adulthood has also been linked with intra-uterine rubella infection (Bedford & Elliman, 1998).

Clinical manifestation of congenital rubella syndrome

The clinical manifestations of the congenital rubella syndrome are divided into three broad groups. First there are those conditions that are directly due to ongoing viral infection. These are present in the first few weeks of life, do not recur and are not associated with permanent sequelae. Examples of these conditions are low birthweight, bone lesions, thrombocytopaenic purpura ('blueberry muffin' infant), hepatosplenomegaly, generalised lymphodenopathy and meningo-encephalitis. Secondly, there are developmental defects related to the effects of the

Table 5.1. Risk of mother-to-child transmission of rubella resulting in damage to the fetus

First trimester	Risks	Comment
Symptomatic rubella	80%	One or more congenital defects
Asymptomatic rubella	Uncertain, slightly less than 80%	Usually cardiac or ocular defects
After first trimester		
13–16 weeks	17%	Fetus is less severely affected.
17–20 weeks	6%	Retinopathy and learning defects
>20 weeks	2%	are common
Rubella before conception		
Onset of rash before LMP[a]	No risk	The appearance of rash coincides
Onset of rash up to 11 days after LMP	No risk	with immunity in the mother, which should protect the fetus.
Onset of rash from 12 days after LMP	Fetus is usually affected	However, there is a possibility that virus infection may persist in the genital tract and can infect the conceptus.
Maternal reinfection in first trimester	8%. Risk is possibly greater if reinfection is symptomatic	Infection of mothers who have immune responses from previous maternal infection or vaccination

[a] LMP: last menstrual period.

virus on organogenesis. Some manifestations may be delayed and may only become apparent in adolescent or adult life. Examples of permanent defects are sensorineural deafness (the most common manifestation of congenital rubella syndrome (CRS)), ocular defects such as cataracts, congenital glaucoma, severe strabismus and microphthalmia, congenital cardiac abnormalities, especially patent ductus arteriosus, ventricular septal defect and peripheral pulmonary stenosis and central nervous system defects such as mental retardation and microcephaly. The third group of delayed defects includes deafness, insulin-dependent diabetes mellitus, mental retardation, 'late onset disease' manifesting with rash, pneumonitis and diarrhoea and growth retardation. Late onset disease is thought to be due to the formation of immune complexes, which are deposited in the various organs, and can occur several years after delivery.

Diagnosis

It is essential that laboratory tests be used to confirm the clinical diagnosis of rubella because there are a number of illnesses accompanied by rash which may

Table 5.2. Serology in pregnant women

Test result IgM	IgG	Interpretation	Counselling	Further Action
−	−	No rubella but fully susceptible	Reassure about infection but warn about vulnerability to rubella	Repeat 3 weeks after exposure or 1 week after onset of rash. Recommend vaccination after pregnancy
+[a]	−	Primary infection	High risk to infant	
+[a]	+	Primary or second infection	Primary – high risk Second – low risk	Avidity test on IgG
−	+	Immunity	Reassurance	

[a]Non-specific low positive IgM ELISA results are frequent in pregnant women and are not associated with active infection.

resemble rubella. A laboratory diagnosis of rubella is crucial for pregnant women who present with an illness accompanied by rash, those who have been in contact with a case of rubella and for infants born to a mother with rubella during pregnancy or those born with clinical features suggesting CRS.

Serologic testing is the mainstay of rubella diagnosis. The most commonly performed test is the enzyme-linked immuno-sorbent assay (ELISA) for IgM and IgG antibodies (Table 5.2). In this regard IgM capture antibody tests are performed because these are not appreciably affected by IgM antiglobulins, such as rheumatoid factor, nor are they influenced by competition from IgG for antibody binding sites in the test system. Caution is necessary in the interpretation of results, as low positive non-specific IgM results are not uncommon in pregnancy. A follow-up test on a different sample should always be requested for confirmation of a presumptive positive result. It is important to note than IgM antibodies can persist for 10 months or longer following primary infection (Pattison et al., 1975) or for months to years after rubella vaccination (O'Shea et al., 1985; Burke et al., 1985).

A refinement of the ELISA test is the urea avidity test, which is performed on the IgG antibodies. In pregnant mothers who test IgM positive, the avidity test distinguishes primary from secondary rubella (reinfection), an important distinction with respect to the risk of transmission of virus to the fetus. The principle of the test is based on the increasing avidity that IgG antibodies display for their specific antigen with increasing time after infection. Thus, IgG antibodies produced in primary infection have a considerably lower avidity than these produced in reinfection. The avidity differentiation may be demonstrated by incorporating a protein denaturing agent, usually urea, into the washing fluid used in the ELISA test. Primary IgG antibodies are far easier to detach from their antigenic sites than are reinfection IgG antibodies during the ELISA washing process. The difference in the final optical density reading, before and after urea washing, is expressed as an avidity index. Thus, in primary infection, IgG antibodies usually have an avidity index of less than 30%, while those produced in reinfection are usually greater than 70%.

Virus isolation may be useful in confirming the diagnosis of CRS. In these cases rubella virus is readily isolated from nasal, blood, throat, urine and cerebrospinal fluid specimens (Best & O'Shea, 1996). Detection of rubella virus RNA by reverse transcriptase polymerase chain reaction (RT-PCR) can also be carried out (Bosma et al., 1995a). Virus isolation may be useful in determining the duration of virus excretion in infected infants as these infants may excrete virus for many months and thus pose a risk to susceptible individuals. Urine is the most sensitive specimen for determining persistence of viral excretion. Rubella is a fastidious, slow-growing virus and positive results are usually only available after 10 to 11 days.

Prenatal diagnosis

Most congenital infections are diagnosed by investigating the infant with congenital abnormalities. In these instances, rubella infection is diagnosed by the presence of rubella specific IgM in the serum of the infant or by isolating virus. However, the fetus is not always infected and prenatal diagnosis may be useful in certain circumstances, for example, when maternal infection has occurred after the first trimester, in cases of possible reinfection or where there are doubts regarding the maternal diagnosis.

Chorionic virus sampling, amniotic fluid sampling, fetal blood sampling and other techniques can be performed in specialized settings, but these techniques are not without risk to the fetus (D'Alton & De Cherney, 1993). Sensitive and rapid diagnostic tests such as the polymerase chain reaction (PCR) are usually required for the diagnosis in these specimens (Bosma et al., 1995b; Morgan-Capner et al., 1984).

Amniocentesis is done by the transabdominal route and a small amount of fluid (10–20 ml) is aspirated. Amniocentesis is usually performed between 15 and 20 weeks of gestation and the fluid is submitted for virus isolation and testing for viral nucleic acid by RT-PCR. The risk of miscarriage attributable to amniocentesis at 15 to 20 weeks is approximately 0.25% to 0.5% (Table 5.3). If done before 15 weeks, the amount of fluid withdrawn is less and risk to fetal loss can approach 5%. Fetoscopy, a technique for sampling fetal blood, involves direct intrauterine

Table 5.3. Prenatal diagnosis

Sample	Gestational age at sampling (weeks)	Risk of fetal loss
Chorionic villus samples (CVS)	10	0.5–1%
Amniotic fluid (AF)	15	0.25-0.5%
Fetal blood	18	2% above background

From Best (1996).

visualisation of the fetus and is performed in the second trimester when the fetus is small and the amniotic fluid is clear.

Chorionic villus samples (CVS) utilizes either a catheter or needle to biopsy placental cells from which infection may be detected. Ultrasonographic scanning is employed to localize the position of the placenta and the fetus. Thereafter, CVS can be done by either the transcervical or transabdominal route. The transabdominal route is preferable and safer, as various manipulations may be necessary in the transcervical procedure in guiding the needle to the placenta. The miscarriage risk is approximately 0–5% to 1% using the transabdominal route and may be higher when the transcervical route is used. Ascending uterine infection is a further complication of the transcervical route and it is therefore necessary to perform the procedure in an operating theatre. Maternal genital infection is a contraindication to the procedure. Transabdominal procedures may be performed in an ultrasound clinic and can be performed with safety at any stage of pregnancy. Certain congenital defects of the extremities, known as limb deficiencies or limb reduction defects have been reported among infants whose mothers underwent CVS.

Cordocentesis involves the use of ultrasonography to locate the position of the placenta and the junction of the umbilical cord with the placenta. The transabdominal route is employed to introduce a needle which is guided by ultrasonography to the placental origin of the umbilical cord from which blood is removed from the fetal vein. If the placental origin of the cord cannot be identified, a loop of the cord is used. The complication rate is low and has been estimated to be less than 2%. The fetal blood is submitted for serological testing for rubella specific IgM. It must be remembered, however, that up to 23 weeks of gestation false negative results may occur as the immune response of the fetus is unreliable before this time.

Prenatal diagnosis requires skilled operators, specialized and sophisticated equipment including ultrasonography and also requires specialized laboratory support with experience in the interpretation of the results. These factors place

Table 5.4. Postnatal diagnosis by serology

Age of infant	Test result	Interpretation
0–3 months	IgM+	Intrauterine infection
3–12 months	IgM+ IgG+	Probably intrauterine infection although in low socio-economic conditions with widespread early infection, unusually early postnatal infection during the first year of life cannot be ruled out
6 months+	IgM− IgG+	Presence of rubella-specific IgG beyond the time at which maternal antibody disappears – indicates intrauterine infection

prenatal testing by these methodologies beyond the reach of most of the developing world. In these settings, serological testing of the mother remains the cornerstone of prenatal diagnosis.

Postnatal diagnosis

Rubella-specific IgM can be detected in 100% of congenitally infected infants until 3 months of age, 90% of infants 3 to 6 months of age and 50% of infants 6 to 12 months of age (Table 5.4). Detection of low avidity IgG in the infant may assist in the diagnosis up to the age of 3 years as the avidity matures more slowly in congenital rubella than following postnatal infection (Thomas et al., 1993).

Virus isolation and PCR may be performed on specimens from the infant for a definitive diagnosis. Virus can be readily isolated from specimens from neonates with CRS. By 3 months, the proportion of infants excreting virus declines to 50–60%. Those with severe disease, particularly in the first few weeks of life, excrete high concentrations of virus in specimens and pose a risk to susceptible individuals. It is important therefore, for health-care workers dealing with such patients to be immune to rubella.

Radiological examination of the long bones may be a useful additional diagnostic test. Typical radiolucent lesions are seen in the metaphyseal portions of long bones in about one fifth of infected infants. Haematological testing may reveal thrombocytopenia in infants with purpuric spots; the platelet count varies from 3 to $100 \times 10^9/l$.

Rubella reinfection

Breakthrough (secondary) infections are assuming increasing importance probably related to the more widespread use of rubella vaccination. It has been suggested that women with immunity induced by vaccination may be more susceptible to reinfection than those with naturally acquired immunity because of qualitative differences in the immune response (Horstmann et al., 1985; O'Shea et al., 1983). As with any case of rubella infection during pregnancy, gestational age at the time of infection determines the risk of fetal abnormality. This risk has been estimated to be approximately 8% (Morgan-Capner et al., 1991; Best, 1993). Testing should be considered for all pregnant women who have been in contact with rubella or who develop a rubella-like illness, even if they have a history of rubella or rubella vaccination or have a previous documented antibody response to rubella.

Evidence for reinfection includes a significant rise in antibody titre in a woman with pre-existing rubella antibody, and/or a significant IgM response. Where no serum samples are available before the event, two laboratory results showing an antibody concentration greater than 15 000 IU/l or a documented history of vaccination together with one antibody-positive laboratory result are also suggestive of reinfection (Best et al., 1989).

Prevention of fetal infection

All women of child-bearing age should have a serological test for rubella antibodies as part of their routine general medical, gynaecological or family planning examinations. If seronegative, vaccine should be administered, provided pregnancy has been excluded. However, pregnant women have sometimes been immunized, or become pregnant sooner than the recommended interval of 3 months. Follow-up of such cases has shown that, of the 123 births reported to the UK National Congenital Rubella Surveillance Programme between 1980 and 1995, no child was born with defects which could be linked to congenital rubella infection (Bedford & Elliman, 1998). Primary infection during the first 16 weeks of pregnancy would be an indication for advising termination of pregnancy (Table 5.1).

The virtual elimination of rubella and CRS in many countries of the western world is entirely due to the effectiveness of the rubella vaccine. The vaccine is well tolerated and produces immune responses in about 95% of vaccinees. Vaccine virus is excreted by vaccinees but does not appear to be transmitted to susceptible contacts (Best, 1997). The vaccine is live attenuated and is therefore contraindicated in severely immunosuppressed persons and in pregnancy. Women in the child-bearing age group should use adequate contraception for 3 months after receipt of rubella vaccine.

A single vaccine dose should theoretically provide lifelong immunity because re-exposure should stimulate a secondary (anamnestic) antibody response by memory B cells. However, because second ('breakthrough') infections are being recognized with increasing frequency, a second booster dose is generally given.

The first dose should be administered at 12 to 15 months of age and the second dose at school entry (4–6 years of age).

Two vaccination strategies have been advocated: universal childhood immunization aims to interrupt circulation and transmission of rubella virus by vaccinating all preschool children. This would diminish the reservoir pool of the virus and reduce the risk of exposure to all pregnant women. This policy requires a high (at least 85%) uptake of vaccination among preschool children to be completely effective. If there is inadequate vaccination with this strategy, the risk of congenital rubella could be aggravated because larger numbers of susceptibles would reach the child-bearing age group having not been exposed to either wild-type virus or vaccine virus (Anderson & May, 1990). Selective vaccination aims to protect the population at risk, prepubertal girls being the target population. This policy is more suitable for countries that are unlikely to attain high vaccine uptake among preschool children. With this policy, wild-type rubella would continue to circulate.

Rubella vaccine, although it is a live attenuated vaccine, may be given simultaneously with other vaccines without any interference. In developed countries, rubella vaccine is commonly combined with measles and mumps vaccines as the triple MMR vaccine. However, if not administered simultaneously, rubella vaccine should not be given soon after or before other live vaccines – a period of 2 weeks to a month should elapse to avoid reduction of efficacy due to interference. Administration of immunoglobulins may also interfere with the activity of rubella vaccine – at least 3 months should elapse after any immunoglobulin administration before rubella vaccine is administered to allow for the complete elimination of any potentially interfering antibodies.

The prime contraindication to rubella vaccination is pregnancy. Women of child-bearing age should be advised to use contraception for at least 3 months after receiving rubella vaccine. The question that arises not infrequently is that of accidental administration of vaccine in the early stages of pregnancy. Examination of products of conception from pregnancy terminations have shown that rubella vaccine virus does indeed cross the placenta and has been shown to infect the developing fetus. However, there is no evidence that the vaccine virus is teratogenic or that it causes any fetal damage. Several registries have been established worldwide and collectively a few thousand such cases have been followed up and investigated – none has revealed any evidence of any pathological effect due to vaccine virus (Bedford & Elliman, 1998). Thus, cases of accidental vaccination in early pregnancy should not warrant consideration of termination and these women can be reassured. Rubella vaccine virus can be isolated from breast milk in lactating women who have received rubella vaccine. However, breastfeeding is not a contraindication to rubella vaccination as there is no evidence that the vaccine virus is harmful in any way to the suckling infant.

In principle caution must be exercised when any live viral vaccine is administered to immunosuppressed individuals and this also holds true for rubella vaccine. Cognisance should also be taken of the reduced efficacy of vaccines in immunosuppressed persons. However, because rubella vaccine virus is so attenuated, it is only in severely immunocompromised (non-HIV infected) individuals where consideration should be given to withholding the vaccine. This would include severe congenital immunodeficiency disorders, patients with leukaemia, lymphoma, generalized malignancy or therapy with alkylating agents, antimetabolites, irradiation or large doses of corticosteroids. With regard to the latter, steroid therapy on its own does not constitute a contraindication to live virus vaccination. This would apply if the therapy is short term (less than 2 weeks), low to moderate dosage, long-term alternate-day treatment with short-acting preparations, maintenance physiological doses as replacement therapy, or if it is administered topically (skin or eyes), by aerosol, or intra-articularly or into a tendon or bursa. What would be considered a 'large dose' is difficult to define but would generally be equivalent to 2 mg/kg or a total of 20 mg/day of prednisolone. If possible it would be preferable to wait for at least 3 months after discontinuing treatment before administration of rubella vaccine. Rubella vaccine is not contraindicated in HIV infection even in symptomatic patients.

Rubella vaccines are prepared in RA27/3 cell lines, a human diploid fibroblast cell culture. The vaccine therefore contains no egg components and is not contraindicated in individuals who are hypersensitive to egg protein (as may be the case with measles and mumps vaccines). Caution should be exercised with individuals who are severely hypersensitive to neomycin, which is used as a preservative and traces of which are found in the vaccine.

There is no evidence that rubella vaccine virus is transmissible from a vaccine recipient to a susceptible contact even though the virus may be detected in respiratory secretions postvaccination. There is therefore no reason not to vaccinate family members or other household contacts of pregnant women, and indeed in an outbreak situation it may be advisable to vaccinate children of susceptible pregnant women if they have not yet been vaccinated, to prevent the introduction of the virus into a household. Although hyperimmune globulin preparations are available there is no evidence that any immunoglobulin preparation is effective in preventing infection when given after exposure to rubella. There is, similarly, no evidence that rubella vaccine itself is effective for post-exposure prophylaxis.

Conclusion

Rubella and the congenital rubella syndrome have been virtually eliminated in most developed countries which have implemented energetic immunization programmes. In theory rubella could be eradicated from the planet by adopting the same kind of global strategies that are presently being carried out for polio and measles and which were so successful in eradicating smallpox. The burden of the congenital rubella syndrome in the developing world is largely unknown – undoubtedly it remains a significant cause of illness and mortality. However, the disease receives relatively scant public health attention when weighed against other competing health priorities and only some 28% of developing countries have national rubella vaccination programmes (Banatvala, 1998). Nevertheless, the successes which have been achieved with other vaccine preventable diseases such as smallpox, polio and measles have motivated the WHO to advocate vaccine control programmes for rubella for the developing world in an effort to ultimately eradicate this disease from the world (Cutts et al., 1997; Robertson et al., 1997).

REFERENCES

Anderson, R. M. & May R. M. (1990). Immunisation and herd immunity. *Lancet*, **335**, 641–5.

Banatvala, J. E. (1998). Rubella – could do better. *Lancet*, **351**, 849–50.

Bedford, H. & Elliman, D. (1998). *Childhood Immunisation: A Review For Parents and Carers.* London: Health Education Authority.

Best, J. M. (1993). Rubella reinfection. *Current Medical Literature. Virology*, **2**, 35–40.

Best, J. M. (1996). Laboratory diagnosis of intrauterine and perinatal virus infections. *Clin. Diag. Virol.*, **5**, 121–9.

Best, J. M. (1997). Rubella vaccines: past, present and future. *Epidemiol. Infect.* **107**, 17–30.

Best, J. M. & O'Shea, S. (1996). Rubella virus. In *Diagnostic Procedures for Viral, Rickettsial and Chlamydial Infection.* 7th edn, ed. E. H. Lennette, D. A. Lennette & E. T. Lennette, pp. 583–600. Washington DC, USA: American Public Health Association.

Best, J. M., Banatvala, J. E., Morgan-Capner, P. & Miller, E. (1989). Foetal infection after maternal reinfection with rubella: criteria for defining reinfection. *Br. Med. J.*, **299**, 773–5.

Bosma, T. J., Corbett, K. M., Ecksteen, M. B., Vijayalakshmi, P., Banatvala, J. E., Morton, K. & Best, J. M. (1995). Use of PCR for prenatal and postnatal diagnosis of congenital rubella. *J. Clin. Microbiol.*, **33**, 2881–7.

Bosma, T. J., Corbett, K. M., O'Shea, S., Banatvala, J. E. & Best, J. M. (1995a). PCR for detection of rubella virus RNA in clinical samples. *J. Clin. Microbiol.*, **33**, 1075–9.

Burke, J. P., Henman, A. R. & Krugman, S. (1985). International symposium on prevention of congenital rubella infection. *Rev. Infect. Dis.*, **7**, Suppl. 1.

Cutts, F. T., Robertson, S. E., Diaz-Ortega, J-L. & Samuel, R. (1997). Control of rubella and congenital rubella syndrome (CRS) in developing countries, part 1: burden of disease from CRS. *Bull. World Health Org.*, **75**, 55–68.

D'Alton, M. E. & De Cherney, A. H. (1993). Prenatal diagnosis. *N. Engl. J. Med.*, **328**, 114–20.

Gregg, N.McA. (1941). Congenital cataract following German measles in the mother. *Trans. Ophth. Soc. Aust.*, **3**, 35–46.

Horstmann, D. M., Schluederberg, A., Emmons, J. E., Evans, B. K. & Randolph, M. F. & Andiman, W. A. (1985). Persistence of vaccine induced immune responses to rubella: comparison with natural infection. *Rev. Infect. Dis.*, **7**, S80–5.

Miller, C. (1991). Rubella in the developing world. *Epidemiol. Infect.*, **107**, 63–8.

Miller, E., Cradock-Watson, L. E. & Pollock, T. M. (1982). Consequences of confirmed rubella at successive stages of pregnancy. *Lancet*, **i**, 871–4.

Morgan-Capner, P., Rodick, C. H., Nicolaides, K. & Cradock-Watson, J. E. (1984). Prenatal diagnosis of rubella. *Lancet*, **ii**, 343.

Morgan-Capner, P., Miller, E., Vurdien, J. E. & Ramsay, M. E. B. (1991). Outcome of pregnancy after maternal reinfection with rubella. *CDR 1*, No. 6, R57–59.

Morgan-Capner, P. (1999). Rubella. In *Viral Infections in Obstetrics and Gynaecology*, ed. D. J. Jeffries & C. N. Hudson. London: Arnold.

O'Shea, S., Best, J. M. & Banatvala, J. E. (1983). Viraemia, virus excretion and antibody responses after challenge in volunteers with low levels of antibody to rubella virus. *J. Infect. Dis.*, **148**, 639–47.

O'Shea, S., Best, J. M., Banatvala, J. E. & Shepherd, W. M. (1985). Development and persistence of class-specific antibodies in the serum and nasopharyngeal washings of rubella vaccinees. *J. Infect. Dis.*, **151**, 89–98.

Pattison, J. R., Dane, D. S. & Mace, J. E. (1975). Persistence of specific IgM after natural infection with rubella virus, *Lancet*, **i**, 185–7.

Plotkin, S. A, Mortimer, E. A. (eds). (1994). Rubella vaccine. *Vaccines*. Philadelphia: W. B. Saunders.

Robertson, S. E., Cutts, F. T., Samuel, R. & Diaz-Ortega, J-L. (1997). Control of rubella and congenital rubella syndrome (CRS) in developing countries, part 2: vaccination against rubella. *Bull. World Health Organ.*, **75**, 69–80.

Thomas, H. I., Morgan-Capner, P., Cradock Watson, J. E., Enders, G., Best, J. M. & O'Shea, S. (1993). Slow maturation of IgG1 avidity in congenital rubella: implications for diagnosis and immunopathology. *J. Med. Virol.*, **41**, 196–200.

Tookey, P. A. & Peckham, C. S. (1999). Surveillance of congenital rubella in Great Britain, 1971–1996. *B.M.J.*, **318**, 769–70.

6

Perinatal group B streptococcal infections

Vibhuti Shah and Arne Ohlsson

Introduction

Infection is a major cause of perinatal morbidity and mortality (Christensen, 1982; Ohlsson et al., 1987). The aetiology of neonatal septicemia varies with geographical location and changes over time (Nyhan & Fousek, 1958; Ohlsson & Serenius, 1981; Ohlsson et al., 1986). From the 1960s onwards, Group B beta-haemolytic streptococcus (GBS) has been one of the most common causes of neonatal infectious morbidity and mortality in the USA (Eickhoff et al., 1964; Franciosi et al., 1973; McCracken, 1973), Canada (Allardice et al., 1982), the UK (Reid, 1975; Lloyd & Reid, 1976), Europe (Cayeux, 1972, Bergqvist, 1974; Bergqvist et al., 1978; Schroder & Paust, 1979; Speer et al., 1985; Vesikari et al., 1989) and Australia (Fliegner & Garland, 1990). GBS causes significant maternal perinatal morbidity (Institute of Medicine, 1985), bacteriuria in pregnancy (Hastings et al., 1986) as well as urinary tract (Munoz et al., 1992) and other infections in the adult non-pregnant population (Opal et al., 1988; Schwartz et al., 1991).

Historical background

Rebecca Lancefield described in 1933 a serological method for differentiating the haemolytic streptococci into a number of groups (Lancefield, 1933). At that time most severe streptococcal infections in the puerperium were caused by streptococci belonging to Group A (Charles & Larsen, 1986). In 1935 GBS was reported as a cause of mild puerperal infection (Lancefield & Hare, 1935), followed by a report of three cases of fatal GBS puerperal infection (Fry, 1938). GBS was subsequently confirmed as an important pathogen in the perinatal period (Nyhan & Fousek, 1958; Eickhoff et al., 1964; Franciosi et al., 1973; Hood et al., 1961).

The organism

The GBS, or *Streptococcus agalactiae*, is a Gram-positive diplococcus. The majority of strains (99%) are beta-haemolytic. The organism contains two polysaccharide antigens, the group-B specific 'C' substance and the type-specific 'S' substance, on the basis of which GBS strains are divided into serotypes Ia, Ib, Ia/c, II, III, IV, V and VI (Baker & Edwards, 1990; Schuchat, 1998). The serotype Ic contains a protein antigen. The type specific antigens are located in the capsule and are important virulence factors. Serotypes III, II and Ic are the most common for early onset disease (EOD) whereas serotype III predominates in late onset disease (LOD) (Baker & Edwards, 1990). Recently a new type V polysaccharide has been found in isolates from neonates infected or colonized with GBS (Rench & Baker, 1993; Blumberg et al., 1996). Serotypes VI and VIII predominate among group B streptococci isolated from pregnant women in Japan (Lachenauer et al., 1999).

Epidemiology

Colonization

The reservoir for GBS in humans is the gastrointestinal tract, with the genito-urinary loci (vagina and urethra) being the major additional sites of colonization in females. GBS colonizes the genitourinary tract of 10–40% of all pregnant women (Baker & Edwards, 1995; Gordon & Sbarra, 1976; Anthony et al., 1981). Colonization rates vary among ethnic groups, geographic locations, age, and sexual habits; however, rates are similar for pregnant and non-pregnant women (Yow et al., 1980). Ohlsson reported in 1992 on maternal and neonatal coloniz-ation rates as well as attack rates for early and late onset neonatal disease from a number of different populations (Ohlsson, 1992). More recently Schimmel et al. surveyed the literature and reported on maternal GBS colonization rates in different locales: USA: 20–40%, Brazil 26%, India 6%, Italy 7%, Australia 12%, Israel 2–3%, Jerusalem 10% (Schimmel et al., 1998). In an individual mother, colonization varies throughout pregnancy and results obtained at 35–37 weeks' gestation correlate best with culture status at birth (Boyer et al., 1983a,b; Gotoff & Boyer, 1997). Sexual transmission occurs, with the father identified as a reservoir. This may explain the difficulty in eradicating the organism during pregnancy (Weindling et al., 1981). In a study by Yancey et al. (1996) the sensitivity and specificity of colonization at 35–37 weeks' gestation in predicting colonization status at term was 87% and 96% as compared with 43% and 85% in patients cultured 6 or more weeks before delivery. This study supports the recommenda-tions from Centers for Disease Control and Prevention (CDC) to perform antena-tal GBS cultures optimally at 35–37 weeks' gestation (Centers for Disease Control and Prevention, 1996).

The isolation rate of GBS from clinical specimens depends on several factors. As bacteria colonize the genital tract from the lower digestive tract intermittently, culture specimens taken both from the anorectal region and vagina increases the likelihood of GBS isolation from 5% to 27% over vaginal cultures alone (Boyer et al., 1983b; Dillon et al., 1982; Badri et al., 1977; Philipson et al., 1995). The use of selective media (i.e. broth containing antimicrobial agents to inhibit competing organisms) increases the yield by as much as 50% (Philipson et al., 1995; Baker et al., 1977; Ferrieri & Blair, 1977; Altaie & Dryja, 1994; Silver & Struminsky, 1996).

Several factors increase the risk of neonatal GBS disease including GBS bacteriuria during pregnancy, gestational age <37 weeks, prolonged rupture of membranes (>18 hours), and maternal intrapartum pyrexia (temperature >38 °C) (Schuchat et al., 1994; Anonymous, 1996; Bramer et al., 1997). These perinatal risk factors have usually been identified from investigators using univariate analysis. Additional perceptible risk factors such as risk of neonatal GBS disease complicating subsequent pregnancies were derived from anecdotal reports (Carstensen et al., 1988; Faxelius et al., 1988).

Screening tests

Chemoprophylaxis strategies that involve identification of colonized women require tests with high sensitivity and specificity. The optimal technique for GBS screening is obtaining a single vaginal–anorectal swab and use of selective broth medium. The disadvantage is that it requires 18–24 hours before the result is available which is an issue for women presenting in labour. Two rapid antigen detection methods, latex particle agglutination test (LPA) (Wald et al., 1987; Isada & Grossman, 1987; Stiller et al., 1989; Brady et al., 1989; Lotz-Nolan et al., 1989; Kontnick & Edberg, 1990; Clark et al., 1992; Quentin et al., 1993; Green et al., 1993) and enzyme-linked immunosorbent assay (ELISA) (Towers et al., 1990; Granato and Petosa, 1991; Hagay et al., 1993; Armer et al., 1993; Wust et al., 1993; Schimmel et al., 1994; Hordnes et al., 1995; Park et al., 1996; Baker, 1996) have been evaluated against the culture tests. The sensitivities and specificities for LPA tests range from 19% to 91.8% and 93.2% to 99.7%, respectively. Similarly for ELISA tests the sensitivities and specificities vary from 7.4% to 89% and 92% to 100%. These tests have been performed in a wide variety of clinical situations: (i) high risk patients presenting with preterm labour or prelabour rupture of the membranes preterm, (ii) women in labour at both preterm and term gestations and (iii) during the second trimester of pregnancy prior to delivery to avoid contamination of blood, amniotic fluid and mucus which could lower the sensitivity of an antigen test. Thus, none of the currently available rapid antigen detection methods appears to be sufficiently sensitive to replace standard culture methods for routine use in selection of women for intrapartum chemoprophylaxis (IPC).

Clinical presentation

Maternal disease

Maternal perinatal GBS disease includes chorioamnionitis, endometritis, sepsis and urinary tract infection. Other rare maternal complications are meningitis, abdominal abscess, endocarditis and necrotizing fascitis. In the USA, endometritis/paraendometritis due to GBS infection has been estimated to occur in 12/1000 deliveries and maternal GBS bacteraemia in 0.8/1000 deliveries (Institute of Medicine, 1985). The presenting signs and symptoms in the mother are fever, malaise, uterine tenderness, lochia and chills. Fatal infection in the offspring of these mothers may occur and it is important that evidence of maternal disease is communicated to alert the paediatric caregivers of the possibility of an infection in the neonate. There is an increased risk for endometritis and bacteraemia if the delivery was by caesarean section (Institute of Medicine, 1985). GBS is isolated in 20% of cases of bacteraemia postpartum. GBS may also cause bacteriuria/urinary tract infection in pregnancy (Hastings et al., 1986; Thomsen et al., 1987; Wood & Dillon, 1981).

Fetal disease

Infection of the fetus with GBS may result in stillbirth (Bergqvist et al., 1978; Fliegner & Garland, 1990; Wood & Dillon, 1981). There are presently no ideal antenatal tests available to predict chorioamnionits or neonatal sepsis of bacterial origin (Ohlsson & Wang, 1990). Christensen et al., (1983) found that severe changes in heart rate during the first stage of labour were typical characteristics of fetuses with congenital GBS pneumonia. The non-stress test was found to have no value in identifying fetuses with congenital sepsis in a retrospective study (Gonen et al., 1991). GBS sepsis has been associated with metabolic acidosis both in an animal model (Barefield et al., 1992) and in human neonates (Hocker et al., 1992) and therefore a low arterial cord pH could be expected in neonates infected in utero. In a retrospective study Montgomery et al. (1991) tested this hypothesis and their results suggest that a mild metabolic acidosis may serve as an indicator of increased risk of EOD.

Neonatal early onset disease (EOD)

Early onset disease (EOD) occurs, by definition, during the first 7 days of life and the vast majority of cases (approximately 90%) present during the first 24 hours of life (Yagupsky et al., 1991; Garland, 1991). In one study neonates with EOD presented with respiratory disease (54%), sepsis without focus (27%) and meningitis (15%) (Yagupsky et al., 1991). The diagnosis of sepsis should be suspected in the neonate who is born with severe respiratory distress (Christensen et al., 1983) or with an abnormal cord pH (Montgomery et al., 1991), who develops acidosis /and or hypotension (Hocker et al., 1992), or who has leukopenia/neutropenia/left shift on differential white blood cell count (Hocker et al., 1992; Yagupsky et al., 1991). Neonates with congenital GBS infection may be born with skin pustules (Ohlsson, 1992). The pustules are 2–3 mm in size and usually have no erythema surrounding their edges. These pustules are most frequently seen in the scalp, neck and upper part of the torso, but may occur on the hands. The presumptive diagnosis of GBS infection in these cases can be supported by Gram stain from aspirates of the pustules.

Neonatal late onset disease (LOD)

Neonatal late onset disease (LOD) occurs beyond 7 days of life and can develop beyond 3 months of age (Yagupsky et al., 1991). Risk factors for late onset disease include non-white race and preterm birth (Yagupsky et al., 1991). Neonates with LOD, present with sepsis (46%), meningitis (37%), urinary tract infection (7%), osteoarthritis (6%), respiratory disease (4%) and cellulitis (4%) (Yagupsky et al., 1991).

Diagnosis of GBS infection

The diagnosis of GBS infection is based on clinical symptoms and the isolation of GBS from specimens obtained using sterile technique from blood, cerebrospinal fluid, urine or endotracheal aspirates. A high proportion of neonates evaluated for sepsis (18%) demonstrate a positive latex particle agglutination (LPA) test for GBS (Harris et al., 1989). The significance of a positive urine GBS LPA-test in the absence of a positive blood culture has been questioned in the light of a high false-positive rate possibly due to contamination of the specimen with GBS (Sanchez et al., 1990), to maternal treatment with antibiotics in labour for GBS colonization or disease (Harris et al., 1989) or to ingestion in utero of bacteria or antigen (Ascher et al., 1991). Neonates born to mothers treated with antibiotics in labour are more likely to have a negative blood culture making the LPA test un-interpretable and the diagnosis of GBS disease most difficult to confirm (Harris et al., 1989; Ascher et al., 1991). There is presently no test available to substitute for a positive GBS culture obtained from normally sterile body fluids in the diagnosis of GBS systemic infection. This makes it very difficult to define an appropriate neonatal outcome measure for studies of maternal chemoprophylaxis to reduce neonatal GBS infection. GBS pneumonia can be diagnosed by clinical and radiographic signs compatible with pneumonia and the presence of GBS on a tracheal aspirate specimen, or the presence of GBS and an inflammatory reaction in lung tissue at autopsy.

Early onset sepsis including GBS sepsis is commonly associated with neutropenia (Yagupsky et al., 1991; Ohlsson & Vearncombe, 1987), but a single early complete blood count may not be adequate as a screening tool for early GBS sepsis. Optimal screening for GBS requires a repeat complete blood count within the first 24 hours of age (Greenberg & Yoder, 1990). Gerdes (1991) reviewed adjunctive non-specific tests to identify the septic neonate. The positive predictive values for these tests (WBC, C-reactive protein, micro-ESR, haptoglobin, fibronectin, C3d, acridine orange cytospin) were all extremely poor and a great variability in test characteristics were shown between different studies (Gerdes, 1991). Other groups performing systematic reviews of diagnostic tests to predict neonatal infections have reached the same conclusions (Da Silva & Ohlsson, 1995; Fowlie & Schmidt, 1998).

Treatment

Antibiotic therapy (penicillin or ampicillin) should be started for any GBS-positive woman who becomes febrile during labour. Erythromycin or clindamycin may be used for mothers who are allergic to penicillin or ampicillin. Broader antibiotic regimens should be considered when treating chorioamnionitis in order to cover both GBS and anaerobic and Gram-negative bacilli (Committee on Technical Bulletins, 1992). Postpartum endometritis should be treated with antibiotics until the patient has been afebrile and free of symptoms for at least 24 hours (Committee on Technical Bulletins, 1992).

For the neonate with systemic GBS infection, the treatment of choice is penicillin G for 10 days. Septic arthritis, osteomyelitis and endocarditis will require longer treatment of up to 4 weeks. As the causative organism of neonatal sepsis is not always known at the onset of symptoms, the recommended initial treatment is ampicillin in combination with gentamicin. A number of adjunctive therapies have been suggested including indomethacin, ibuprofen, dazmegrel, corticosteroids, granulocyte transfusion, human immune globulin, fibronectin, complement, and plasma transfusion (Baker & Edwards, 1990). Further randomized controlled trials (RCTs), which include long-term follow-up, are required to prove whether any of these therapies will be of benefit.

Chemoprophylaxis of the asymptomatic GBS carrier mother in labour makes it very difficult to evaluate the asymptomatic neonate for the possibility of infection. There are presently no published RCTs providing guidelines with regard to interpretation of culture results or treatment for the neonate in this situation (Baley & Fanaroff, 1992). Experts advocate that the term, asymptomatic infant born to a GBS-colonized mother given ampicillin before delivery should not be treated at all (Baker, 1990; Gibbs et al., 1992). Asymptomatic preterm infants should be treated with ampicillin and gentamicin after a complete blood cell count, blood culture and a chest radiograph has been done (Baker, 1990; Gibbs et al., 1992). The treatment can be stopped after 48 hours if the neonate remains asymptomatic and there has been no growth in blood specimen.

Outcome of neonatal infection

There is a paucity of reports on short and long-term outcome on neonates infected with GBS at birth. The mortality from neonatal GBS disease has been reported at 54% for preterm and 15% for term infants in the US (Baker & Edwards, 1990). Vesikari et al. (1989) reported on a decreased mortality from GBS infections from 23% in the early 1970s to 13% in the early 1980s in Finland. A mortality rate of 10% was reported from Sweden in 1983 with a handicap rate of 30% (Bennet et al., 1989). A 22% mortality rate was reported in early-onset group B meningitis from Toronto, Canada in 1985; 70% of the survivors were considered normal and 15% had major handicaps (Chin & Fitzhardinge 1985). In a more recent study from Rochester, New York, the case-fatality rate was 13% in EOD and 0% in LOD (Yagupsky et al., 1991). Population-based surveillance data from US in the 1990s indicate a further reduction in mortality to between 4 and 6% (Centers for Disease Control, 1997; Zangwill et al., 1992).

Burden of illness

GBS case-fatality rates are now much lower than they were in the 1970s ($>50\%$) and 1980s (15–25%); this reduction is attributed to the prompt recognition and initiation of antibiotic therapy as well as improvements in neonatal intensive care. Recently, the mortality rate in a large multistate population was reported to be 6% (Zangwill et al., 1992), with higher rates in preterm infants, which account for about 25% of the infections (Faxelius et al., 1988). On the basis of age- and race-adjusted projections for the entire US population in 1990, 7600 cases of neonatal GBS sepsis (1.8/1000 live births) were estimated to occur resulting in 310 deaths (Centers for Disease Control, 1996). At a population level rates for EOD in the USA range from 0.76 to 5.46 cases per 1000 live births (Benitz et al., 1999).

Prevention strategies

In 1996, CDC developed and published guidelines for the prevention of EOD in conjunction with the American Academy of Pediatrics (AAP) and American College of Obstetricians and Gynecologists (ACOG) (Centers for Disease Control, 1996). The recommended strategies are an extension of the guidelines previously published by AAP and ACOG. An algorithm for management of a newborn whose

Table 6.1. Summary of guidelines for prevention of early onset neonatal GBS infections

Prevention strategy	Group endorsements for strategy
(a) Universal antenatal screening at 26-28 weeks' gestation with a single vaginal–anorectal swab and selective intrapartum chemoprophylaxis[a] of GBS colonized women with identified risk factors	(i) American Academy of Pediatrics (AAP), 1992 (ii) Society of Obstetricians and Gynecologists of Canada (SOGC), Canadian Paediatric Society (CPS),1994
(b) No universal screening but intrapartum chemoprophylaxis for all women with identified risk factors[b]	(i) American College of Obstetrics and Gynecologists (ACOG), 1993 (ii) SOGC, CPS,1994 (iii) Centers for Disease Control (CDC) and Prevention (CDC), ACOG and AAP, 1996; AAP, 1997 (106), SOGC, 1997
(c) Universal antenatal screening at 35–37 weeks' gestation with a single combined vaginal–anorectal swab, and the offer of intrapartum chemoprophylaxis to all GBS carriers. If the results of culture unknown at the time of labour intrapartum chemoprophylaxis administered to all women with risk factors	(i) CDC, ACOG and AAP, 1996; AAP, 1997; SOGC, 1997

[a] Intrapartum chemoprophylaxis is defined as follows. CDC defines adequate treatment as at least one dose of intravenous penicillin given at least 4 hours prior to delivery. AAP considers adequate treatment to be two doses of intravenous penicillin, given at least 4 hours apart, prior to delivery.
[b]Risk factors include (i) labour (<37 weeks' gestation), (ii) prolonged rupture of membranes ≥ 18 hours, (iii) maternal fever $> 38.0\,°C$, (iv) GBS bacteriuria during pregnancy and (v) previous delivery of a newborn with GBS disease regardless of current GBS colonization status.

mother received IPC is provided. Table 6.1 summarizes the major prevention strategies recommended over the past decade (American Academy of Pediatrics et al., 1992, 1997; Society of Obstetricians and Gynaecologists et al., 1994; American College of Obstetricians and Gynecologists 1993; Society of Obstetricians and Gynecologists, 1997). Since the CDC publication, AAP has withdrawn its initial recommendations for 28-week screening and selective intrapartum chemoprophylaxis (IPC) and endorsed the CDC guidelines. The ACOG and CDC recommend that obstetric practices should choose a single protocol from two alternatives to establish consistent management of patients. Perusal of the table suggests that the screening at 35–37 weeks with risk factor approach is the most logical and practical of the strategies. The potential advantages of this strategy include: (i) high concordance between prenatal and intrapartum GBS carriage status and potentially justifying exposure of this group to antibiotics and its associated adverse effects, (ii) women who begin prenatal care late in the gestation would be eligible, and (iii) clinicians would not have to wait for the development of risk factors in women during labour to administer antibiotics.

Cost-effective analysis

More than a dozen approaches to selection for prophylaxis have been evaluated theoretically using decision analysis, although most have not been tested for efficacy (Yancey & Duff, 1994; Strickland et al., 1990; Mohle-Boetani et al., 1993; Rouse et al., 1994). In their analysis Yancey and Duff (1994) concluded that universal screening and treatment of all GBS positive mothers is cost-effective, however Strickland et al., (1990) calculated that universal screening programmes are not cost efficient when the prevalence is <10%. Mohle-Boetani et al. (1999) suggest that implementation of risk factor strategy and universal screening with selective IPC of colonized women with risk factors is not cost effective unless the incidence of EOD is greater than 0.6/1000 live births and 1.2/1000 live births respectively. Rouse et al., (1994) analysed 19 different preventive strategies and concluded that universal intrapartum maternal treatment, treatment based on risk factors and antenatal screening at 36 weeks and intrapartum treatment of all GBS positive mothers and all preterm deliveries were the optimal strategies. Fargason et al. (1997) noted that, for the risk-based strategy, the CDC paediatric algorithm increased the cost of averting one case by 94–112% as compared to 51% for the screening-based strategy. Similarly Mohle-Boetani et al. (1993) in their analysis of the risk-based strategy suggested that cost savings occurred only if the hospital stay of the neonate is not extended beyond 24 hours. Thus, the paediatric costs of longer hospital stays and therapies may have a major impact on the cost-effectiveness analysis of these strategies.

Table 6.2 provides a comparison of the cost-effectiveness of the AAP (1992), ACOG (risk factor based) and the CDC (screening based) protocol. The ACOG protocol was found to be least expensive, while the AAP approach was most expensive per case of disease averted. The CDC and ACOG recognize that these protocols are not adequately tested clinically and therefore one protocol is not superior to the other. The projected estimates are the result of the decision analyses and are based on a series of assumptions that are not universally accepted. The economic estimates have not been verified and some potential costs (e.g. care of newborns whose mothers received IPC) have not been accounted for (Boyer &

Table 6.2. Comparison of the cost-effectiveness of the AAP, ACOG and CDC protocols

	AAP (initial)	ACOG (risk-based) CDC (risk-based)	CDC (screening-based)
Antenatal culture (gestational weeks)	26-28	None	35-37
Intrapartum treatment and risk factors	Treat women in labour if positive culture and risk factor(s) present	Treat if risk factors present	Treat if preterm labour or if positive culture and risk factor(s) present and offer treatment if cultures positive and no risk factors
Treated (%)	3-4	18[a]	28[a]
GBS disease reduction (%)	50	70[a]	85[a]
Cost per case GBS disease prevented (US$)	$148 200[a]	$69 800[a]	$85 600[a]
Advantages	Low use of antibiotics Clinical effectiveness proven	Simple Best cost–benefit ratio. No cost of antenatal culture Avoids culture, logistic and accuracy issues	Most effective Allows for treatment of a colonized woman in the absence of risk factors Improved correlation with colonisation status at delivery
Disadvantages	Complex Dependent on compliance with screening Culture cost, accuracy, and logistic issues Not effective for women who do not receive prenatal care	High antibiotic use (80% of women treated unnecessarily) Protection not provided for term infants born to GBS colonised women following uncomplicated pregnancy Has not been adequately tested	Highest antibiotic use, may lead to selection of resistant bacteria Increased risk of penicillin allergy Clinically untested Time consuming as low risk women need to be informed about options

[a]Estimates based on decision analysis (Rouse et al., 1994).

Table 6.3. Theoretical model comparing 'No antibiotics' with three preventive strategies[a]

Protocol	Incidence of early onset neonatal disease	Case reduction factor	Cases per year per 400 000 births	Number of women treated with antibiotics per year	Number of women treated with antibiotics per case prevented	Number of neonatal deaths per year	Number of women treated with antibiotics per neonatal death prevented
No antibiotics[b]	2/1000		800		6%	48	
AAP	2/1000	0.5	400	16 000	40	24	667
ACOG (risk based)	2/1000	0.7	240	72 000	129	14	2 118
CDC (screening based)	2/1000	0.85	120	112 000	165	7	2,732

[a] Modified from Glantz et al. (1998).
[b] Mortality rate 6%.

Gotoff, 1985). They are at best speculative, and can serve as a guide to policy makers but not necessarily for the individual physician.

To estimate the number of women who need to be treated to prevent one case of EOD (Table 6.3), a theoretical model was created based on the disease incidence of 2/1000, mortality rate of 6% and case reduction factors used from Table 6.2 (Glantz & Kedley, 1998). In Canada, per $\simeq$ 400 000 births (364 732 births in 1996) (Guyer et al., 1998), 800 cases of EOD are expected when no IPC is administered to women in labour. Based on our model, we need to treat 40 women using the initial AAP strategy, 130 women for the risk-based approach and 165 women for CDC screening-based approach, respectively, to prevent one case of EOD. To prevent one death from EOD we need to treat 667 women in the AAP strategy, 2118 for the risk-based approach and 2732 for the CDC screening-based approach. However, the number needed to treat will vary depending on the incidence of the disease, the prevalence of colonization rate and risk factor(s).

Thus, within a given health care system the choice of a preventive strategy depends on the incidence of the EOD, the patient characteristics, available clinical resources and possibly maternal infection rates. Ongoing surveillance of all cases of early onset bacterial infections is important for timely detection of increase in the rate of sepsis from other causes or an increase in infections with antibiotic-resistant pathogens.

Prophylaxis/prevention

Several interventions are potentially available to reduce early onset GBS disease. These include vaginal antisepsis, immunoprophylaxis and chemoprophylaxis: in the antepartum, intrapartum and postpartum period.

Vaginal antisepsis

Several studies have evaluated the effect of vaginal wash or wipe with chlorhexidine solutions or gel on peripartum infection, vertical transmission of GBS, neonatal infection and rate of admission to neonatal intensive care unit. No reduction in the rate of peripartum or neonatal infection was noted (Sweeten et al., 1997; Henrichsen et al., 1994). In a RCT (Adriaanse et al., 1995) no reduction was noted in the rate of vertical transmission of GBS to neonates. Burman et al. (1992), however, reported that chlorhexidine prophylaxis was associated with a reduction in the rate of admission for infants born to carrier mothers. Similarly, Taha et al. (1997) have reported a reduction in neonatal and maternal postpartum infections following the use of chlorhexidine. The effect on the rate of early onset GBS disease has not been evaluated.

Immunoprophylaxis

Administration of GBS hyperimmune globulin or monoclonal antibodies to colonized pregnant women at delivery might prevent maternal and neonatal disease but would not prevent other pregnancy complications possibly associated with GBS such as preterm prelabour rupture of membrane or preterm delivery (Thomsen et al., 1987; Regan et al., 1981; Walsh & Hutchins, 1989; Newton & Clark, 1988). As most neonates acquire the infection in utero and are born symptomatic, administration of hyperimmune and monoclonal preparations to the neonate at birth most likely would not prevent EOD but could possibly favourably alter the course of the disease and possibly prevent LOD. Further studies in this area are needed (Fischer et al., 1990; Baker & Noya, 1990; Coleman et al., 1992).

GBS vaccines would have the potential of preventing both perinatal infections and infections in the non-pregnant population. An ideal vaccine is not presently available (Institute of Medicine, 1985; Walsh & Hutchins, 1989; Coleman et al., 1992; Baker & Kasper, 1985; Baker et al., 1988). Coleman et al. (1992) conclude that 'the development of a vaccine for prevention of neonatal GBS sepsis is an attainable goal' and 'further study of the immunogenic properties of bacterial-cell wall polysaccharides and their conjugates, C proteins, and the potential universal antigen is required'. It has been estimated that maternal immunization would be able to prevent 90% of neonatal GBS disease (Institute of Medicine, 1985). Research in this area continues but the progress has been slow.

Chemoprophylaxis
Antepartum

Several studies have evaluated the role of antibiotics in decreasing the incidence of maternal and neonatal colonization at birth with GBS. A significant reduction in maternal colonization was noted within 3 weeks of completion of therapy, however the difference was no longer apparent at delivery (Hall et al., 1976; Gardner et al., 1979). Oral antibiotic therapy for GBS bacteriuria is associated with a decrease in preterm delivery and prelabour rupture of membranes (Thomsen et al., 1987; McDonald et al., 1989).

Intrapartum

Ablow et al. (1976) were the first to suggest IPC for prevention of EOD. Systematic reviews agree on a statistically significant reduction in neonatal colonization rate following IPC. Allen et al., (1993) combined the results of RCTs and cohort studies, and concluded that IPC is effective. Ohlsson & Myrh (1994) thought that, because of serious concerns regarding the quality of RCTs and the study heterogeneity with regards to interventions, it was inappropriate to combine the studies. However, they concluded that there is a trend towards reduction in neonatal infection with IPC.

We systematically reviewed the effectiveness of IPC based on three different strategies: (i) universal screening and IPC to all colonized women (ii) universal screening and selective IPC of colonized women with risk factors and (iii) IPC based on risk factors only.

(i) Effectiveness of universal screening and IPC of all colonized women

Four RCTs (Tuppurainen & Hallman, 1989; Matorras et al., 1991; Easmon et al., 1983; Morales et al., 1986) and four cohort studies (Allardice et al., 1982; Morales et al., 1986; Jeffery & Lahra, 1998; Garland & Fliegner, 1991) have evaluated the effectiveness of universal screening and IPC for all colonized women either on neonatal colonization or EOD or both. Two trials were excluded because the patient population were subsets of subsequent studies (Lim et al., 1986; Tuppurainen et al., 1986).

On the basis of these RCTs and cohort studies we conclude that neonatal colonization is significantly reduced by IPC. Because of the heterogeneity in the study design, the patient population, and antibiotic regimens studies cannot be combined. A meta-analysis of two RCTs with EOD as an outcome gives a RR of 0.21 (95% CI: 0.04,1.17) (Table 6.4). Similarly, a meta-analysis of cohort studies

Table 6.4. Effectiveness of universal screening and IPC on EOD (RCTs)

Comparison: Effectiveness of Universal screening and IPC

Outcome: Early onset GBS disease

Study	Experimental n/N	Control n/N	Relative risk (95% Cl fixed)	Weight (%)	RR (95% Cl fixed)
Matorras (1991)	0/60	3/65		43.2	0.15 (0.01, 2.93)
Tuppurainen (1989)	1/88	5/111		56.8	0.25 (0.03, 2.12)
Total (95% Cl)	1/148	8/176		100.0	0.21 (0.04, 1.17)
Chi-square 0.07 (df=1) z=1.78					

```
          1   2   1   5   10
        Favours treatment   Favours control
```

Table 6.5. Effectiveness of universal screening and IPC on EOD (cohort studies)

Comparison: Effectiveness of universal screening and IPC

Outcome: Early onset GBS disease

Study	Experimental n/N	Control n/N	Relative risk (95% Cl fixed)	Weight (%)	RR (95% Cl fixed)
Allardice (1982)	0/57	9/136		11.1	0.12 (0.01, 2.10)
Garland (1991)	16/30917	27/26915		56.7	0.52 (0.28, 0.96)
Jeffery (1998)	8/36342	8/5732		27.1	0.16 (0.06, 0.42)
Morales (1986)	0/135	2/128		5.0	0.19 (0.01, 3.91)
Total (95% Cl) (1986)	24/67451	46/32911		100.0	0.36 (0.22, 0.591)
Chi-square 4.74 (df=3) z=3.98					

```
          1   2   1   5   10
        Favours treatments   Favours control
```

gives a RR of 0.36 (95% CI: 0.22,0.59) (Table 6.5).

Randomized controlled trials provide the most valid data on which to base all measures of the benefits and risks of particular therapies. Interestingly, none of the randomized controlled trials evaluating the effectiveness of universal screening and IPC (Tuppurainen & Hallman, 1989; Matorras et al., 1991) has shown a statistically significant reduction in EOD. Although they show a trend towards reduction in EOD, none of these studies has enough power to demonstrate a significant difference in EOD between the treatment and control group (Type II error). There is cumulative evidence from cohort studies that universal screening and IPC of all women is effective in preventing EOD (Allardice et al., 1982; Morales et al., 1986; Garland & Fleigner, 1991; Jeffery & Lahra, 1998).

Table 6.6. Effectiveness of selective IPC on EOD (RCT)

Comparison: Effectiveness of selective IPC
Outcome: Early onset GBS disease

Study	Experimental n/N	Control n/N	Relative risk (95% Cl fixed)	Weight (%)	RR (95% Cl fixed)
Boyer (1986)	0/85	4/79	⟵————————	100.0	0.10 (0.01, 1.89)
Total (95% Cl)	0/85	4/79	◁▬▬—	100.0	0.10 (0.01, 1.89)
Chi-square 0.00 (df=0) z=1.53					

1 2   1   5 10
Favours treatment Favours control

Table 6.7. Effectiveness of selective IPC on EOD (cohort studies)

Comparison: Effectiveness of selective IPC
Outcome: Early onset GBS disease

Study	Experimental n/N	Control n/N	Relative risk (95% Cl fixed)	Weight (%)	RR (95% Cl fixed)
Gibbs (1994)	0/114	5/28	⟵———	33.0	0.02 (0.00, 0.40)
Morales (1987)	0/36	13/48	⟵————	43.7	0.05 (0.00, 0.80)
Pylipow (1994)	0/70	5/54	⟵————	23.3	0.07 (0.00, 1.25)
Total (95% Cl)	0/220	23/130	◁▬▬—	100.0	0.05 (0.01, 0.24)
Chi-square 0.31 (df=2) z=3.65					

1 2   1   5 10
Favours treatment Favours control

(ii) Selective IPC (Universal screening and selective treatment with IPC of colonized women with risk factors)

One randomized controlled trial (Boyer & Gotoff, 1986) and three-cohort studies (Morales & Lim, 1987; Pylipow et al., 1994; Gibbs et al., 1994) were included in the review. One prospective study was excluded, as data extraction was not possible (Poulain et al., 1997).

Neonatal colonization is reduced by universal screening and IPC of women with risk factors as demonstrated by Boyer and Gotoff (1986); however, the study was unable to demonstrate a statistically significant reduction in EOD (RR (95%CI): 0.10 (0.01,1.89)) (Table 6.6). A meta-analysis based on cohort studies was performed to assess the effectiveness of universal screening and selective IPC based on risk factors on EOD. There was a significant reduction in EOD with the use of IPC (RR (95%CI): 0.05 (0.01,0.24)) (Table 6.7).

Table 6.8. Number needed to treat based on preventive strategies (point estimate, 95% CI)

Outcomes (study design)	Universal screening and IPC NNT (95% CI)	Selective IPC NNT (95% CI)
Neonatal colonization (RCT)	3 (2, 4)	2.4 (2,4)
Neonatal colonization (Cohort studies)	2 (2, 3)	Not available
EOD (Cohort studies)	1000[a]	6 (4,10)

[a] Not estimatable.

(iii) IPC based on risk factors only

There have been no prospective studies to date evaluating the effectiveness of the risk-based strategy. Two retrospective reviews describing the authors' experience with the risk-based strategy were identified.

Lieu et al. (1998) demonstrated a reduction in the incidence of EOD from 1.3/1000 to 0.8/1000 live births in their population following the implementation of the risk factor based strategy. Approximately 18% of the mothers were noted to have risk factors: 7.7% had preterm delivery and 10.6% had delivery with fever and/or rupture of membranes for ≥ 18 hours. Even though there was a reduction in the incidence of EOD, this finding did not reach statistical significance ($P = 0.08$). Similarly, Factor et al. (1998) showed a decline in the incidence of GBS from 1.7/1000 in 1992 to 0.2/1000 live births in 1995 ($P = 0.002$), following the initiation of risk based strategy in 1992. However, the decrease in EOD was disproportionate to the increase in IPC use. The investigators speculate several possible explanations for this: (i) women with the highest risk were most easily identified by this protocol, (ii) this trend may represent natural fluctuation in the disease rates, (iii) antibiotic masking of culture results and (iv) the small number of EOD cases and women with high risk sampled in this study may reduce the precision of the estimates for decline in incidence of the disease.

Based on observational studies there has been a reduction in EOD following the implementation of risk factor based strategy. However, to date there have been no prospective studies evaluating the effectiveness of IPC using this strategy.

The effectiveness of a therapeutic manoeuvre can be assessed by the number of patients requiring treatment (number needed to treat) to prevent one adverse event (Laupacis et al., 1988). Based on our analysis of the data from RCTs and cohort studies, the following numbers of women need to be treated to prevent one case of EOD (Table 6.8). Two to three women need to be treated with IPC to prevent one infant from colonization in both universal and selective IPC strategy.

Based on cohort studies 1000 women need to be treated if the universal screening strategy and IPC to all colonized women is used, while six colonized women (95% CI: 4,10) need treatment with selective IPC to prevent one case of EOD. A much larger proportion of women will receive antibiotics if universal screening and IPC is adopted as a preventive strategy compared to universal screening and selective IPC based on risk factors. The potential change in antibiotic resistance of GBS strains as a result of intrapartum prophylaxis is of major concern (Morales et al., 1999). The results of these analyses favour universal screening and risk factor-based IPC over universal screening and IPC to all colonized women.

Postpartum

Neonatal prophylaxis has been evaluated to prevent EOD. In a RCT Pyati et al. (1983) found that penicillin given at birth to neonates weighing $\leq 2000\,g$ does not prevent EOD or reduce mortality associated with disease. Siegel et al. (1982) and Siegel and Cushion (1996) demonstrated that neonatal colonization and EOD were reduced following administration of a single dose of penicillin within 60 minutes of birth. The concerns with this study were: (i) blood cultures were not obtained prior to antibiotic administration, (ii) use of antibiotics may predispose to an increased incidence of infection with penicillin resistant organism and (iii) as most of the cases of EOD begin in utero, intervention is required prior to delivery. Therefore, this form of prophylaxis is currently not recommended.

Conclusions

Perinatal GBS infections remain a major health problem. Until an effective vaccine has been developed, all cases of perintal GBS infections cannot be prevented. An efficient rapid test for GBS has still not been developed. The results of our analyses of different strategies for prevention currently favour universal screening and risk factor-based IPC over universal screening and IPC to all colonized women. In view of the concerns about the quality and heterogeneity of the studies, it is likely that the point estimates for effectiveness for the different interventions have been overestimated. Conducting RCTs with a placebo group is currently not possible, but large RCTs comparing the different strategies head to head could be undertaken using institutions or health regions as the unit of randomization. Surveillance for GBS perinatal infections is necessary and should include measures to ascertain the potential change in antibiotic resistance of GBS strains.

REFERENCES

Ablow, R. C., Driscoll, S. G., Effmann, E. L., Gross, I., Jolles, C. J., Uauy, R. & Warshaw, J. B. (1976). A comparison of early-onset group B streptococcal neonatal infection and the respiratory-distress syndrome of the newborn. *N. Engl. J. Med.*, **294**, 65–70.

Adriaanse, A. H., Kollee, L. A., Muytjens, H. L., Nijhuis, J. G., de Haan, A. F. & Eskes, T. K. (1995). Randomized study of vaginal chlorhexidine disinfection during labor to prevent vertical transmission of group B streptococci. *Eur. J. Obstet. Gynecol. Reprod. Biol.*, **61**, 135–41.

Allardice, J. G., Baskett, T. F., Seshia, M. M. K., Bowman, N. & Malazdrewicz, R. (1982). Perinatal group B streptococcal colonization and infection. *Am. J. Obstet. Gynecol.*, **142**, 617–20.

Allen, U. D., Navas, L. & King, S. M. (1993). Effectiveness of intrapartum penicillin prophylaxis in preventing early-onset group B streptococcal infection: results of a meta-analysis. *Can. Med. Assoc. J.*, **149**, 1659–65.

Altaie, S. S. & Dryja, D. (1994). Detection of group B Streptococcus: comparisons of solid and liquid culture medium with and without selective antibiotics. *Diagn. Microbiol. Infect. Dis.*, **18**, 141–4.

American Academy of Pediatrics (AAP), Committee on Infectious Diseases and Committee on Fetus and Newborn (1992). Guidelines for prevention of group B streptococcal (GBS) infection by chemoprophylaxis. *Pediatrics*, **90**, 775–78.

American Academy of Pediatrics (AAP), Committee on Infectious Diseases and Committee on Fetus and Newborn (1997). Revised guidelines for prevention of early-onset group B streptococcal (GBS) infection. *Pediatrics*, **99**, 489–96.

American College of Obstetricians and Gynecologists (ACOG) (1993). Group B streptococcal infections in pregnancy: ACOG's recommendations. *ACOG Newsletter*, **37**, 1.

Anonymous (1996). Prevention of perinatal group B streptococcal disease: a public health perspective. Adapted February 1997. *M.M.W.R.*, **45**(RR-7).

Anthony, B.F., Eisenstadt, R., Carter, J., Kim, K. S., & Hobel, C. J. (1981). Genital and intestinal carriage of group B streptococci during pregnancy. *J. Infect. Dis.*, **143**, 761–6.

Armer, T., Clark, P., Duff, P. & Saravanos, K. (1993). Rapid intrapartum detection of group B streptococcal colonization with an enzyme immunoassay. *Am. J. Obstet. Gynecol.*, **168**, 39–43.

Ascher, D. P., Wilson, S., Mendiola, J. & Fischer, G. W. (1991). Group B streptococcal latex agglutination testing in neonates. *J. Pediatr.*, **119**, 458–61.

Badri, M. S., Zawaneh, S., Cruz, A. C., Mantilla, G., Baer, H., Spellacy, W. N. & Ayoub, E. M. (1977). Rectal colonization with group B streptococcus: relation to vaginal colonization in pregnant women. *J. Infect. Dis.*, **135**, 308–12.

Baker, C. J. (1990). Antibiotic therapy in neonates whose mothers have received intrapartum group B streptococcal chemoprophylaxis. *Pediatr. Infect. Dis. J.*, **9**, 149–50.

Baker, C. J. (1996). Inadequacy of rapid immunoassays for intrapartum detection of group B streptococcal carriers. *Obstet. Gynecol.*, **88**, 51–5.

Baker, C. J. & Edwards, M. S. (1990). Group B streptococcal infections. In *Infectious Diseases of the Fetus and Newborn Infant* 3rd edn., ed. J. S. Remington & J. O. Klein, pp. 742–811. Philadelphia: W. B. Saunders Company.

Baker, C. J. & Noya, F. J. (1990). Potential use of intravenous immune globulin for group B streptococcal infection. *Rev. Infect. Dis.*, **12**, S476–82.

Baker, C. J. & Edwards, M. S. (1995). Group B streptococcal infections. In *Infectious Disease of the Fetus and Newborn Infant.* 4th edn., ed. J. S. Remington & J. O. Klein, pp. 980–1054.

Philadelphia: W. B. Saunders Company.

Baker, C. J., Clark, D. J. & Barrett, F. F. (1973). Selective broth medium for isolation of group B streptococci. *Appl. Microbiol.*, 26, 884–5.

Baker, C. J., Goroff, D. K., Alpert, S., Crockett, V. A., Zinner, S. H., Evrard, J. R., Rosner, B., & McCormack, W. M. (1977). Vaginal colonization with group B streptococcus: a study in college women. *J. Infect. Dis.*, 135, 392–7.

Baker, C. J. & Kasper, D. L. (1985). Group B streptococcal vaccines. *Rev. Infect. Dis.*, 7, 458–67.

Baker, C. J., Rench, M. A., Edwards, M. S., Carpenter, R. J., Hays, B. M. & Kasper, D. L. (1988). Immunization of pregnant women with a polysaccharide vaccine of group B streptococcus. *N. Engl. J. Med.*, **319**, 1180–5.

Baley, J. E. & Fanaroff, A. A. (1992). Neonatal infections, Part 2, specific infectious diseases and therapies.(2.Group B streptococcal infections). In *Effective Care of the Newborn Infant*, ed. J. C. Sinclair & M. B. Bracken, pp. 480–3. Oxford: Oxford University Press.

Barefield, E. S., Oh, W. & Stonestreet, B. S. (1992). Group B streptococcus-induced acidosis in newborn swine: regional oxygen transport and lactate flux. *J. Appl. Physiol.*, **72**, 272–7.

Benitz, W. E., Gould, J. B. & Druzin, M. L. (1999). Risk factors for early-onset group B streptococcal sepsis: estimation of odds ratios by critical literature review. *Pediatrics*, **103**, e77.

Bennet, R., Bergdahl, S., Eriksson, M. & Zetterstrom, R. (1989). The outcome of neonatal septicemia during fifteen years. *Acta Paediatr. Scand.*, **78**, 40–3.

Bergqvist, G. (1974). Neonatal infections caused by group B streptococci 3. Incidence in Sweden 1970–71. *Scand. J. Infect. Dis.*, **6**, 29–31.

Bergqvist, G., Holmberg, G., Rydner, T. & Vaclavinkova, V. (1978). Intrauterine death due to infection with group B streptococci. *Acta Obstet. Gynecol. Scand.*, **57**, 127–8.

Blumberg, H. M., Stephens, D. S., Modansky, M., Erwin, M., Elliot, J., Facklam, R. R., Schuchat, A., Baughman, W. & Farley, M. M. (1996). Invasive group B streptococcal disease: the emergency of serotype V. *J. Infect. Dis.*, **173**, 365–73

Boyer, K. M. & Gotoff, S. P. (1986). Prevention of early-onset neonatal group B streptococcus disease with selective intrapartum chemoprophylaxis. *N. Engl. J. Med.*, **314**, 1665–9.

Boyer, K. M., Gadzala, C. A., Burd, L. I., Fisher, D. E., Paton, J. B. & Gotoff, S. P. (1983a). Selective intrapartum chemoprophylaxis of neonatal group B streptococcal early-onset disease. I. Epidemiologic rationale. *J. Infect. Dis.*, **148**, 795–801.

Boyer, K. M., Gadzala, C. A., Kelly, P. D., Burd, L. I. & Gotoff, S. P. (1983b). Selective intrapartum chemoprophylaxis of neonatal group B streptococcal early-onset disease. II. Predictive value of prenatal cultures. *J. Infect. Dis.*, **148**, 802–9.

Boyer, K. M. & Gotoff, S. P. (1985). Strategies for chemoprophylaxis of GBS early onset infections. *Antibiot. Chemother.*, **35**, 267–80.

Brady, K., Duff, P., Schilhab, J. C. & Herd, M. (1989). Reliability of a rapid latex fixation test for detecting group B streptococci in the genital tract of parturients at term. *Obstet. Gynecol.*, **73**, 678–81.

Bramer, S., van Wijk, F. H., Mol, B. W. & Adriaanse, A. H. (1997). Risk indicators for neonatal early-onset GBS-related disease. A case-control study. *J. Perinat. Med.*, **25**, 469–75.

Burman, L. G., Christensen, P., Christensen, K., Fryklund, B., Helgesson, A. M., Svenningsen, N. E. & Tullus, K. (1992). Prevention of excess neonatal morbidity associated with group B streptococci by vaginal chlorhexidine disinfection during labour. *Lancet*, **340**, 65–9.

Carstensen, H., Christensen, K. K., Grennert, L., Persson, K. & Polberger, S. (1988) Early-onset neonatal group B septicemia in siblings. *J. Infect.*, **17**, 201–4.

Cayeux, P. (1972). Infections neonatales a streptocques du groupe B constatations etiologiques. A propos de 77 observations. *Arch. Franc. Pediatr.*, **29**, 391–6.

Centers for Disease Control and Prevention (1996). Prevention of perinatal group B streptococcal disease: a public health perspective. *M.M.W.R.*, **45**(No.RR-7), 1–24.

Centers for Disease Control and Prevention (1997). Decreasing incidence of perinatal group B streptococcal disease – United States, 1993–1995. *M.M.W.R.*, **46**, 473–7.

Charles, D. & Larsen, B. (1986). Streptococcal puerperal sepsis and obstetric infections: a historical perspective. *Rev. Inf. Dis.*, **8**, 411–22.

Chin, K. C. & Fitzhardinge, P. M. (1985). Sequelae of early-onset group B haemolytic streptococcal neonatal meningitis. *J. Pediatr.*, **106**, 819–22.

Christensen, K. K. (1982). Infection as a predominant cause of perinatal mortality. *Obstet. Gynecol.*, **59**, 499–508.

Christensen, K. K., Christensen, P., Dahlander, K., Linden, V., Lindroth, M. & Svenningsen, N. (1983). The significance of group B streptococci in neonatal pneumonia. *Eur. J. Pediatr.*, **140**, 118–22.

Clark, P., Armer, T., Duff, P. & Davidson, K. (1992). Assessment of a rapid latex agglutination test for group B streptococcal colonization of the genital tract. *Obstet. Gynecol.*, **79**, 358–63.

Coleman, R. T., Sherer, D. M. & Maniscalco, W. M. (1992). Prevention of neonatal group B streptococcal infections: advances in maternal vaccine development. *Obstet. Gynecol.*, **80**, 301–9.

Committee on Technical Bulletins of the American College of Obstetricians and Gynaecologists. (1992). Group B streptococcal infections in pregnancy. Number 170.

Da Silva, O., Ohlsson, A. & Kenyon, C. (1995). Accuracy of leukocyte indices and C-reactive protein for diagnosis of neonatal sepsis: a critical review. *Pediatr. Infect. Dis. J.*, **14**, 362–6.

Dillon, H. C. Jr, Gray, E., Pass, M. A. & Gray, B. M. (1982). Anorectal and vaginal carriage of group B streptococci during pregnancy. *J. Infect. Dis.*, **145**, 794–9.

Easmon, C. S. F., Hastings, M. J. G., Deeley, J., Bloxham, B., Rivers, R. P. A. & Marwood, R. (1983). The effect of intrapartum chemoprophylaxis on the vertical transmission of group B streptococci. *Br. J. Obstet. Gynaecol.*, **90**, 633–5.

Eickhoff, T. C., Klein, J. O., Daly, A. K., Ingall, D. & Finland, M. (1964). Neonatal sepsis and other infections due to group B beta-haemolytic streptococci. *N. Engl. J. Med.*, **271**, 1221–8.

Factor, S. H., Levine, O. S., Nassar, A., Potter, J., Fajardo, A., O'Sullivan, M. J. & Schuchat, A. (1998). Impact of a risk-based prevention policy on neonatal group B streptococcal disease. *Am. J. Obstet. Gynecol.*, **178**, 1568–71

Fargason, C. A., Peralta-Carcelen, M., Rouse, D. J., Cutter, G. R. & Goldenberg, R. L. (1997). The pediatric costs of strategies for minimizing the risk of early-onset group B streptococcal disease. *Obstet. Gynecol.*, **90**, 347–52.

Faxelius, G., Bremme, K., Kvist-Christensen, K., Christensen, P. & Ringertz, S. (1988). Neonatal septicemia due to group B streptococci – perinatal risk factors and outcome of subsequent pregnancies. *J. Perinat. Med.*, **16**, 423–30.

Ferrieri, P. & Blair, L. L. (1977). Pharyngeal carriage of group B streptococci: detection by three methods. *J. Clin. Microbiol.*, **6**, 136–9.

Fischer, G. W., Hemming, V. G., Gloser, H. P., Bachmayer, H., von Pilar, C. E., Wilson, S. R. & Baron, P. A. (1990). Polyvalent group B streptococcal immune globulin for intravenous administration: overview. *Rev. Infect. Dis.*, **12**, S483–91.

Fliegner, J. R. & Garland, S. M. (1990). Perinatal mortality in Victoria, Australia: role of group B streptococcus. *Am. J. Obstet. Gynecol.*, **163**, 1609–11.

Fowlie, P. W. & Schmidt, B. (1998). Diagnostic tests for bacterial infection from birth to 90 days – a systematic review. *Arch. Dis. Child Fetal Neonat. Ed.*, **78**, F92–9.

Franciosi, R. A., Knostman, J. D. & Zimmerman, R. A. (1973). Group B streptococcal neonatal and infant infections. *J. Pediatr.*, **82**, 707–18.

Fry, R. M. (1938). Fatal infections by haemolytic streptococcus group B. *Lancet*, **i**, 199–201.

Gardner, S. E., Yow, M. D., Leeds, L. J., Thompson, P. K., Mason, E. O. & Clark, D. J. (1979). Failure of penicillin to eradicate group B streptococcal colonization in the pregnant women. A couple study. *Am. J. Obstet. Gynecol.*, **135**, 1062–5.

Garland, S. M. (1991). Early onset neonatal group B streptococcus (GBS) infection: associated obstetric risk factors. *Aust. NZ J. Obstet. Gynaecol.*, **31**, 117–18.

Garland, S. M. & Fliegner, J. R. (1991). Group B streptococcus (GBS) and neonatal infections: the case for intrapartum chemoprophylaxis. *Aust. NZ J. Obstet. Gynecol.*, **31**, 119–22.

Gerdes, J. S. (1991). Clinicopathologic approach to the diagnosis of neonatal sepsis. *Clin. Perinatol.*, **18**, 361–81.

Gibbs, R. S., Hall, R. T., Yow, M. D., McCracken, G. H. & Nelson, J. D. (1992). Consensus: perinatal prophylaxis for Group B streptococcal infection. *Pediatr. Infect. Dis. J.*, **11**, 179–83.

Gibbs, R. S., McDuffie, R. S., McNabb, F., Fryer, G. E., Miyoshi, T. & Merenstein, G. (1994). Neonatal group B streptococcal sepsis during 2-years of a universal screening program. *Obstet. Gynecol.*, **84**, 496–500.

Glantz, J. C. & Kedley, K. E. (1998). Concepts and controversies in the management of group B streptococcus during pregnancy. *Birth*, **25**, 45–53.

Gonen, R., Ohlsson, A., Farine, D. & Milligan, J. E. (1991). Can the nonstress test predict congenital sepsis? *Am. J. Perinatol.*, **8**, 91–3.

Gordon, J. S. & Sbarra, A. J. (1976). Incidence, technique of isolation, and treatment of group B streptococci in obstetric patients. *Am. J. Obstet. Gynecol.*, **126**, 1023–6.

Gotoff, S. P. & Boyer, K. M. (1997). Prevention of early-onset neonatal group B streptococcal disease. *Pediatrics*, **99**, 866–9.

Granato, P. A. & Petosa, M. T. (1991). Evaluation of a rapid screening test for detecting group B streptococci in pregnant women. *J. Clin. Microbiol.*, **29**, 1536–8.

Green, M., Dashefsky, B., Wald, E. R., Laifer, S., Harger, J. & Guthrie, R. (1993). Comparison of two antigen assays for rapid intrapartum detection of vaginal group B streptococcal colonization. *J. Clin. Microbiol.*, **31**, 78–82.

Greenberg, D. N. & Yoder, B. A. (1990). Changes in the differential white blood cell count in screening for group B streptococcal sepsis. *Pediatr. Infect. Dis. J.*, **9**, 886–9.

Guyer, B., MacDorman, M. F., Martin, J. A., Peters, K. D. & Strobino, D. M. (1998). Annual summary of vital statistics – 1997. *Pediatrics*, **102**, 1333–49.

Hagay, Z. J., Miskin, A., Goldchmit, R., Federman, A., Matzkel, A. & Mogilner, B. M. (1993). Evaluation of two rapid tests for detection of maternal endocervical group B streptococcus: enzyme-linked immunosorbent assay and gram stain. *Obstet. Gynecol.*, **82**, 84–7.

Hall, R. T., Barnes, W., Krishnan, L., Harris, D. J., Rhodes, P. G., Fayez, J. & Miller, G. L. (1976). Antibiotic treatment of parturient women colonized with group B streptococcus. *Am. J. Obstet. Gynecol.*, **124**, 630–4.

Harris, M. C., Deuber, C., Polin, R. A. & Nachamkin, I. (1989) Investigation of apparent false-positive urine latex particle agglutination tests for the detection of group B streptococcus antigen. *J. Clin. Microbiol.*, **27**, 2214–17.

Hastings, M. J. G., Easmon, C. S. F., Neill, J., Bloxham, B. & Rivers, R. P. A. (1986). Group B streptococcal colonisation and the outcome of pregnancy. *J. Infect.*, **12**, 23–29.

Henrichsen, T., Lindemann, R., Svenningsen, L. & Hjelle, K. (1994). Prevention of neonatal infections by vaginal chlorhexidine disinfection during labour. *Acta Paediatr.*, **83**, 923–6.

Hocker, J. R., Simpson, P. M., Rabalais, G. P., Stewart, D. L. & Cook, L. N. (1992). Extracorporeal membrane oxygenation and early-onset group B streptococcal sepsis. *Pediatrics*, **89**, 1–4.

Hood, M., Janney, A. & Dameron, G. (1961). Beta haemolytic streptococcus group B associated with problems of the perinatal period. *Am. J. Obstet. Gynecol.*, **82**, 809–18.

Hordnes, K., Eide, M., Ulstein, M., Digranes, A. & Haneberg, B. (1995). Evaluation of a rapid enzyme immunoassay for detection of genital colonization of group B streptococci in pregnant women: own experience and review. *Aus. NZ J. Obstet. Gynaecol.*, **35**, 251–3.

Institute of Medicine (1985). Prospects for immunizing against Streptococcus Group B. In *New Vaccine Development. Establishing Priorities*, Vol. 1. Diseases of importance in the United States, pp. 424–39. Washington, DC: National Academy Press.

Isada, N. B. & Grossman, J. H. (1987). A rapid screening test for the diagnosis of endocervical group B streptococci in pregnancy: microbiologic results and clinical outcome. *Obstet. Gynecol.*, **70**, 139–41.

Jeffery, H. E. & Lahra, M. (1998). Eight-year outcome of universal screening and intrapartum antibiotics for maternal group B streptococcal carriers. *Pediatrics*, **101**, E2.

Kontnick, C. M. & Edberg, S. C. (1990). Direct detection of group B streptococci from vaginal specimens compared with quantitative culture. *J. Clin. Microbiol.*, **28**, 336–9.

Lachenauer, C. S., Kasper, D. L., Shimada, J., Ichiman, Y., Ohtsuka, H., Kaku, M., Paoletti, L. C., Ferrieri, P. & Madoff, L. C. (1999). Serotypes VI and VIII predominate among group B streptococci isolated from pregnant Japanese women. *J. Infect. Dis.*, **179**, 1030–3.

Lancefield, R. C. (1933). A serological differentiation of human and other groups of haemolytic streptococci. *J. Exp. Med.*, **57**, 571–95.

Lancefield, R. C. & Hare, R. (1935). The serological differentiation of pathogenic and non-pathogenic strains of haemolytic streptococci from parturient women. *J. Exp. Med.*, **61**, 335–49.

Laupacis, A., Sackett, D. L. & Roberts, R. S. (1988). An assessment of clinically useful measures of the consequences of treatment. *N. Engl. J. Med.*, **318**, 1728–33.

Lieu, T. A., Mohle-Boetani, J. C., Ray, T., Ackerson, L. M. & Walton, D. G. (1998). Neonatal group B streptococcal infection in a managed care population. *Obstet. Gynecol.*, **92**, 21–7.

Lim, D. V., Morales, W. J., Walsh, A. F. & Kazanis, D. (1986). Reduction of morbidity and mortality rates for neonatal group B streptococcal disease through early diagnosis and chemoprophylaxis. *J. Clin. Microbiol.*, **23**, 489–92.

Lloyd, D. J. & Reid, T. M. (1976). Group B streptococcal infection in the newborn. Criteria for early detection and treatment. *Acta Paediatr. Scand.*, **65**, 585–91.

Lotz-Nolan, L., Amato, T., Iltis, J., Wallen, W. & Packer, B. (1989). Evaluation of a rapid latex agglutination test for detection of group B streptococci in vaginal specimens. *Eur. J. Clin. Microbiol. Infect. Dis.*, **8**, 289–93.

McCracken, G. H. (1973). Group B streptococci: the new challenge in neonatal infections. *J. Pediatr.*, **82**, 703–6.

McDonald, H., Vigneswaran, R. & O'Loughlin, J. A. (1989). Group B streptococcal colonization and preterm labour. *Aust. NZ J. Obstet. Gynaecol.*, **29**, 291–3.

Matorras, R., Garcia-Perea, A., Omenaca, F., Diez-Enciso, M., Madero, R. & Usandizaga, J. A. (1991). Intrapartum chemoprophylaxis of early-onset group B streptococcal disease. *Eur. J. Obstet. Gynecol. Reprod. Biol.*, **40**, 57–62.

Mohle-Boetani, J. C., Lieu, T. A., Ray, G. T. & Escobar, G. (1999). Preventing neonatal group B streptococcal disease: cost-effectiveness in a health maintenance organisation and the impact of delayed hospital discharge for newborns who received intrapartum antibiotics. *Pediatrics*, **103**, 703–10.

Montgomery, D. M., Stedman, C. M., Robichaux, A. G., Joyner, J. C. & Scariano, S. M. (1991). Cord blood gas patterns identifying newborns at increased risk of group B streptococcal sepsis. *Obstet. Gynecol.*, **78**, 774–7.

Morales, W. J. & Lim, D. (1987). Reduction of group B streptococcal maternal and neonatal infections in preterm pregnancies with premature rupture of membranes through a rapid identification test. *Am. J. Obstet. Gynecol.*, **157**, 13–16.

Morales, W. J., Lim, D. V. & Walsh, A. F. (1986). Prevention of neonatal group B streptococcal sepsis by the use of a rapid screening test and selective intrapartum chemoprophylaxis. *Am. J. Obstet. Gynecol.*, **155**, 979–83.

Morales, W. J., Dickey, S. S., Bornick, P. & Lim, D. V. (1999). Change in antibiotic resistance of group B streptococcus: Impact on intrapartum management. *Am. J. Obstet. Gynecol.*, **181**, 310–4.

Munoz, P., Coque, T., Rodriguez Creixems, M., Bernaldo de Quiros, J. C., Moreno, S. & Bouza, E. (1992). Group B streptococcus: a cause of urinary tract infection in non-pregnant adults. *Clin. Infect. Dis.*, **14**, 492–6.

Newton, E. R. & Clark, M. (1988). Group B streptococcus and preterm rupture of membranes. *Obstet. Gynecol.*, **71**, 198–202.

Nyhan, W. L. & Fousek, M. D. (1958). Septicemia of the newborn. *Pediatrics*, **22**, 268–78.

Ohlsson, A. (1992). Perinatal group B streptococcal infections. *Can. J. Obstet. Gynaecol. & Women's Health Care*, 455–63.

Ohlsson, A. & Serenius, F. (1981). Neonatal septicemia in Riyadh, Saudi Arabia. *Acta Paediatr. Scand.*, **70**, 825–9.

Ohlsson, A. & Vearncombe, M. (1987). Congenital and nosocomial infection sepsis in infants born in a regional perinatal unit: cause, outcome and white blood cell response. *Am. J. Obstet.*

Gynecol., **156**, 407–13.

Ohlsson, A. & Wang, E. (1990). An analysis of antenatal tests to detect infection in preterm premature rupture of the membranes. *Am. J. Obstet. Gynecol.*, **162**, 809–18.

Ohlsson, A. & Myhr, T. L. (1994). Intrapartum chemoprophylaxis of perinatal group B streptococcal infections: a critical review of randomized controlled trials. *Am. J. Obstet. Gynecol.*, **170**, 910–7.

Ohlsson, A., Bailey, T. & Takieddine, F. (1986). Changing etiology and outcome of neonatal septicemia in Riyadh, Saudi Arabia. *Acta Paediatr. Scand.*, **75**, 540–4.

Ohlsson, A., Shennan, A. T. & Rose, T. H. (1987). Review of causes of perinatal mortality in a regional perinatal center, 1980–1984. *Am. J. Obstet. Gynecol.*, **157**, 443–5.

Opal, S. M., Cross, A., Palmer, M. & Almazan, R. (1988). Group B streptococcal sepsis in adults and infants. Contrasts and comparisons. *Arch. Intern. Med.*, **148**, 641–5.

Park, C. H., Ruprai, D., Vandel, N. M., Hixon, D. L. & Mecklenburg, F. E. (1996). Rapid detection of group B streptococcal antigen from vaginal specimens using a new optical immunoassay technique. *Diagn. Microbiol. Infect. Dis.*, **24**, 125–8.

Philipson, E. H., Palermino, D. A. & Robinson, A. (1995). Enhanced antenatal detection of group B streptococcus colonization. *Obstet. Gynecol.*, **85**, 437–9.

Poulain, P., Betremieux, P., Donnio, P. Y., Proudhon, J. F., Karege, G. & Giraud, J. R. (1997). Selective intrapartum anti-bioprohylaxy of group B streptococci infection of neonates: a prospective study in 2454 subsequent deliveries. *Eur. J. Obstet. Gynecol. Reprod. Biol.*, **72**, 137–40.

Pyati, S. P., Pildes, R. S., Jacobs, N. M., Ramamurthy, R. S., Yeh, T. F., Raval, D. S., Lilien, L. D., Amma, P. & Metzger, W.I. (1983). Penicillin in infants weighing two kilograms or less with early-onset group B streptococcal disease. *N. Engl. J. Med.*, **308**, 1383–9.

Pylipow, M., Gaddis, M. & Kinney, J. S. (1994). Selective intrapartum prophylaxis for group B streptococcus colonization: management and outcomes of newborns. *Pediatrics*, **93**, 631–5.

Quentin, R., Dubarry, I., Gignier, C., Saulnier, M., Pierre, F. & Goudeau, A. (1993). Evaluation of a rapid latex test for direct detection of streptococcus agalactiae in various obstetrical and gynaecological disorders. *Eur. J. Clin. Microbiol. Infect. Dis.*, **12**, 51–4.

Regan, J. A., Chao, S. & James, L. S. (1981). Premature rupture of the membranes, preterm delivery, and group B streptococcal colonization of mothers. *Am. J. Obstet. Gynecol.*, **141**, 184–6.

Reid, T. M. (1975). Emergence of group B streptococci in obstetric and perinatal infections. *Bri. Med. J.*, 2, 533–5.

Rench, M. A. & Baker, C. J. (1993). Neonatal sepsis caused by a new group B streptococcal serotype. *J. Pediatr.*, **122**, 638–40.

Rouse, D. J., Goldenberg, R. L., Cliver, S. P., Cutter, G. R., Mennemeyer, S. T. & Fargason, C. A. (1994). Strategies for the prevention of early-onset neonatal group B streptococcal sepsis: a decision analysis. *Obstet. Gynecol.*, **83**, 483–94.

Sanchez, P. J., Siegel, J. D., Cushion, N. B. & Threlkeld, N. (1990). Significance of a positive urine group B streptococcal latex agglutination test in neonates. *J. Pediatr.*, **116**, 601–6.

Schimmel, M. S., Eidelman, A. I., Rudensky, B. & Isacsohn, M. (1994). Value of a rapid enzyme linked immunosorbent assay for maternal vaginal group B streptococcus colonization.

J. Perinatol., **14**, 198–200.

Schimmel, M. S., Samueloff, A. & Eidelman, A. I. (1998). Prevention of neonatal group B streptococcal infections. Is there a rationale prevention strategy? *Clin. Perinatol.*, **25**, 687–97.

Schroder, H. & Paust, H. (1979). B-Streptokokken als haufigste Erreger der Neugeborenensepsis. Einleitung, Haufigkeit. *Monatsschr Kinderheilkd.*, **127**, 720–3.

Schuchat, A. (1998). Epidemiology of group B streptococcal disease in the United States: shifting paradigms. *Clin. Microbiol. Rev.*, **11**, 497–513.

Schuchat, A., Deaver-Robinson, K., Plikaytis, B. D., Zangwill, K. M., Mohle-Boetani, J. & Wegner, J. D. (1994). Multistate case-control study of maternal risk factors for group B streptococcal disease. The Active Surveillance Study Group. *Pediatr. Infect. Dis. J.*, **13**, 623–9.

Schwartz, B., Schuchat, A., Oxtoby, M. J., Cochi, S. L., Hightower, A. & Broome, C. V. (1991). Invasive group B streptococcal disease in adults. A population-based study in metropolitan Atlanta. *J.A.M.A.*, **266**, 1112–14.

Siegel, J. D. & Cushion, N. B. (1996). Prevention of early-onset group B streptococcal disease: another look at single-dose penicillin at birth. *Obstet. Gynecol.*, **87**, 692–8.

Siegel, J. D., McCracken, G. H., Threlkeld, N., DePasse, B. M. & Rosenfeld, C. R. (1982). Single-dose penicillin prophylaxis of neonatal group-B streptococcal disease. Conclusion of a 41 month controlled trial. *Lancet*, **i**, 1426–30.

Silver, H. M. & Struminsky, J. (1996). A comparison of the yield of positive antenatal group B streptococcus cultures with direct inoculation in selective growth medium versus primary inoculation in transport medium followed by delayed inoculation in selective growth medium. *Am. J. Obstet. Gynecol.*, **175**, 155–7.

Society of Obstetricians and Gynaecologists of Canada and the Canadian Pediatric Society. (1994). National consensus statement on the prevention of early-onset group B streptococcal infections in the newborn. *J. Soc. Obstet. Gynaecol. Can.*, **16**, 2271–8.

Society of Obstetricians and Gynecologists. (1997). Statement on the prevention of early-onset group B streptococcal infections in the newborn. *J. Soc. Obstet. Gynaecol. Can.*, **19**, 751–8.

Speer, C. P., Hauptmann, D., Stubbe, P. & Gahr, M. (1985). Neonatal septicemia and meningitis in Gottingen, West Germany. *Pediatr. Infect. Dis.*, **4**, 36–41.

Stiller, R. J., Blair, E., Clark, P. & Tinghitella, T. (1989). Rapid detection of vaginal colonization with group B streptococci by means of latex agglutination. *Am. J. Obstet. Gynecol.*, **160**, 566–8.

Strickland, D. M., Yeomans, E. R. & Hankins, G. D. (1990). Cost-effectiveness of intrapartum screening and treatment for maternal group B streptococci colonization. *Am. J. Obstet. Gynecol.*, **163**, 4–8.

Sweeten, K. M., Eriksen, N. L. & Blanco, J. D. (1997). Chlorhexidine versus sterile water vaginal wash during labor to prevent peripartum infection. *Am. J. Obstet. Gynecol.*, **176**, 426–30.

Taha, T. E., Biggar, R. J., Broadhead, R. L., Mtimavalye, L. A., Justesen, A.B., Liomba, G. N., Chiphangwi, J. D. & Miotti, P. G. (1997). Effect of cleansing the birth canal with antiseptic solution on maternal and newborn morbidity and mortality in Malawi: clinical trial. *Br. Med. J.*, **315**, 216–20.

Thomsen, A. C., Morup, L. & Brogaard Hansen K. B. (1987). Antibiotic elimination of group-B streptococci in urine in prevention of preterm labour. *Lancet*, **i**, 591–3.

Towers, C. V., Garite, T. J., Friedman, W. W., Pircon, R. A. & Nageotte, M. P. (1990).

Comparison of a rapid enzyme-linked immunosorbent assay test and the gram stain for detection of group B streptococci in high-risk antepartum patients. *Am. J. Obstet. Gynecol.*, **163**, 965–7.

Tuppurainen, N. & Hallman. M. (1989). Prevention of neonatal group B streptococcal disease: intrapartum detection and chemoprophylaxis of heavily colonized parturients. *Obstet. Gynecol.*, **73**, 583–7.

Tuppurainen, N., Osterlund, K. & Hallman, M. (1986). Selective intrapartum penicillin prophylaxis of early onset group B streptococcal disease. *Pediatr. Res.*, **20**, 403A.

Vesikari, T., Isolauri, E., Tuppurainen, N., Renlund, M., Koivisto, M., Janas, M., Ikonen, R. S., Kero, P., Heinonen, K., Nyman, R., et al., (1989) Neonatal septicaemia in Finland 1981–85. Predominance of Group B streptococcal infections with very early onset. *Acta. Paediatr. Scand.*, **78**, 44–50.

Wald, E. R., Dashefsky, B., Green, M., Harger, J., Parise, M., Korey, C. & Byers, C. (1987). Rapid detection of group B streptococci directly from vaginal swabs. *J. Clin. Microbiol.*, **25**, 573–4.

Walsh, J. A. & Hutchins, S. (1989). Group B streptococcal disease: its importance in developing world and prospect for prevention with vaccines. *Pediatr. Infect. Dis. J.*, **8**, 271–6.

Weindling, A. M., Hawkins, J. M., Coombes, M. A. & Stringer, J. (1981). Colonisation of babies and their families by group B streptococci. *Brit. Med. J.*, **283**, 1503–5.

Wood, E. G. & Dillon, H. C. (1981). A prospective study of group B streptococcal bacteriuria in pregnancy. *Am. J. Obstet. Gynecol.*, **140**, 515–20.

Wust, J., Hebisch, G. & Peters, K. (1993). Evaluation of two enzyme immunoassays for rapid detection of group B streptococci in pregnant women. *Eur. J. Clin. Microbiol. Infect. Dis.*, **12**, 124–7.

Yagupsky, P., Menegus, M. A. & Powell, K. R. (1991). The changing spectrum of group B streptococcal disease in infants: an eleven-year experience in a tertiary care hospital. *Pediatr. Infect. Dis. J.*, **10**, 801–8.

Yancey, M. K. & Duff, P. (1994). An analysis of the cost-effectiveness of selected protocols for the prevention of neonatal group B streptococcal infection. *Obstet. Gynecol.*, **83**, 367–71.

Yancey, M. K., Schuchat, A., Brown, L. K., Lee Ventura, V. & Markenson, G. R. (1996). The accuracy of late antenatal screening cultures in predicting genital group B streptococcal colonization at delivery. *Obstet. Gynecol.*, **88**, 811–15.

Yow, M. D., Mason, E. O., Leeds, L. J., Thompson, P. K., Clark, D. J. & Gardner, S. E. (1979). Ampicillin prevents intrapartum transmission of group B streptococcus. *J.A.M.A.*, **241**, 1245–7.

Yow, M. D., Leeds, M. J., Thompson, P. K., Mason, E. O. Jr, Clark, D. J. & Beachler, C. W. (1980). The natural history of group B streptococcal colonization in the pregnant woman and her offspring. I. Colonization studies. *Am. J. Obstet. Gynecol.*, **137**, 34–8.

Zangwill, K. M., Schuchat, A. & Wenger, J. D. (1992). Group B streptococcal disease in the United States, 1990: report from a multistate active surveillance system. CDC Surveillance Summaries. *M.M.W.R.*, **41**(SS-6), 25–32.

7

Mother-to-child transmission of cytomegalovirus

Marie-Louise Newell

The virus

Cytomegalovirus (CMV) is an enveloped DNA virus and a member of the herpes family which also includes herpes simplex, Epstein–Barr and varicella-zoster viruses. Like other herpes viruses, once primary infection has occurred the virus establishes itself in the host in a latent form, possibly in peripheral blood mono-nuclear cells, and may periodically reactivate (Jafari et al., 1995). During active infection CMV is found in epithelial cells (Griffiths & Grundy, 1998). Infection is controlled by cellular and humoral immune responses, with the cellular responses being the most important and much of the tissue damage associated with CMV infection is probably due to the immune mediated inflammatory reaction to infected cells expressing CMV antigen (Griffiths & Grundy, 1998). CMV is probably transmitted through infected secretions coming into contact with mucous membranes, but not through intact skin. Droplet infection seems to play a minor role. The virus is unstable outside the body and is vulnerable to ordinary soaps, detergents, commonly used disinfectants and heat. Normal hygienic procedures should thus substantially reduce, or eliminate, the risk of transmission of infection.

Both primary and recurrent (with the same or a different strain) infections are associated with viral shredding in body fluids, including urine, saliva, semen, cervical secretions and breast milk. In healthy individuals symptoms of CMV infection are usually mild or not apparent and rarely cause serious illness. However, infection can be life threatening in immunocompromised individuals and in very premature infants, and when acquired in pregnancy it can result in fetal damage (Fig. 7.1).

CMV infection affects the central nervous system in a substantial proportion of infected neonates. CMV infection is the leading cause of intrauterine infections with an incidence of congenital infection ranging from 0.5% to 2% of all live

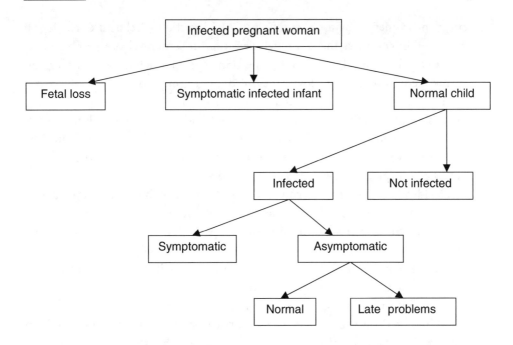

Figure 7.1   The consequences of maternal CMV infection.

births, depending on the rate of primary and recurrent infection in the population studied (Ahlfors et al., 1984; Peckham et al., 1983a; Schopfer et al., 1978; Stagno et al., 1982). In addition to intrauterine infection, infants born to seropositive mothers may acquire infection during delivery or in early life as a result of breastfeeding or prolonged close contact with an infected individual. In the UK about 20% of children become infected by 12 months (Peckham et al., 1987a, b), but infection acquired after birth is rarely associated with adverse outcome, except in the very premature infant.

Prevalence

Infection with CMV occurs throughout the world. As it is usually asymptomatic and harmless, infection is only recognized by the detection of serum antibodies. Prevalence of CMV antibodies increases with age, but the increment varies between populations (Stagno, 1996). A number of antenatal prevalence studies have been conducted, suggesting a prevalence between 50% and 95%, depending on the population. In non-industrialized countries of Africa and Asia, most women of childbearing age are seropositive, probably having acquired infection in early life, whilst in industrialized countries in Europe and America about 50% of pregnant women remain susceptible to CMV infection (Peckham et al., 1983). Even within countries there is much variation in seroprevalence. For example, studies in Chile, Brazil, Japan and in the USA report more than 80% of pregnant women seropositive among lower socio-economic groups (Kamada, 1983; Stagno et al., 1982; Yow et al., 1987), and between 40 and 50% among middle income groups. Generally, the prevalence of CMV antibodies correlates with non-white race, socio-economic and educational status, being breastfed as an infant, the presence of young children at home, sexual activity and maternal age (Chandler et al., 1985; Murph et al., 1998; Preece et al., 1986).

Worldwide most people acquire CMV during childhood, and the rate of acquisition of CMV in the first few years of life is high, especially in non-industrialized countries and in selected groups in developed countries (Stagno, 1996). In a prospective study in the USA, 14% of children developed CMV antibody before 1 year of age, 12% in the second year of life, and between 1.5% and 5% annually thereafter. By age 10 years, 33% of children were CMV antibody positive, but infection was more common in non-white, lower socio-economic class children (Yow et al., 1988). The seroprevalence rate at age 1 year depends on the duration of breastfeeding, for example in Sweden, about 30% of 1 year olds are seropositive. Day care centre or nursery attendance can be a source of acquisition of CMV infection in early childhood, as after primary infection children excrete the virus for a long time. Although it has been suggested that about 50% of susceptible children under the age of 3 years who attend a day care centre of reasonable size will acquire CMV infection (Adler, 1988; Bale et al., 1999), this has not been confirmed in other studies (Ahlfors et al., 1999; Grillner & Strangert 1986) and may reflect differences in the organization of day care and the background from which these children come (Nelson et al., 1987; Tookey & Peckham, 1991).

Between one and four in every one hundred women found to be susceptible in early pregnancy will acquire a primary infection during pregnancy, with higher rates observed in women younger than 20 years of age, single, non-white and from lower socio-economic classes (Preece et al., 1986). Sexual transmission of CMV may be important in young women, whereas infection in susceptible pregnant women probably occurs predominantly from contact with young children (Pass et al., 1995; Preece et al., 1986; Tookey et al., 1992).

Pregnancy and vertical transmission

CMV can be transmitted in utero, during delivery or postpartum through breast-feeding. Viraemia occurs during a primary infection and the virus can cross the placenta. After primary infection virus is shed for weeks or months in pharyngeal

Table 7.1. Rate of CMV secretion in pregnant and non-pregnant women from similar background

Site	Pregnant women		Non-pregnant women	
	Number tested	Number positive (%)	Number tested	Number positive (%)
Cervix	1552	134 (8.6)	398	43 (10.8)
Urine	684	27 (3.9)	230	6 (2.6)
Throat	562	16 (1.8)		

From Stagno et al. (1982).

and cervical secretions, with periodic reactivations of latent infections occurring throughout the life of the host. Although pregnancy was initially said to favour virus shedding in cervical secretions, this was not confirmed in studies which adequately controlled for the characteristics of the women involved (Stagno et al., 1982, Table 7.1).

Up to 40% of women with a primary CMV infection during pregnancy are likely to transmit the infection to their fetus: transmission can occur at any stage of pregnancy (Ahlfors et al., 1999; Stagno et al., 1982). Transmission is especially likely to occur in infants born to women who shed CMV from the cervix or the vagina around the time of delivery and an estimated 50% of infants born to these mothers acquire CMV infection. Between 10% and 30% of seropositive pregnant women have a reactivation of the infection during pregnancy and although mother-to-child transmission in these cases is rare, it can occur: 1–3% of infants of seropositive mothers are infected in utero, and about 10% of infants of women excreting CMV at delivery (Rutter et al., 1985). It could be expected that in populations where reactivation of infection is frequent, similar numbers of children with congenital CMV acquired infection after primary maternal infection than after reactivation (Stagno et al., 1982).

CMV can be present in breastmilk (Hayes et al., 1972), with between 25 and 70% of seropositive women shedding CMV in milk at some stage. CMV is rarely found in colostrum, and duration of breastfeeding has been associated with the risk of acquisition of infection in the infant (Peckham et al., 1987a). If CMV is isolated in the milk, the risk of acquisition of infection is high.

Biological risk factors for congenital CMV are not well defined, but could include high maternal viral load, maternal infection with a virulent type of virus and gestational age at acquisition. Limited indirect evidence suggests an important role of the maternal immune response in reducing the risk of vertical transmission and also fetal damage, which could explain the different risk in primary as opposed to recurrent infection. For example, in a study of nearly 200 infants, a quarter of those born to mothers who acquired infection in the first trimester of pregnancy had one or more sequelae, compared with only 8% of those born to mothers with immunity to CMV and recurrent infection. The infants born to mothers with primary infection during pregnancy were not only more likely to be infected, but also at increased risk of mental retardation and sensorineural hearing loss (Fowler et al., 1992). In a study of vertical transmission of CMV involving 325 mother–child pairs, in 150 of whom the mother was also HIV-infected, CMV transmission was not more common in the presence of HIV-co-infection (Mussi-Pinhata et al., 1998).

Congenital infection

An estimated 2400 infants with congenital CMV infection, acquired in utero, are born each year in England, Scotland and Wales (based on 800 000 births annually), of whom about 200–300 will suffer some long-term damage (Peckham, 1991). In the USA an estimated 40 000 cases of congenital CMV infection (or about 1% of all live births) occur annually: of these between 7000 and 8000 will suffer from significant neurological deficits such as hearing loss, mental retardation and motor disability (Boppana et al., 1997; Demmler, 1991). In Sweden there are between 50 and 100 infants with congenital infection per 100 000 births (Ahlfors et al., 1999).

Although both primary and recurrent maternal infection during pregnancy can result in fetal infection, the risk of damage following maternal recurrent infection appears to be low, although defects compatible with congenital CMV infection have been reported (Ahlfors et al., 1999; Rutter et al., 1985; Stagno et al., 1982). In the UK about two-thirds of congenital infections result from primary infection and in Sweden one-half. The prevalence of in utero infection varies in different populations and the rate of congenital CMV ranges from 0.2 to 2.2% of live births depending on the population studied (Peckham, 1991; Stagno et al., 1983). Higher rates are found in women living in developing countries, those of lower socio-economic groups, younger age, single and those with other sexually transmitted diseases (Fowler et al., 1993). Infants born to non-white, adolescent, low-income mothers are not only more likely to acquire CMV infection, but also to develop long-term damage (Fowler et al., 1993). It is not known whether the higher vertical transmission rates in these groups are due to a higher incidence in the small number of susceptible women or to recurrent infection.

Although CMV can be isolated from colostrum and breastmilk (Hayes et al., 1972; Pass et al., 1995; Stagno et al., 1980), and transmission through this route can occur (Peckham et al., 1987a), acquisition of CMV from the mother through the birth canal or breast milk rarely causes clinical symptoms such as hepato-splenomegaly, anaemia or low weight gain. However, premature infants who receive breastmilk from a CMV positive woman are at risk of acquiring CMV infection, which in some cases can lead to pneumonia (Vochem et al., 1998).

Diagnosis of congenital infection

The classical method for detecting CMV is visualization of cytopathic effects (cytomegaly) of the virus in tissue specimens. The isolation of CMV from a throat swab or urine sample obtained in the first 2 or 3 weeks of life indicates congenital infection; it is easy to detect CMV in newborns with congenital infection because large amounts of virus are present. Viraemia can be demonstrated by PCR and seems to be present in nearly all cases (Barbi et al., 1998; Fischler et al., 1999; Johansson et al., 1997). Virus isolation from samples taken after the neonatal period would not distinguish congenital from acquired infection, which commonly occurs in the early months of life and is not associated with complications. Virus isolation in tissue culture is the standard against which other methods are assessed. More recently developed tests include the centrifugation-enhanced rapid techniques which use monoclonal antibody to CMV immediate or early antigens to provide results in 24 hours compared with several days to weeks for tissue culture (Gleaves et al., 1984). Polymerase chain reaction (PCR) and other methods to detect CMV DNA in urine or saliva can also be used, although their use for routine diagnosis needs to be confirmed (Nelson et al., 1995; Pass et al., 1995; Demmler et al., 1988). The CMV PCR assay uses primers that are common to nearly all CMV strains. Detection of CMV DNA on blood spots collected routinely for the diagnosis of metabolic disorders in neonates (Guthrie cards) has been used in a limited number of studies to diagnose congenital infection with high sensitivity and specificity (Barbi et al., 1998; Fischler et al., 1999; Johansson et al., 1997). Direct antigen detection in leukocytes may also confirm diagnosis (Barbi et al., 1998).

Antibody assays for CMV document past CMV infection. Because maternal IgG antibody crosses the placenta, all infants of CMV seropositive women will be IgG positive. Detection of CMV IgM antibody, formed during fetal life and presence of which would indicate congenital infection, is less reliable than virus isolation and not recommended for the diagnosis of congenital infection in isolation. Any newborn with clinical signs and symptoms of a suspected CMV infection should be investigated for IgM anti-CMV antibodies and cultured for virus for CMV from fresh urine. CMV infected children may excrete the virus in saliva and urine for many years.

Table 7.2. Clinical signs and symptoms associated with congenital CMV infection

Microcephaly
Cerebral palsy
Mental retardation
Sensorineural deafness
Pneumonitis
Hepatosplenomegaly
Jaundice
Thrombocytopenic purpura
Virus shedding

Burden of disease

The incidence and clinical severity of congenital CMV infection depend on the incidence and nature (primary or reactivation) of CMV infection in pregnancy. Congenitally infected infants, as those who acquire CMV after birth, shed virus for prolonged periods, and CMV is detectable in the urine and pharynx for months or even years. Sensorineural hearing loss is the most common single defect attributable to congenital CMV (Fowler et al., 1997). It has been estimated that 12% of bilateral congenital sensorineural hearing loss is due to CMV (Peckham et al., 1987b), and this has replaced congenital rubella as the most common viral cause of congenital deafness. In addition, an estimated 7% of cerebral palsy is due to congenital CMV (Stagno et al., 1982).

CMV causes multiorgan disease, and clinical manifestations include hepatomegaly, splenomegaly, thrombocytopenia, prolonged neonatal jaundice, pneumonitis, growth retardation, chorioretinitis, microcephaly and occasionally cerebral calcification (Table 7.2). The prognosis differs greatly between infants with congenital CMV infection who are asymptomatic at birth and those who are symptomatic (Jones & Isaacs, 1995). Fewer than 10% of congenitally infected infants are symptomatic at birth, but half of these have only mild disease. Most children with signs of infection at birth suffer long-term complications which are often multiple and may include cerebral palsy, mental retardation, optic atrophy and sensorineural deafness (Anderson et al., 1996; Pass et al., 1980; Ramsey et al., 1991). The severity of handicap varies, but about 10% of infected symptomatic children die. In contrast most of the 90% infants who are asymptomatic at birth develop normally (Ivarsson et al., 1997; Kashden et al., 1998), although a small proportion (about 5–15%) will have long-term neurological sequelae, sensorineural hearing loss being the most frequent problem (Ahlfors et al., 1979; Peckham, 1991; Saigal et al., 1982). However, more severe neurodevelopmental deficits, including microcephaly and spastic quadriparesis have been described in rare cases (Stagno, 1995).

The long-term prognosis for a CMV infected symptomatic neonate varies with the type of symptoms present at birth, but there is a lack of information from large prospective studies. Chorioretinitis, found in 10–15% of symptomatic neonates, has the greatest association with neurological damage (Boppana et al., 1987). In a small and retrospective study of 32 infants with symptomatic CMV at birth, all children with chorioretinitis had significant mental retardation (Boppana et al., 1987). Microcephaly is also predictive of later neurological sequelae, although the absence of microcephaly at birth does not necessarily predict normal outcome. The presence of atypical symptoms or signs at birth, such as hepato- or splenomegaly, jaundice and prematurity, are less strongly associated with long-term outcome (Boppana et al., 1987). The predictive value of elevated protein or detection of CMV-DNA in the cerobrospinal fluid or radiographic abnormalities have yet to be determined (Jones & Isaacs, 1995; Troendle Atkins et al., 1994).

Treatment and prevention

Antiviral agents are commonly used to treat disseminated CMV infection in immunocompromised people, such as those with advanced HIV infection (Hebart & Einsele, 1998; Mussi-Pinhata et al., 1998). However, none of these antiviral agents has been licensed for use during pregnancy. Indeed, all three commonly used drugs (ganciclovir, foscarnet and cidofovir) are known to have teratogenic or embryotoxic effects in animals, although evidence for teratogenicity in humans is absent. Antiviral therapy during pregnancy to reduce the risk of congenital CMV infection is thus not currently an option.

There is no established treatment for congenital CMV infection, although ganciclovir or foscarnet have been suggested for use to inhibit disease progression. However, there are no approved antivirals for use in neonates to prevent progression of CMV disease, and only anecdotal reports of the use of ganciclovir to treat infants with symptomatic congenital CMV infection. In a phase I/II trial in the USA, intravenous ganciclovir was given intravenously for 6 weeks to infants with symptomatic CMV, and shown to repress CMV replication, but viral shedding resumed once treatment stopped (Whitley et al., 1997). A randomized trial in newborns with symptomatic congenital CMV infection is under way.

There is as yet no vaccine available with a protective effect against CMV (Boppana & Pass, 1999). Cell-mediated immunity plays a major protective role, which suggests that a vaccine boosting this part of the immune system could be used to either prevent primary CMV infection in pregnant women or to prevent development of the serious sequelae in a congenitally infected neonate. In one study, it was estimated that routine immunization of all women between 15 and 25 years of age would be cost-effective even if only 15% of them were seronegative and susceptible. With a seroprevalence of 55–70% and between 30 and 45% of pregnant women susceptible to a primary infection, 24 cases of symptomatic congenital infection would be prevented for every 100 000 women immunized (Porath et al., 1990).

Screening policy

Both professionals and the public have raised the question of whether antenatal or neonatal screening should be carried out, but most authorities agree that routine antenatal screening is not indicated at present. As most maternal infections are asymptomatic, repeated serological screening of all susceptible seronegative women would be required throughout pregnancy. For women who are initially seropositive, the presence of CMV-specific IgM might indicate infection early in pregnancy, but as IgM may persist for 3 to 6 months after a primary infection or even longer, it is not possible to exclude infection before conception. There is no effective treatment for either mother or infant, and the only intervention that could be offered to a woman with a primary infection is termination of the pregnancy. Given that the risk for a woman with a primary infection giving birth to an infant with congenital CMV damage is about 5% or less, it is unlikely that this could justify routine screening.

Since about a third of primary maternal infections lead to fetal infection and most infected infants are normal, prenatal diagnosis of intrauterine CMV infection by amniocentesis and isolation of CMV from amniotic fluid has been proposed (Grose et al., 1992). However, this procedure does not distinguish normal from affected fetuses and indeed, isolation of virus in the amniotic fluid is not proof of fetal infection, and negative results do not exclude fetal infection. Unlike rubella, where the risk of damage is restricted to early fetal exposure to infection, infants of women who acquire CMV infection at any stage of pregnancy are at risk of fetal damage. Infections very early in pregnancy may be missed and, if a seroconversion occurs, in a primary maternal infection, there is no treatment to offer. In view of the low risk of fetal damage, therapeutic abortion is unlikely to be an acceptable alternative.

Neonatal screening has been proposed to identify children potentially at risk of neurological problems, particularly sensorineural hearing loss. However, as fewer than 10% of asymptomatic infants identified as congenitally infected would subsequently develop a CMV-related problem and there is at present no treatment to offer, there would be little benefit from this approach. Neonatal screening could have serious and unnecessary psychological consequences for parents and children, most of whom will be normal. The only advantage for those affected would be the benefit derived from an earlier diagnosis of a problem such as hearing impairment. Universal viral culture for all live births is not feasible and serological screening is not sufficiently sensitive. However, the development regarding CMV DNA PCR (Demmler, 1991), which can be carried out on routinely collected neonatal bloodspots, could offer scope for investigating the contribution of congenital CMV to mental retardation or hearing problems in children (Fischler et al., 1999).

REFERENCES

Adler, S. P. (1988). Molecular epidemiology of cytomegalovirus, viral transmission among children attending a day care center, their parents and caretakers. *J. Pediatr.*, **112**, 366– 72.

Ahlfors, K., Ivarsson, S., Johnsson, T. & Svanberg, L. (1979). A prospective study on congenital and acquired cytomegalovirus infections in infants. *Scand. J. Infect. Dis.*, **11**, 177– 8.

Ahlfors, K., Ivarsson, S. A., Harris, S., Svanberg, L., Holmquist, R., Lernmark, R. & Theander, G. (1984). Congenital cytomegalovirus infection and disease in Sweden and the relative importance of primary and secondary maternal infections, preliminary findings from a prospective study. *Scand. J. Infect. Dis.*, **16**, 129– 37.

Ahlfors, K., Ivarsson, S. A. & Harris, S. (1999). Longterm study of maternal and congenital cytomegalovirus infection in Sweden. *Scand. J. Infect. Dis.*, **31**, 433–57.

Anderson, K. S., Amos, C. S., Boppana, S. & Pass, R. (1996). Ocular abnormalities in congenital cytomegalovirus infection. *J. Am. Optom. Assoc.*, **67**, 273– 8.

Bale, J. F., Zimmerman, B., Petheram, S. L. & Murph, J. R. (1999). Cytomegalovirus transmission in child care homes. *Arch. Pediatr. Adolesc. Med.*, **153**, 75– 9.

Barbi, M., Binda, S., Primache, V. & Clerici, M. (1998). Congenital cytomegalovirus infection in a northern Italian region. NEOCMV group. *Eur. J. Epidemiol.*, **14**, 791– 6.

Boppana, S. & Pass, R. F. (1999). Cytomegalovirus. In *Viral Infections in Obstetrics and Gynaecology*, ed. D. J. Jeffries, C. N. Hudson, pp. 35–56. London: Arnold.

Boppana, S. B., Pass, R. F. & Britt, W. J. (1987). Early clinical manifestations and intellectual outcome in children with symptomatic congenital cytomegalovirus infection, neonatal morbidity and mortality. *J. Pediatr.*, **111**, 343– 8.

Boppana, S. B., Fowler, K. B. & Vaid, Y. (1997). Neuroradiographic findings in the newborn period and long-term outcome in children with symptomatic congenital cytomegalovirus infection. *Pediatrics*, **99**, 409–14.

Chandler, S. H., Holmes, K. K. & Wentworth, B. B. (1985). The epidemiology of cytomegaloviral infection in women attending a sexually transmitted disease clinic. *J. Infect. Dis.*, **152**, 597–605.

Demmler, G. J. (1991). Summary of a workshop on surveillance for congenital cytomegalovirus disease. *Rev. Infect. Dis.*, **13**, 315–29.

Demmler, G. J., Buffone, G. J., Schimbor, C. M. & May, R. A. (1988). Detection of cytomegalovirus in urine from newborns by using polymerase chain reaction DNA amplification. *J. Infect. Dis.*, **158**, 1177–84.

Fischler, B., Rodensjo, P., Nemeth, A., Forsgren, M. & Lewensohn-Fuchs, I. (1999). Cytomegalovirus DNA detection on Guthrie cards in patients with neonatal cholestasis. *Arch. Dis. Child.*, **80**, F130–4.

Fowler, K. B., Stagno, P. H. S., Pass, R. F., Britt, W. J., Boll, T. J. & Alford, C. A. (1992). The outcome of congenital cytomegalovirus infection in relation to maternal antibody status. *N. Engl. J. Med.*, **326**, 663–7.

Fowler, K. B., Stagno, S. & Pass, R. F. (1993). Maternal age and congenital cytomegalovirus infection, screening of two diverse newborn populations. *J. Infect. Dis.*, **168**, 552–6.

Fowler, K. B., McCollister, F. P., Dahle, A. J., Boppana, S., Britt, W. J. & Pass, R. F. (1997). Progressive and fluctuating sensorineural hearing loss in children with asymptomatic congenital cytomegalovirus infection. *J. Pediatr.*, **130**, 624–30.

Gleaves, C. A., Smith, T. F., Shuster, E. A. & Pearson, G. R. (1984). Rapid detection of cytomegalovirus in MRC-5 cells innoculated with urine specimens by using low-speed centrifugation and monoclonal antibody to an early antigen. *J. Clin. Microbiol.*, **19**, 917–9.

Griffiths, P. D. & Grundy, J. E. (1998). The status of CMV as a human pathogen. *Epidemiol. Infect.*, **100**, 1–15.

Grillner, L. & Strangert, K. (1986). Restriction endonuclease analysis of cytomegalovirus DNA from strains isolated in day care centers. *Pediatr. Infect. Dis. J.*, **5**, 184–7.

Grose, C., Meehan, T. & Weiner, C. (1992). Prenatal diagnosis of congenital cytomegalovirus infection by virus isolation after amniocentesis. *Pediatr. Infect. Dis. J.*, **11**, 605–7.

Hayes, C., Danks, D. M., Gila, S. H. & Jack, I. (1972). Cytomegalovirus in human milk. *N. Engl. J. Med.*, **287**, 177–8.

Hebart, H. & Einsele, H. (1998). Diagnosis and treatment of cytomegalovirus infection. *Curr. Opin. Hematol.*, **5**, 483–7.

Ivarsson, S. A., Lernmark, B. & Svanberg, L. (1997). Ten-year clinical, developmental and intellectual follow-up of children with congenital cytomegalovirus infection without neurologic symptoms at one year of age. *Pediatrics*, **99**, 800–3.

Jafari, H. S., Schuchat, A., Hilsdon, R., Whitney, C. G., Toomey, K. E. & Wenger, J. D. (1995). Barriers to prevention of perinatal group B streptococcal disease. *Pediatr. Infect. Dis. J.*, **14**, 662–7.

Johansson, P. J., Jonsson, M., Ahlfors, K., Ivarsson, S. A., Svanberg, L. & Guthenberg, C. (1997). Retrospective diagnostics of congenital cytomegalovirus infection performed by polymerase chain reaction in blood stored on filter paper. *Scand. J. Infect. Dis.*, **29**, 465–8.

Jones, C. A. & Isaacs, D. (1995). Predicting the outcome of symptomatic congenital cytomegalovirus infection. *J. Pediatr. Child Health*, **31**, 70–1.

Kamada, M. (1983). A prospective study of congenital cytomegalovirus infection in Japan. *Scand. J. Infect. Dis.*, **15**, 227–32.

Kashden, J., Frison, S., Fowler, K. B., Pass, R. F. & Boll, T. J. (1998). Intellectual assessment of children with asymptomatic congenital cytomegalovirus infection. *J. Dev. Behav. Pediatr.*, **19**, 254–9.

Murph, J. R., Souza, I. E., Dawson, J. D., Benson, P., Petheram, S. J., Pfab, D., Gregg, A., O'Neill, M. E., Zimmerman, B. & Bale, J. F. (1998). Epidemiology of congenital cytomegalovirus infection, maternal risk factors and molecular analysis of cytomegalovirus strains. *Am. J. Epidemiol.*, **147**, 940–7.

Mussi-Pinhata, M. M., Yamamoto, A. Y., Figueiredo, L. T., Cervi, M. C. & Duarte, G. (1998). Congenital and perinatal cytomegalovirus infection in infants born to mothers infected with human immunodeficiency virus. *J. Pediatr.*, **132**, 285–90.

Nelson, D. B., Peckham, C. S., Pearl, K. N., Chin, K. S., Garrett, A. J. & Warren, D. E. (1987). Cytomegalovirus infection in day nurseries. *Arch. Dis. Child.*, **62**, 329–32.

Nelson, C. T., Istas, A. S., Wilkerson, M. K. & Demmler, G. J. (1995). PCR detection of cytomegalovirus DNA in serum as a diagnostic test for congenital cytomegalovirus infection. *J. Clin. Microbiol.*, **33**, 3317–8.

Pass, R. F., Stagno, S., Myers, G. J. & Alford, C. A. (1980). Outcome of symptomatic congenital cytomegalovirus infection, results of long-term longitudinal follow-up. *J. Pediatr.*, **66**, 758–62.

Pass, R. F., Little, E. A., Stagno, S. & Britt, W. J. (1987). Young children as a probable source of maternal and congenital cytomegalovirus infection. *N. Engl. J. Med.*, **316**, 1366–70.

Pass, R. F., Duliege, A. M. & Boppana, S. B. (1995). Immunogenicity of a recombinant CMV gB vaccine (abstract). *Pediatr. Res.*, **37**, 185A.

Peckham, C. S. (1991). Cytomegalovirus infection, congenital and neonatal disease. *Scand J. Infect. Suppl.*, **78**, 82–7.

Peckham, C., Chin, K. S., Coleman, J. C., Henderson, K., Hurley, R. & Preece, P. M. (1983). 7Cytomegalovirus infection in pregnancy, preliminary findings from a prospective study. *Lancet*, **i**, 1352–5.

Peckham, C. S., Johnson, C., Ades, A., Pearl, K. & Chin, K. S. (1987a). The early acquisition of cytomegalovirus infection. *Arch. Dis. Child.*, **62**, 780–5.

Peckham, C. S., Stark, O., Dudgeon, J. A., Martin, J. A. M. & Hawkins, G. (1987b). Congenital cytomegalovirus infection, a cause of sensorineural hearing loss. *Arch. Dis. Child.*, 62, 1233–7.

Porath, A., McNutt, R. A., Smiley, L. M. & Weigle, K. A. (1990). Effectiveness and cost benefit of a proposed live cytomegalovirus vaccine in the prevention of congenital disease. *Rev. Infect. Dis.*, **12**, 31–40.

Preece, P. M., Tookey, P., Ades, A. & Peckham, C. S. (1986). Congenital cytomegalovirus infection, predisposing maternal factors. *J. Epidemiol. Community Health*, **40**, 205–9.

Ramsey, M. E. B., Miller, E. & Peckham, C. S. (1991). Outcome of confirmed symptomatic congenital cytomegalovirus infection. *Arch. Dis. Child.*, **66**, 1068–9.

Rutter, D., Griffiths, P. D. & Trompeter, R. S. (1985). Cytomegalic inclusion disease after recurrent maternal infection. *Lancet*, **ii**, 1182.

Saigal, S., Lunyk, O., Larke, R. P. B. & Chernesky, M. A. (1982). The outcome in children with congenital cytomegalovirus infection. *Am. J. Dis. Child.*, **136**, 896–905.

Schopfer, K., Lauber, E. & Krech, U. (1978). Congenital cytomegalovirus infection in newborn infants of mothers infected before pregnancy. *Arch. Dis. Child.*, **53**, 536–9.

Stagno, S. (1995). Cytomegalovirus. In *Infectious Diseases of the Foetus and Newborn Infant*. 3rd edn, ed. J. S. Remington & J. O. Klein. Philadelphia: W.B. Saunders Company.

Stagno, S. (1996). Cytomegalovirus. In *Oxford Textbook of Medicine*, 3rd edn, Volume 1, ed. D. J. Weatherall, J. G. G. Ledingham & D. A. Warrell. Oxford, UK. Oxford University Press.

Stagno, S., Reynolds, D. W., Pass, R. F. & Alford, C. A. (1980). Breast milk and the risk of cytomegalovirus infection. *N. Engl. J. Med.*, **302**, 1073–6.

Stagno, S., Pass, R. F. & Dworsky, M. E. (1982). Congenital cytomegalovirus infection, the relative importance of primary and recurrent maternal infection. *N. Engl. J. Med.*, **306**, 945–9.

Stagno, S., Pass, R. F., Dworsky, M. E. & Alford, C. A. (1983). Congenital and perinatal cytomegalovirus infections. *Semin. Perinatol.*, **7**, 31–42.

Tookey, P. A. & Peckham, C. S. (1991). Does cytomegalovirus present an occupational risk? *Arch. Dis. Child.*, **66**, 1009–10.

Tookey, P. A., Ades, A. E. & Peckham, C. S. (1992). Cytomegalovirus prevalence in pregnant women, the influence of parity. *Arch. Dis. Child.*, **67**, 779–83.

Troendle Atkins, J., Demmler, G. J., Williamson, W. D., McDonald, J. M., Istas, A. S. & Buffone, G. J. (1994). Polymerase chain reaction to detect cytomegalovirus DNA in cerebrospinal fluid of neonates with congenital infection. *J. Infect. Dis.*, **169**, 1334–7.

Vochem, M., Hamprecht, K., Jahn, G. & Speer, C. P. (1998). Transmission of cytomegalovirus to preterm infants through breast milk. *J. Infect. Dis.*, **17**, 53–8.

Whitley, R. J., Cloud, G. & Gruber, W. (1997). A pharmacokinetic and pharmacodynamic evaluation of ganciclovir for the treatment of symptomatic congenital cytomegalovirus infection, results of a phase II study. *J. Infect. Dis.*, **175**, 1080–6.

Yow, M. D., White, N. H., Taber, L. H., Frank, A. L., Gruber, W. C., May, R. A. & Norton, H. J. (1987). Acquisition of cytomegalovirus infection from birth to 10 years, a longitudinal serologic study. *J. Pediatr.*, **110**, 37–41.

Yow, M. D., Williamson, D. W. & Leeds, L. J. (1988). Epidemiologic characteristics of cytomegalovirus infection in mothers and their infants. *Am. J. Obstet. Gynecol.*, **158**, 1189–95.

8

Varicella

G. Justus Hofmeyr

Introduction

Historically, varicella (chicken-pox) infection in pregnancy has received less attention than other causes of congenital infection (such as the 'STORCH' group, syphilis, toxoplasmosis, rubella, cytomegalovirus and herpes virus). Recent work has highlighted the importance of varicella as a cause of both congenital and perinatal infections. Recognition of the ultrasound features of congenital varicella infection has contributed to a rational approach to maternal varicella infections during pregnancy.

Prevalence

Varicella is a common childhood infection caused by the varicella-zoster virus (VZV). The historical events spanning the first half of the twentieth century which led to the recognition that varicella and zoster are caused by the same virus, have recently been summarized by Weller (1996). Varicella is relatively uncommon in adults but the proportion of infections reported in adults is increasing, and is particularly high in tropical countries.

Varicella is highly infectious, with attack rates of up to 90% in household settings. Respiratory secretions and the skin lesions are infective, and the infective period is from 2 days before appearance of the skin lesions until the lesions have crusted. The incubation period is 10 to 21 days (mean 15 days). The rash may be preceded by a 1 to 2 day prodromal illness with fever, headache, malaise and anorexia. The fever lasts 1 to 3 days if present. The severity of these symptoms increases with age. The rash affects the trunk, scalp, face and extremities, and progresses over the period of a week from macules to papules, vesicles, pustules then crusted lesions.

Zoster may occur months to years after primary varicella infection. Immune system compromise may precipitate an attack. The rash appears in a unilateral dermatomal distribution, and severe neuralgic pain may persist for months after the skin lesions have healed.

Maternal varicella infection occurs in 0.5 to 3/1000 pregnancies. The exact frequency of congenital infections is not known, but is considered to be 'low' – in the region of 2% of second trimester maternal varicella infections (Pastuszak et al., 1994; Enders et al., 1994). Shingles (zoster) in the mother is not associated with fetal infection, as there is no viraemia, and the fetus is protected by maternal antibodies from the preceding infection.

Risk factors

Women without previous varicella infection are at risk. Recall of previous infection has been found to be unreliable, with about one-third false-positive and false-negative recall when compared with serological evidence of previous exposure. Second infections do occur but are rare. Contact with a person with a current varicella infection carries a high risk of transmission if living in the same household or exposed to face-to-face contact for 5 minutes or indoor contact for 1 hour. Casual transient contact does not pose a high risk. Up to 20% of infected individuals are unaware of the source of the infection.

Consequences of the infection

Consequences for the mother

Varicella is a more serious infection in adults than in children. Mortality in the USA has been estimated at 1 per 100 000 in children and 31 per 100 000 in adults. Infections are more severe in immunocompromised and possibly also in pregnant adults. Prognostic clinical signs for severe disease include the extent of the rash (which is related to the viral load and the immune response) and haemorrhage into rash elements. Complications include pneumonitis, encephalitis, generalized spread to internal organs, hepatitis, arthritis, pericarditis, glomerulonephritis and Reye's syndrome and haemorrhagic varicella. Secondary bacterial infection may cause cellulitis. Pneumonitis is the commonest cause of serious morbidity or death (Feldmann, 1994). Risk factors for pneumonitis include smoking, chronic lung disease, immunosuppression, including the use of systemic steroids, and possibly ventilatory restriction by the enlarged uterus in late pregnancy. Clinical signs and symptoms of pneumonitis include dry cough, tachypnoea, dyspnoea, haemoptysis, chest pain and cyanosis. Diffuse nodular shadowing is seen on X-ray.

Consequences for the fetus

The fetal varicella syndrome is now well documented. The risk is low. In the prospective study of Enders et al. (1994), nine cases of congenital varicella syndrome were diagnosed, all in women with varicella in the first half of pregnancy. The incidence was 2 of 472 women with varicella before 13 weeks' gestation (0.4%), and 7 of 351 between 13 and 20 weeks (2%). No cases of congenital varicella syndrome were diagnosed in 366 women diagnosed with zoster during pregnancy. The clinical effects of congenital varicella syndrome vary in severity, and several organ systems may be involved. Low birthweight is almost invariable. Cicatricial skin lesions may be the only manifestation, and are not always present. They appear pale yellow and pox-like, in a dermatomal distribution. Scarring may become apparent only after weeks or months. Skeletal abnormalities include most commonly limb hypoplasia, and occasionally other bones such as the mandible, clavicle, scapula, ribs, fingers and toes may be involved. These deformities may be secondary to cicatricial lesions, or may be atrophic changes following denervation of limbs. Neurological abnormalities include mental retardation, microcephaly, cortical atrophy, central nervous system calcifications, ventriculomegaly, paralysis and atrophy of limbs, and deafness. Eye abnormalities include choreoretinitis, microphthalmia, cataracts, corneal opacities, optic atrophy and strabismus. Gastrointestinal abnormalities include gastro-oesophageal reflux, duodenal stenosis, jejunal dilatation, microcolon and atresia of the sigmoid colon. They are probably due to damage to the autonomic nervous system and spinal cord. Genitourinary damage may present as a neurogenic bladder (Gilstrap & Sebastian, 1990, Pastuszak et al., 1994).

The dermatomal distribution of the skin lesions and the neurological effects suggest that the congenital varicella syndrome, like herpes zoster, may represent a reactivation of a primary fetal infection. The very short latency period may be due to the immaturity of the fetal immune system. Mortality has been reported to be between 40% and 100%, and survivors may be affected by psychomotor retardation, blindness, seizures, cataracts and limb deformities (Hanshaw, 1985).

Dystrophic calcification occurs much more rapidly in utero than at any other time, and in congenital varicella infection occurs in the multiple small foci of visceral necrosis resulting from the disseminated infection (Wigglesworth & Singer, 1991).

In the study of Enders et al. (1994), zoster during early childhood was diagnosed in ten infants who were asymptomatic at birth.

Consequences for the neonate

Maternal varicella infection in the last 3 weeks of pregnancy may be associated, in about 24 to 50% of cases, with intrauterine or neonatal varicella. This presents with a typical varicella rash in the neonate. The condition may be serious if the presentation in the mother occurs between 5 days before and 2 days after birth. In one series, the mortality rate for this period was 4 out of 13 neonates (31%) (Meyers, 1974). Maternal infection presenting more than 5 days before birth results in a benign form of neonatal varicella. Anti-VZV antibodies are detected in the maternal circulation 4–5 days after the appearance of the rash. The IgG antibodies readily cross the placenta, and presumably provide protection for the neonate. The larger the time lapse between the maternal infection and delivery, the less severe the clinical manifestations in the neonate (Sison & Sever, 1993).

Diagnosis

Fetal varicella infection may be confirmed by detection of viral DNA by polymerase chain reaction in amniotic fluid, fetal blood or chorionic villi, or by detection of IgM antibodies in fetal blood. However, both these tests may give false negative results. Unlike the situation for rubella, the prenatal laboratory diagnosis of fetal varicella infection is not reliable (Lecuru et al., 1994).

Thorough sonographic examination at 5 or more weeks after the initial infection, with particular attention to the possible sonographic anomalies listed in Table 8.1, and generalized dystrophic calcification, should detect most cases of varicella embryopathy (Hofmeyr et al., 1996).

Pretorius et al. (1992) evaluated prenatal sonographic findings in determining fetal congenital abnormalities in maternal varicella infection and found sonography to be useful in establishing the normalcy of a fetus at risk, and in diagnosing affected fetuses. In their study 37 cases of maternal varicella infection were reviewed, 28 in the first trimester and 9 in the second trimester. Of five cases of confirmed varicella embryopathy, prenatal diagnosis was made sonographically in all of them. None of the 32 unaffected infants demonstrated in utero ultrasonographic abnormalities. Ultrasound findings of the five affected cases and an additional five cases from the literature (Scharf et al., 1990; Cuthbertson et al., 1987; Alexander, 1979; Harding & Baumer, 1988; Hofmeyr et al., 1996) are summarized in Table 8.1. Maternal infection in these ten cases occurred at 10 weeks gestation (1), 13–16 weeks' gestation (8) and 20 weeks' gestation (1). The time interval between maternal infection and sonography was between 5 and 19 weeks. The outcome of those affected included two intrauterine fetal deaths, two therapeutic abortions, four neonatal deaths at less than 36 hours, one death at 8 days and one death at 4 months. The abnormalities revealed by postmortem examination are summarized in Table 8.2. The findings at autopsy suggest that additional sonographic abnormalities might have been detected with a more thorough ultrasound examination.

Table 8.1. Summary of prenatal sonographic findings of congenital varicella infection in ten reported cases

Polyhydramnios	7
Hydrops fetalis	3
Liver hyperechogenicities	4
Lung and cardiac hyperechogenicities	1
Two vessel cord	1
Flexed limbs and decreased motion	1
Short lower limb	1
Bilateral clubbed feet	1
Neurogenic bladder	1
Meningocoele	1
Ventriculomegaly	2
Impaired fetal growth	1
Oligohydramnios	1
Malpositioned hands	1

Burden of disease

Maternal varicella is uncommon. In the USA, the incidence is estimated as 7 in 10 000 pregnancies (Balducci et al., 1992), giving an annual disease burden of 3000 cases (Keyserling, 1997).

Prevention

Prepregnancy medical evaluations may include history and testing for varicella immunity and immunization of susceptible women, or vaccination may be done as part of a policy of universal screening and vaccination of adults. The cost-effectiveness of a policy of universal testing and immunization prior to pregnancy may vary from one socio-economic situation to another (Seidman et al., 1996, Coyle et al., 1997).

Routine antenatal screening of pregnant women for varicella immunity, with a view to treating susceptible women with hyperimmune varicella zoster immuno-globulin in the event of varicella exposure, has been found to be not cost-effective (Glantz & Mushlin, 1998).

Treatment/management

Pregnant women exposed to varicella

A careful history of the exposure is important. Casual, transient exposure would not normally require further action. Following high-risk exposure (living in the

Table 8.2. Summary of postmortem findings in nine reported cases of congenital varicella infection

Skin lesions/vasculitis	5
Cerebral atrophy/necrosis	3
Hydrocephalus	1
Necrotizing chorioretinitis	1
Hypoplastic thorax/lungs	2
Hydrops fetalis	1
Hypoplastic heart	1
Dextrocardia	1
Sigmoid atresia	3
Club feet	3
Flexed limbs	1
Paralysis of arm	1
Micrognathia	1
Cryptorchidism	1
Dystrophic calcification, brainstem	1
liver	4
lungs	3
thyroid	1
kidneys	2
colon	1
adrenals	2
pancreas	1
diaphragm	1
myocardium	1
Vesico-urethral fusion	1

same household or exposed to face-to-face contact for 5 minutes or indoor contact for 1 hour), susceptibility to infection should be determined on history, confirmed by serological testing for anti-VZV antibodies (Steinberg & Gershon, 1991). As 85% of women with unknown immune status have been found to be immune (Pastuszak et al., 1994), testing rather than routine passive immunization is cost-effective (Rouse et al., 1996). If non-immune and at risk for infection (but no evidence yet of current infection), hyperimmune varicella-zoster immunoglobulin should be administered intramuscularly (Enders et al., 1994, Innocencion et al., 1998, Whitley & Kimberlin, 1997), preferably within 72 to 96 hours of exposure, although there may be benefit up to 10 days after exposure. Apart from reduction of risks to the mother, there is some evidence that the risk of fetal infection is reduced. In a prospective study conducted in the UK and in Germany, no cases of congenital varicella syndrome or zoster in infancy were identified in 97 women who received postexposure varicella zoster immune globulin. Specific IgM antibody was detected in one of 89 cord blood samples tested, compared with 76 of 615 (12.3%) in women who had not received immune globulin (Enders et al., 1994).

The effectiveness and safety in pregnancy of postexposure prophylaxis with antiviral agents such as acyclovir have not been established. Postexposure prophylaxis with varicella vaccine has been shown to be effective in children exposed to varicella, but the vaccine is a live attenuated virus and should not be used in pregnancy. However, immunization is important for susceptible household contacts of pregnant women who have themselves been exposed to varicella, to limit their chance of carrying the infection to the pregnant woman.

Pregnant women with varicella infection

Absolute indications for hospitalization are chest or abdominal pain, neurological symptoms other than headache, haemorrhagic rash or bleeding tendency, severe rash or immunosuppression. Relative indications are late pregnancy, poor obstetric history, smoking, chronic lung disease, poor social background, and inability to monitor adequately at home or excessive anxiety.

The use of antiviral therapy is based on an evaluation of the risks and benefits. Acyclovir crosses the placenta unchanged, by passive diffusion, and is concentrated in the amniotic fluid. It is excreted by the fetal kidneys. Breast milk levels are about three times those in the plasma. It has not been approved for use in pregnancy because the possibility of adverse fetal effects cannot be ruled out, although no animal nor human studies have to date shown evidence of toxic effects (Andrews et al., 1988). It is preferably administered by intravenous infusion as oral absorption is poor. Valacyclovir is better absorbed orally. It is converted in the intestine and absorbed as acyclovir. Toxic effects on the fetus have also not been demonstrated, although the number of pregnant women studied is smaller for valacyclovir than for acyclovir. Famcyclovir has the least documentation of use in pregnancy.

In weighing up the benefits and risks of antiviral treatment, an important factor is the presence of, or risk of developing, pneumonitis. In the presence of complicated varicella infection, acyclovir therapy has been advocated (Gilbert, 1995, Paryani & Arvin, 1986; Brown & Baker, 1989; Prober et al., 1990). Most authors have advocated intravenous acyclovir (400–500mg or 10mg/kg or 500mg/m², 8-hourly), although the oral route has also been advocated, 200mg 5-hourly (Mutalik et al., 1997) to 800mg 5 times daily (Whitley & Kimberlin, 1997).

Because secondary bacterial pneumonia is a major complication of pneumonitis, antibiotic prophylaxis is often administered, particularly if risk factors for developing pneumonitis are present. The value to the mother of hyperimmune globulin and corticosteriod therapy have not been established. Once the maternal infection is established, neither hyperimmune globulin nor treatment with acyclovir has been shown to prevent intrauterine transmission or alleviate fetal infection (Seidman et al., 1996).

Perinatal maternal infection

If a mother develops the varicella rash from 5 days before to 2 days after delivery, the neonate should receive hyperimmune varicella zoster immune globulin (125 units) as soon as possible after birth, as this may prevent or attenuate the infection (Report of the Committee on Infectious Diseases, 1994). The infant should be monitored for 14 days as the presentation of the illness may be delayed. In two studies the attack rates were 51% of 41 (Hanngren et al., 1985) and 45% of 132 infants (Preblud, 1986). There was only one fatality, which may not have been due to varicella. There is insufficient evidence for the prophylactic use of acyclovir, but if there is evidence of neonatal infection, therapeutic acyclovir should be administered intravenously (10–15 mg per kg 8-hourly for 7 days).

Postnatal varicella infection

Postnatal varicella infection is rare, as antibodies from the mother protect most neonates. Postnatal infections are usually no more severe than childhood varicella, as droplet infection via the respiratory tract exposes the infant to a far smaller viral load than does transplacental infection. There may be a case for treatment with acyclovir for preterm neonates, and for neonates whose mothers have no varicella immunity.

Conclusion

Maternal varicella infection is uncommon, and the proportion of fetuses or infants affected is small. However, in rare cases the infection may have devastating effects on the mother, fetus or neonate. Public awareness of the risks of varicella in pregnancy is important. Health workers need a clear understanding of the disease in order to take prompt preventive measures, counsel exposed or infected women appropriately, and undertake appropriate diagnostic and therapeutic measures.

REFERENCES

Alexander, I. (1979). Congenital varicella. *Br. Med. J.*, **2**, 1074.
Andrews, E. B., Tilson, H. H., Hurn, B. A. & Cordero, J. F. (1988). Acyclovir in pregnancy

registry. *Am. J. Med.*, **85**, 123.

Balducci, J., Rodis, J. F., Rosengren, S., Vintzileos, A. M., Spivey, G. & Vosseller, C. (1992). Pregnancy outcome following first-trimester varicella infection. *Obstet. Gynecol.*, **79**, 5–6.

Brown, Z. & Baker, D. (1989). Acyclovir therapy during pregnancy. *Obstet. Gynecol.*, **73**, 526–31.

Coyle, P. V., McCaughey, C., Wyatt, D. E. & O'Neill, H. J. (1997). Varicella vaccine in pregnancy. *Br. Med. J.*, **314**, 226.

Cuthbertson, G., Weiner, C. P. & Giller, R. H. (1987). Prenatal diagnosis of second trimester congenital varicella syndrome by virus-specific immunoglobulin. *J. Pediatr.*, **111**, 592–5.

Enders, G., Miller, E., Craddock-Watson, J., Bailey, I. & Ridehalgh, M. (1994). Consequences of varicella and herpes zoster in pregnancy, prospective study of 1739 cases. *Lancet*, **343**, 1548–51.

Feldmann, S. (1994). Varicella-zoster virus pneumonia. *Chest*, **106**, S22–S27.

Gilbert, G. (1995). Infectious diseases. In *Preventive Care in Obstetrics,* ed. S. A. Steegers, T. K. Eskes & E. M. Symonds, pp. 529–43. New York: Balliére's Clinical Obstetrics and Gynaecology.

Gilstrap, L. C. & Sebastian, F. (1990). *Infections in Pregnancy*, p. 177. New York: Wiley-Liss.

Glantz, C. & Mushlin, A. I. (1998). Cost-effectiveness of routine antenatal varicella screening. *Obstet. Gynecol.*, **91**, 519–28.

Hanngren, K., Grandien, M. & Granstrom, G. (1985). Effect of zoster immunoglobulin for varicella prophylaxis in the newborn. *Scand. J. Infect. Dis.*, **17**, 343–7.

Hanshaw, J. B., (1985). Varicella-zoster infections. In *Viral Diseases of the Fetus and Newborn.* 2nd edn., p. 161. Philadelphia: W. B. Saunders Company.

Harding, B. & Baumer, J. A. (1988). Congenital varicella-zoster. A serologically proven case with necrotising encephalitis and malformation. *Acta Neuropathol.*, **76**, 311–15.

Hofmeyr, G. J., Moolla, S. & Lawrie, T. (1996). Prenatal sonographic diagnosis of congenital varicella infection – a case report. *Prenat. Diagn.*, **16**, 1148–51.

Innocencion, G., Loebstein, R., Lalkin, A., Geist, R., Petric, M. & Koren, G. (1998). Managing exposure to chickenpox during pregnancy. *Can. Fam. Physician*, **44**, 745–7.

Keyserling, H. L. (1997). Other viral agents of perinatal importance: Varicella, parvovirus, respiratory syncytial virus, and enterovirus. *Clin. Perinatol.*, **24**, 193–211.

Lecuru, F., Taurelle, R., Bernard, J. P., Parrat, S., Lafay-pillet, M. C., Rozenberg, F., Lebon, P. & Dommergues, M. (1994). Varicella zoster infection during pregnancy, the limits of prenatal diagnosis. *Eur. J. Obstet. Gynecol.*, **56**, 67–8.

Meyers, J. (1974). Congenital varicella in term infants, risk reconsidered. *J. Infect. Dis.*, **129**, 215–7.

Mutalik, S., Gupte, A. & Gupte, S. (1997). Oral acyclovir therapy for varicella in pregnancy. *Int. J. Dermatol.*, **36**, 49–51.

Paryani, C. & Arvin, A. (1986). Intrauterine infection with varicella-zoster virus after maternal varicella. *N. Engl. J. Med.*, **314**, 1541–6.

Pastuszak, A. L., Levy, M., Schick, B., Zuber, C., Feldkamp, M., Gladstone, J., Bar-Levy, F., Jackson, E., Donnefeild, A. & Meschino, W. (1994). Outcome after maternal varicella infection in the first 20 weeks of pregnancy. *N. Engl. J. Med.*, **330**, 901–5.

Preblud, S. R. (1986). Varicella: complications and costs. *Paediatrics*, **78**, 728–35.

Pretorius, D. H., Hayward, I., Jones, K. L. & Stamm, E. (1992). Sonographic evaluation of pregnancies with maternal varicella infection. *J. Ultrasound Med.*, **11**, 459–63.

Prober, C. G., Gershon, A. A., Grose, C., McCracken, G. H. Jr & Nelson, J. D. (1990). Consensus: varicella-zoster infections in pregnancy and the perinatal period. *Pediatr. Infect. Dis. J.*, **9**, 865–9.

Report of the Committee on Infectious Diseases, 1994 Red Book, edn 23, p. 10 (1994). Elk Grove Village, IL: American Academy of Pediatrics.

Rouse, D., Gardner, M., Allen, S. & Goldenberg, R. (1996). Management of the presumed susceptible varicella (chickenpox)-exposed gravida, a cost-effectiveness/cost–benefit analysis. *Obstet. Gynecol.*, **87**, 932–6.

Scharf, A., Scherr, O. & Enders, G. (1990). Virus detection in the fetal tissue of a premature delivery with congenital varicella syndrome, a case report. *J. Perinat. Med.*, **18**, 317–22.

Seidman, D. S., Stevenson, D. K. & Arvin, A. M. (1996). Varicella vaccine in pregnancy. *B. M. J.*, **313**, 701–2.

Sison, A. & Sever, J. (1993). Viral infections. In *Obstetrics and Perinatal Infections*, ed. D. Charles, pp. 111–48. St Louis: Mosby Year Book.

Steinberg, S. & Gershon, A. (1991). Measurement of antibodies to varicella-zoster virus by using a latex agglutination test. *J. Clin. Microbiol.*, **29**, 1527–9.

Weller, T. H. (1996). Varicella, historical perspective and clinical overview. *J. Infect. Dis.*, **174**, S306–S309.

Whitley, R. J. & Kimberlin, D. W. (1997). Treatment of viral infections during pregnancy and the neonatal period. *Clin. Perinatol.*, **24**, 267–83.

Wigglesworth, J. & Singer, D. (1991). *Textbook of Fetal and Perinatal Pathology*, p. 556. London: Blackwell Scientific Publications.

9

Herpes simplex

Marianne Forsgren and Gunilla Malm

Introduction

Herpes simplex type 1 (HSV-1) and 2 (HSV-2) infections are common in pregnant women; the symptoms – if any – are generally mild. However, HSV infection during pregnancy can result in transmission of the virus to the neonate, sometimes with serious disease and severe sequelae in the child (Nahmias et al., 1983; Koskiniemi et al., 1989; Malm et al., 1991; Azazi et al., 1990; Whitley & Arvin, 1995). Prevention is difficult, as the majority of HSV infections during pregnancy are atypical or silent. Furthermore, in the neonate vague symptoms are often not recognizable as herpes simplex disease, and early treatment of an infected child is therefore usually not an option.

Transmission of herpes simplex virus infection to the neonate is rare, which makes identification of risk factors for transmission and evaluation of preventive strategies difficult. Although results from large multicentre studies and the use of improved virological diagnostic tools have contributed to knowledge, formulation of evidence-based recommendations for prevention and management is still not possible. Management of HSV infection in pregnant women and children may also be influenced by non-medical factors, such as anxiety.

The prevalence of herpes infection – genital and oral – varies by populations of pregnant women and so does the risk of neonatal herpes. Preventive strategies should be guided by the incidence of neonatal infections. For an estimate of the real rate of neonatal herpes, surveillance studies based on active search for neonatal infections have to be undertaken in collaboration between neonatologists and virological laboratories.

The virus and spread of virus

Herpes simplex virus (HSV) belongs to the human herpes viruses and is an enveloped DNA virus. The infectivity of the virus is easily destroyed by soap and other disinfectants, heat ($>50\,°C$) or desiccation. There are two types of herpes simplex viruses – type 1 and type 2 (HSV-1 and HSV-2). Within the types additional variations between HSV strains can be used to identify transmission routes: only strains directly transmitted from one individual to another are identical (Buchman et al., 1978).

HSV is usually acquired after close contact and transmission of infectious genital and/or oral secretions to mucous membranes or abraded skin of a susceptible individual. The incubation time is 1–7 days. Whether or not clinical symptoms occur, viral replication in the cells of epidermis and dermis allows retrograde spread via neurones to the regional ganglia (trigeminal or sacral ganglia) where lifelong latency is established. Subsequently, after stimulation, virus is again transported to skin or mucous membranes appearing as vesicles, ulcers or virus excretion with no or only vague clinical signs. The rate of recurrence varies between individuals but is generally more frequent during the first year(s) after a first apparent infection (Benedetti et al., 1994).

Past infection with HSV-1 does not protect against acquisition of HSV-2, although the clinical picture is modified. Exogenous reinfection with strains of the same HSV type may also occur, but its significance in the normal individual is not clear (Buchman et al., 1979; Lakeman et al., 1986; Sakaoka et al., 1995). In a primary infection in an individual with no past experience of either herpes virus type, the amount of excreted virus is very high, the entire oral or genital tract is nearly always involved. The risk of transmission may persist for weeks or months after the lesions have healed. If someone is infected for the first time with one HSV type, and has past experience of the other type, the symptoms are milder and excretion is shorter. In recurrent infection in the normal host, the risk of infection is usually localized and lasts only a few days (Corey & Spear, 1986a,b; Corey et al., 1988).

Prevalence of herpes infections in pregnant women

Rates of acquisition of HSV-1 and 2 vary in different populations, and the spread is largely influenced by socio-economic factors (Nahmias et al., 1990). In developing countries and in lower socio-economic populations in Western countries most people have acquired HSV-1 by 15 years of age and few pregnant women are susceptible. In industrialized countries the acquisition rate is much slower and a substantial number of adults remain susceptible to HSV-1.

An estimated 20–40% of pregnant women are susceptible and at risk of primary HSV-1 infection. Estimated HSV-2 seroprevalence rates in pregnant women range from 10–30% in higher socio-economic and 40–65% in lower socio-economic populations (Ades et al., 1989; Löwhagen et al., 1990; Nahmias et al., 1990; Forsgren et al., 1994; Whitley & Arvin, 1995; Enders et al., 1999). A considerable proportion of pregnant women are thus susceptible and at risk of primary HSV-1 or -2 infection. The incidence of HSV-2 has been estimated at 2.4 to 20 in studies from USA, and for HSV-1 at 1.8 per 1000 pregnancies (Boucher et al., 1990; Mertz et al., 1992; Bryson et al., 1993; Brown et al., 1997). However, few prospective studies have been carried out. In discordant couples, where the woman is seronegative, there is a significant risk of acquisition of HSV infection during pregnancy, even after a long monogamous sexual relationship (Brown et al., 1997; Bryson et al., 1993; Kulhanjian et al., 1992; Mertz et al., 1992).

A slower acquisition rate has been observed for type 2 infection in women with previous HSV-1 infection. HSV-2 has been the more common type to cause genital herpes in most countries (Whitley & Arvin, 1995). Although there has been an increase in primary genital infections caused by type 1, overall HSV recovery by pregnant women remains dominated by type 2 (Whitley & Arvin, 1995; M. Forsgren et al., personal communication, 1999).

Clinical symptoms and history of genital herpes

Primary genital infection in an individual with no prior experience of herpes may be symptomatic with bilateral blistering and ulceration of external genitalia and cervix with vulvar pain, dysuria, vaginal discharge and local lymphadenopathy. Infection may be accompanied by systemic symptoms, such as fever, myalgia and occasionally urinary retention and meningitis. Serious disease in the pregnant woman may occasionally occur: necrotizing cervicitis, hepatitis (Young et al., 1996) or widely disseminated disease. The high rate of HSV-2 seropositive individuals compared to the rate of individuals with a clinical history of genital herpes (Mertz et al., 1992; Koutsky et al., 1992; Frenkel et al., 1993; Brown et al., 1995; Cowan et al., 1996) again indicates that the majority of genital herpes infections are subclinical or run an unrecognized course. Also during pregnancy most cases of primary genital HSV infection are not accompanied by symptoms or herpes-like signs, and an even higher rate of HSV-2 infections are silent in pregnant women with prior HSV-1 infection (Brown et al., 1997).

Education of doctors, midwives and women, and the use of viral diagnostics to trace atypical herpes presentations (urinary tract infections unresponsive to therapy, itching, minor fissures, often combined with vaginal discharge at recurrent intervals, with or without concomitant candidosis or non-specific vulvar eythema), may increase awareness and recognition of genital herpes.

Differentiation between primary and recurrent infection in a first episode of genital herpes is not possible simply by history-taking. An asymptomatic primary infection may be followed by subsequent symptomatic disease. Thus in a clinically apparent first herpes episode the infection might be a true primary infection (no prior HSV-1 or HSV-2), a first infection with genital herpes in an individual with antibodies to the alternate HSV type, or in the majority of cases a recurrent infection (prior infection of the same type) (Frenkel et al., 1993; Hensleigh et al., 1997). The type of infection can only be correctly classified by isolation and typing of the virus in combination with herpes type specific serology.

Routes and risk of transmission of herpes simplex to the child

The placenta appears to be an effective barrier in preventing infection of the fetus in utero, and congenital infections are rare (Whitley & Arvin, 1995). Transmission across the placenta may occur in the later stages of pregnancy and could explain infection in infants delivered by caesarean section (Peng et al., 1993). Ascending infection from an infected cervix after preterm rupture of the amniotic membranes is another route of intrauterine transmission. More than 80% of all HSV infected infants acquire infection intrapartum (Whitley & Arvin, 1995). Lesions in the skin and/or mucous membranes, acting as a port of viral entrance, may increase the transmission risk. HSV infection starting in lesions after scalp electrode or vacuum extraction have repeatedly been demonstrated (Malm et al., 1991, 1995; Whitley & Arvin, 1995; Hagadorn et al., 1996).

The risk of transmission to the child is increased in the absence of maternal antibodies to the infecting HSV-type. Protection correlates with the presence of neutralizing antibodies or other type-specific antibodies to the infecting virus type transmitted from the mother before birth (Yeager & Arvin, 1984; Ashley et al., 1992; Whitley & Arvin, 1995). Moreover, preterm labour has been associated with primary infection (Whitley & Arvin, 1995; Brown et al., 1996). The most dangerous situation for the neonate is thus a primary genital herpes infection in the mother with either herpes virus type a few weeks before or in the first days after delivery (Brown et al., 1997).

Once seroconversion to HSV-2 has occurred in the mother some weeks after onset of infection, transmission is less common. However, even then it has been documented (Malm et al., 1995) in the following circumstances: inefficient protection by the early maternal antibody response, persisting viral excretion for many weeks beyond clinical healing (Corey, 1988) and a high recurrence rate with viral shedding regardless of initial therapy (Benedetti et al., 1994).

In recurrent genital infection there is a significant, although not complete, protection from maternal antibody in the child. The viral exposure is generally of low intensity and restricted to the external genital tract, although shedding from other sites e.g. the cervix, may occur in 5–10 % (M. Forsgren et al., personal communication, 1999). Virus is shed at intervals between clinical recurrences, 2% of follow-up days has been reported (Wald et al., 1995). The risk of shedding increases with the frequency of symptomatic recurrences after acquisition of a primary genital HSV infection (Benedetti et al., 1994). The duration is similar whether the recurrence is symptomatic or not. The observed rate of asymptomatic shedding of HSV (viral culture) at labour has varied between 0.35 and 1.4% (Brown et al., 1991, 1996). Parallel sensitive analyses of HSV-DNA demonstrate that the real rate of infant exposure in recurrent genital HSV may be considerably higher (Cone et al., 1994; Wald et al., 1997; Boggess et al., 1997), the level of excreted virus seems to correlate with transmission (Cone et al., 1994). The risk of transmission to the child after recurrent herpes infection in the mother is low, even if the virus is shed at labour, probably less than 3% (Prober et al., 1987; Brown et al., 1991, 1996). The overall risk of transmission in a woman who is HSV-2 seropositive at the start of pregnancy is estimated to be of a magnitude below 1:6000 (Forsgren, 1990).

Primary oral infections in the mother can also be transmitted to the child at or after birth. Maternal recurrent oral infection has not been associated with risk to the fetus or child. Individuals (father, relatives and staff) in the acute stage of labial herpes may, however, transmit the infection at close contact with a seronegative mother and/or her unprotected child. An external source of infection was recorded in 5% (USA: Whitley & Arvin, 1995; Sweden: Malm et al., 1995) to 15% (UK: Tookey & Peckham, 1996) of neonatal HSV. Nosocomial spread has been described (Adams et al., 1981).

Neonatal disease

Prevalence

The reported incidence of neonatal HSV differs around the world. In USA the estimated incidence is 20–50 per 100 000 deliveries, (Whitley & Arvin, 1995); in Sweden 6–10 per 100 000 (Forsgren, 1990), in Norway 4 per 100 000 (Norwegian Institute of Public Health) and in the UK around 1.65 per 100 000 live births (Tookey & Peckham, 1996). Although the figures reflect the magnitude of the problem, a true comparison requires active search with standardized clinical criteria and the use of optimal diagnostic tools.

Clinical presentation

Different clinical presentations of neonatal HSV disease have classically been described as the congenital form, the disseminated form, localized encephalitis (without visceral involvement) or a localized form with vesicles in the skin – eye and/or mouth (see Table 9.1) (Nahmias et al., 1983; Whitley & Arvin, 1995). Herpes type-2 is the most common cause of neonatal herpes, and results in the most serious neurological impairments in surviving children. Type 1 infections

Table 9.1. Neonatal herpes: clinical presentation, outcome in relation to type of infection and symptoms in the mother

Children Neonatal disease	DISS	CNS	SEM	Congenital
Definition	Viscera±CNS involved	CNS Viscera not involved	Skin–eye–mouth CNS/viscera not involved	Infected in utero
Age at onset	4–11 days	2–6 weeks (peak 14 days)	7–12 days	≤2 days
Symptoms	Sepsis-like, jaundice, intravascular coagulopathy, irritability, seizures, lethargia	Subfebrility, lethargia, poor feeding, irritability, seizures	Vesicles in skin–eye or mouth, keratoconjunctivitis	Scarring, vesicles at birth, brain damage
Vesicles at onset	80%	50%	90 %	Scars or vesicles
Mortality treated	60%	15%	None	?
Neurological sequelae treated	40%	50–60%	5–10%	100% ?
Mothers				
Most frequent type of infection	Primary genital/oral/ or non-maternal source	Recurrent genital or first genital infection with one HSV-type/ past infection with the other	Recurrent genital	Primary recurrent described
Herpes-like symptoms ongoing or history	Less than half	Less common	Less common	?
Herpes type	HSV-1 or HSV-2	HSV-2 most frequent	HSV-2 most frequent	?

DISS=disseminated disease, CNS=encephalitis or meningitis, SEM=skin–eye–mouth disease.

are often milder and have a better long-term prognosis (Corey et al., 1988; Malm et al., 1991).

The congenital form of HSV-infection in the neonate is rare, representing only 5% of cases in the American Multicenter Study (Whitley & Arvin, 1995). The disseminated form of neonatal herpes is mainly spread from maternal genital or oral herpes infection in a mother with no past experience of any herpes virus type or from an external source of infection (labial herpes in relatives or staff) to a newborn unprotected by maternal herpes antibodies. The pregnancy may end in premature labour (Brown et al., 1996, 1997). The neonate lacks protecting maternal antibodies, and virus is spread via the bloodborne route. As herpes-like vesicles may be lacking the diagnosis may be misdiagnosed as septicaemia.

The CNS-form of neonatal herpes most commonly presents as encephalitis. Pleocytosis with mononuclear dominance (> 20 cells/mm³ in fullterm and > 50 cells/ mm³ in premature neonates), erythrocytes as a sign of haemorrhagic necrosis and proteinosis (> 0.9 g/l in fullterm and 1.2 g/l in preterm babies, sometimes as high as 5–10 g/l) are regular findings in cerebrospinal fluid (Whitley et al., 1991a). The source of infection is herpes in secretions of the birth canal affecting a child partially protected by maternal antibodies. The virus may be transported to the brain via a neurogenous route by retrograde axonal transport from nerve endings in skin or mucosal lesions (scalp-electrode or other lesions), from the eyes or from the nasopharynx (Malm et al., 1991; Whitley, 1995). A milder CNS-form may also present with symptoms of meningitis, often caused by herpes type 1 and with a favourable prognosis (Corey et al., 1988; Englund et al., 1991; Malm et al., 1991). The skin–eye–mouth form of neonatal herpes is the clinical classification of children without recognizable involvement of the viscera or the brain. However, 24% of children have demonstrable HSV-DNA in cerebrospinal fluid by a PCR technique, indicating a potential risk for ongoing infection in the brain (Kimberlin et al., 1996a).

The mortality remains high in disseminated disease, but is lower in encephalitis after the introduction of antiviral therapy (Whitley et al., 1991a). Neurological sequelae of different severity are, however, considerable: microcephaly, spastic quadriplegia, chorioretinitis and even blindness (see Fig. 9.1). HSV-2 encephalitis accounts for a worse prognosis (Corey et al., 1988; Malm et al., 1991). If only one hemisphere of the brain is involved, a spastic hemiplegia may be seen, with or without mental retardation and/or speech disturbances.

The overall long-term prognosis in children with skin–eye–mouth disease is favourable. No mortality has been reported, but 5–10% of cases have neurological sequelae, rising to 30% without therapy (Whitley & Arvin, 1995). The prognosis in the child is dependent on early recognition and initiation of therapy (Whitley et al., 1991b; Whitley, 1995). Thus, a paediatrician must always consider herpes simplex virus not only when vesicles are present but also in combination with other pathogens for the aetiology of unclear septicaemia or an encephalitis in a child in the first 6 weeks of life. Herpes aetiology has to be actively excluded before excluding a clinical suspicion of herpes encephalitis.

Early diagnosis is a challenge. Verification of herpes diagnosis is easily obtained if vesicles or ulcers are present by demonstration of virus by culture and rapid diagnostic methods (if available). The history of herpes in the mother and father may give a hint but the lack of a herpes history does not exclude the diagnosis. In fact, in the majority of cases (in 60–70%) the mother is not aware of previous

(a)

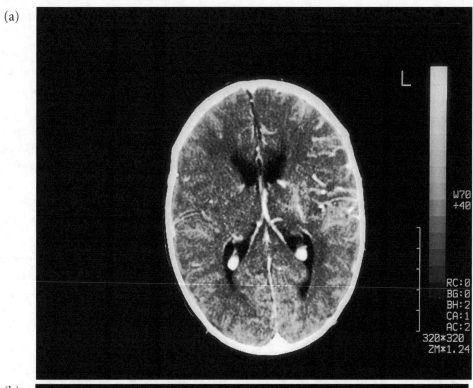

(b)

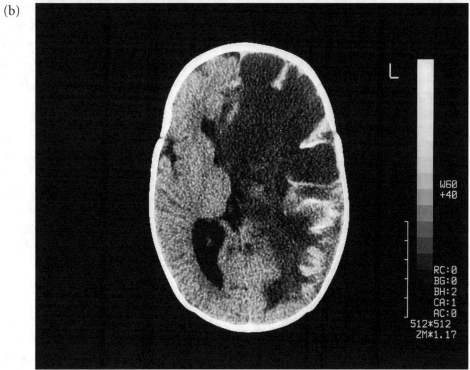

herpes infection (Malm et al., 1991; Whitley & Arvin, 1995). In encephalitis, abnormal EEG patterns with periodic lateral epileptiform discharges appear 2–3 days after the first symptoms, lesions on a CT scan are usually not visible until 4–6 days after first symptom, and on MRI they become visible after 2–3 days (Mizrahi & Tharp, 1985; Sugimoto et al., 1985; Bale et al., 1987; Koskiniemi et al., 1989; Malm et al., 1991). Demonstration of HSV DNA in cerebrospinal fluid and blood by the highly sensitive and reliable PCR technique is possible in the majority, but not all, of cases (Diamond et al., 1999; Kimura et al. 1991b; Kimberlin et al., 1996a; Malm & Forsgren, 1999). Cultivation of virus from samples from oropharynx and conjunctiva should always be carried out. Serological investigation of the mother and the child for type-common and type-specific antibody activity has often been disregarded as a complement to other investigations. Higher antibody levels in the mother than in the child, often seen as a sign of activation of herpes at the time of birth, may alert the clinician to the possibility of a herpes diagnosis (M. Forsgren & G. Malm, unpublished observations). A comparison with an antenatal serum, stored from HIV or rubella testing, can be helpful.

Treatment

Neonates with a confirmed or strongly suspected neonatal herpes virus infection should be treated with intravenous acyclovir, 20 mg/kg three times daily for 14–21 days, irrespective of symptoms or form of neonatal disease (Whitley & Arvin, 1995). The pharmacokinetics of acyclovir, intravenously and orally, in the neonate, have been described (Englund et al., 1991; Frenkel et al., 1991). Toxicity has not been reported, but investigation of renal and liver function is recommended before starting intravenous therapy. In one study of long-term oral therapy with 300 mg/m^2 2–3 times a day, 46% of children had reversible neutropenia (Kimberlin et al., 1996b), also seen in 19% of high dose intravenous treatment. As the prognosis in the CNS infected child is often poor, high dosage acyclovir (20 mg/kg × 3) is now recommended for treatment of all forms of neonatal herpes as the outcome hereby has improved (D. F. Kimberlin et al., personal communication, 1999).

After the completion of the intravenous therapy, long-term oral prophylaxis may be discussed to prevent recurrent CNS disease. In children with neonatal

Figure 9.1   (*a*)   CT of the brain 8 days after first neurological symptoms (seizures) in a 20-day-old girl
(*opposite*)   with herpesencephalitis type 2. Increased attenuation of the brain parenchyma is seen in the
whole left hemisphere.
(*b*)   When the child is 3.5 months old, a widespread destruction is seen.

HSV-2 encephalitis, relapses of the encephalitis have been reported, usually soon after termination of the intravenous therapy, although the underlying pathogenetic mechanism are not yet fully understood (Kimura et al., 1991a,b; Barthez-Carpentier et al., 1995). In children with skin–eye–mouth disease and with ≥ three episodes of recurrent skin HSV-2 vesicles within the first 6 months of life, neurological sequelae are common (Whitley et al., 1991b). Evaluation studies of the preventive effect of long-term oral acyclovir are ongoing (phase I/II Kimberlin et al., 1996b; phase III NIAID Collaborative Antiviral Study Group).

Recurrent skin vesicles occur irrespective of the presence of neonatal vesicles (Malm et al., 1991) in 80% of all children with neonatal herpes, and in 95% of neurologically impaired children. This may cause problems in day care centres during recurrences, and intermittent antiviral therapy may be useful.

Preventive measures

Prevention of acquisition of infection

Prevention of vertical transmission is currently possible only in cases of recognized herpes in the mother. In addition, prevention of acquisition of primary infection during pregnancy can be achieved in a woman without a history of genital herpes whose partner has a history of genital herpes (Boucher et al., 1990; Mertz et al., 1992; Bryson et al., 1993; Brown et al., 1997). Serological investigation of HSV-2 antibodies identifies the women at highest risk and the couple benefits from instruction on the risk and preventive measures.

Detection of HSV in the birth canal

Rapid confirmation of herpes lesions by antigen detection is possible in experienced laboratories, but is not universally available. Methods for bedside detection of asymptomatic HSV infections are not yet available. Antenatal and intrapartum cultures may be of value to monitor viral secretion after a primary genital infection but routine culture on a weekly basis, previously performed in USA for women with recurrent herpes, is not recommended (Arvin et al., 1986; Binkin & Koplan, 1989).

Antiviral therapy

Acyclovir, valaciclovir, famciclovir (and the iv penciclovir) all have an effect on replicating virus with a comparable clinical effect in HSV-infections (Mertz et al., 1997a,b), but do not prevent the establishment of latency nor eradicate latent virus. Drug resistance has not been a problem to date in immunocompetent individuals, but continuous vigilance is required, especially in neonates of acyclovir-treated mothers. Pharmacokinetic data for acyclovir and valaciclovir demonstrate a drug concentration in the blood of the fetus similar to that of the mother (Frenkel et al., 1991; Kimberlin et al., 1998). Follow-up data on pregnancy exposure are presently available for acyclovir (Glaxo Wellcome Acyclovir in Pregnancy Registry). Short-term adverse effects in the fetus and the child attributable to acyclovir have not been reported in this register or in other studies. However, teratogenicity or long-term adverse effects cannot yet be excluded.

Mode of delivery

Caesarean section is used for the prevention of exposure of the child to a HSV-infected birth canal. Based on limited data, it has been suggested that caesarean section performed within 6 hours after rupture of the membranes would prevent transmission (Nahmias et al., 1983). However, neonatal herpes has occasionally occurred despite caesarean section (Peng et al., 1993; Whitley & Arvin, 1995). Given the high risk of transmission, it is generally agreed that caesarean section should be recommended in women with a genital primary HSV infection during the last weeks of pregnancy, but mode of delivery for women with recurrent HSV infection and acute lesions in the birth canal is under debate (van der Meijden & Dumas, 1987; Randolph et al., 1993; van Everdingen et al., 1993; Brocklehurst et al., 1995; Tookey & Peckham, 1996; Fonnest et al., 1997). Further information on the risk to the neonate, the effect of antiviral treatment during delivery, the efficacy of early diagnosis, and pre-emptive therapy or antiviral prophylaxis in the child, is required before evidence-based recommendations can be made. Due to the observed risk of viral entry through lesions in the skin, scalp electrodes and instrumental delivery should only be used when strictly necessary.

Antiviral suppression

If recurrences of genital herpes could be prevented by the use of suppressive antiviral chemotherapy, the number of caesarean sections for symptomatic herpes could be reduced. This has been calculated to be cost-effective as a strategy in the USA (Randolph et al., 1996). The results from reported and ongoing studies are somewhat conflicting. In a Norwegian study (B. Stray-Pedersen, 1990, personal communication, 1999) suppression with acyclovir 200 mg × 4 daily orally was started 10 days before term in 408 women, 30 first-episode genital herpes cases were included; serologic confirmation of the real nature of infection was not available. None shed virus at onset of labour. The rate of caesarean section was the same as the average rate in the hospital. No adverse effects were seen in the mothers or children (3 months' clinical observation time). In a UK study, however, no reduction of the rate of caesarean section was achieved (Brocklehurst et al, 1998). The observed reduction of shedding is hopeful (Wald et al., 1996). Given the very low transmission risk in recurrent HSV infection, studies are,

Table 9.2. Considerations for the management of pregnant women with herpes infections

Herpes infection	Antibody activity to isolated HSV type	Antiviral treatment	Management at term
First episode genital herpes			
First and second trimester	Yes= recurrent infection		See below
	No or unknown[a]	In line with clinical condition	Consider suppressive therapy vaginal delivery if no lesions present
Third trimester	Yes = recurrent infection		See below
before 35 weeks	No or unknown[a]	Yes	Consider suppressive therapy Culture virus from vagina–vulva at start of labour Vaginal delivery if no lesions present
35 weeks and later, puerperium	No or unknown[a]	Yes, continue over birth	High risk if the mother is seronegative Consider caesarean section Clinical and virological observation of the child
Lesions in the birth canal at ongoing labour or preterm rupture of membranes	Yes or no or unknown[a]	Start i.v. continue oral therapy	Clinical and virological observation of the child Low risk in recurrent infection High risk if the mother is seronegative
Recurrent genital herpes	Yes or clear-cut history or previously verified herpes	No	Plan for vaginal delivery Frequent recurrences in last months of pregnancy: Consider suppressive therapy Caesarean section may be considered only with acute lesions within the real birth canal at start of labour
Unclear herpes suspect lesions in the birth canal at the start of labour	Yes, no or unknown[a]	To be considered in line with the clinical findings	Vaginal delivery Culture virus from vagina–vulva, if positive clinical and virological observation of the child

Table 9.2. (*cont.*)

Herpes infection	Antibody activity to isolated HSV type	Antiviral treatment	Management at term
First episode oral herpes 35 weeks and later, puerperium	Yes = recurrent infection	No	See below Vaginal delivery
	No or unknown[a]	Yes	Clinical and virological observation of the child
Recurrent oral herpes	Yes or clearcut history	No	Only hygienic measurement

[a] unknown: only a minority are true first time infection, the majority are recurrent.

A validation of the level of evidence for different suggestions is reviewed by Smith et al., 1998.

Therapy: acyclovir: i.v. 10 mg/kg × 3; oral 200 mg × 5 or 400 mg × 3 for 7–10 days; in verified high risk cases (first infection in the last six weeks) 400 mg × 4 during the first week may be considered. Suppressive therapy: 200 mg × 4 (Stray-Pedersen, 1990, B. Stray-Pedersen, 1999 personal communication) or 400 mg × 3 from 10 days before term until delivery. The choice of drug may be reconsidered as new data appear.

Vaginal delivery: the use of instruments that injure the fetal scalp such as scalp electrodes, fetal blood or vacuum extractor are probably best minimized since skin lesions can be a port of entry.

Isolation: The mother with active genital or oral HSV lesions requires isolation only in case of acute illness, she is allowed to breastfeed and handle her own infant with proper hand hygiene.

An exposed child should be nursed together with the mother rather than in a general ward and followed up for 4–6 weeks. Therapy should promptly be instituted if virological or clinical signs of HSV infection appear. There are at present no data on the value: of acyclovir as prophylaxis to an exposed child. However, anticipatory antiviral therapy may be considered in a child exposed to primary genital herpes infection at delivery or in the last weeks of pregnancy.

however, not yet large enough to demonstrate the prevention of transmission of virus to the child (Brown, 1998; Scott, 1999). One case of neonatal herpes in spite of acyclovir suppression has been reported, but compliance to therapy was not documented (Haddad et al., 1993). Routine antiviral suppression therapy is not currently recommended, but may be considered if an increased risk for shedding is anticipated. Several clinical studies are ongoing.

Observation of an exposed child

Close collaboration between the obstetrician, paediatrician and a qualified virological laboratory, and education of the parents are crucial for the early detection of neonatal herpes in an exposed child. Risk evaluation by characterization of the maternal infection; sampling from skin lesions (if present), eyes, oropharynx in the neonate for virus detection after 24–48 hours and at regular intervals up to 4–6 weeks is essential for the early diagnosis and institution of therapy.

Diagnostic methods

Virus culture

This remains a definitive diagnostic method in the vesicle/ulcer stage and for identifying subclinical shedding. Typing of virus should be performed. In experienced hands, rapid confirmation of herpes lesions in the acute stage by antigen detection (e.g. by immunofluorescence) has a high sensitivity but is not universally available. Parallel cultures are strongly recommended. Demonstration of HSV DNA by PCR, with high-quality techniques in specialized laboratories has a very high sensitivity and specificity to trace low level virus shedding and improves rapid diagnosis of neonatal infection (Diamond et al., 1999; Kimura et al., 1991b; Kimberlin et al., 1996b; Malm & Forsgren, 1999). The technique has also been used to diagnose intrauterine infection (Lanouette et al., 1996).

Serological methods

These are of great value in diagnosing past infections with HSV-1 and/or 2 (Ashley & Wald, 1999). Current type common serologic tests are not sufficient and may even under some circumstances be misleading. Type-specific assays especially type-2 and Western blot as a reference method are required for proper investigation and are available in specialized laboratories. New generation assays with genetically engineered antigens have now been introduced.

Management considerations

While definitive recommendations cannot be made, guidance based on present knowledge for the management of the pregnant woman with herpes is given in Table 9.2. It is recommended that herpes diagnostic tools including type-specific HSV antibody tests are used to optimize the management of first episode herpes, verification of the diagnosis if the clinical picture is unclear and for the follow-up of the exposed child.

Future outlook

It is important to emphasize that even with the best care, many cases of neonatal herpes cannot be prevented. New on site tests for antigen and HSV-type specific antibody are being introduced, but the value in the prevention of neonatal herpes remains to be determined. Large-scale screening programmes with the use of type-specific serology, with the aim of identifying pregnant women at risk for transmitting herpes to their children, have been advocated (Brown, 1998). Experience is being gained from an area with high rate of neonatal herpes and the support of an expert clinical virological laboratory (Ashley & Wald, 1999).

However, efficacy under less optimal conditions also has to be evaluated, and the cost–benefit and psycho-social aspects should be considered. The ultimate solution for the prevention of neonatal herpes is a general vaccination programme. Although no vaccine is presently available, many vaccine development projects are in progress.

REFERENCES

Adams, G., Stover, B.H., Keenlyside R. A., Hooton T. M., Buchman, T. G., Roizman, B. & Stewart J. A. (1981). Nosocomial herpetic infections in a pediatric intensive care. *Am. J. Epidemiol.*, **113**, 126 32.

Ades, A. E., Peckham, C. S., Dale, G. E., Best, J. M. & Jeansson, S. (1989). Prevalence of antibodies to herpes simplex virus types 1 and 2 in pregnant women, and estimated rates of infection. *J. Epidemiol. Community Health*, **43**, 53–60.

Azazi, M., Malm, G. & Forsgren, M. (1990). Late ophthalmologic manifestations of neonatal herpes simplex virus infection. *Am. J. Ophthalmol.*, **109**, 1–7.

Arvin, A. M., Hensleigh, P. A., Prober, C. C., Au, D. S., Yasukawa, L. L., Wittek, A. E., Palumbo, P. E., Paryani, S. G. & Yeager, A. S. (1986). Failure of antepartum maternal cultures to predict the infant's risk of exposure to herpes simplex virus at delivery. *N. Engl. J. Med.*, **315**, 796–800.

Ashley, R. L., Dalessio, J., Burchett, S., Brown, Z., Berry, S., Mohan, K. & Corey L. (1992). Herpes simplex virus-2 (HSV-2) type-specific antibody correlates of protection in infants exposed to HSV-2 at birth. *J. Clin. Investig.*, **90**, 511–4.

Ashley, R. L. & Wald, A. (1999). Genital herpes: review of the epidemic and potential use of type-specific serology. *Clin. Microbiol. Rev.*, **12**, 1–8.

Bale, J. F., Andersen, R.D. & Grose, C. (1987). Magnetic resonance imaging of the brain in childhood herpesvirus infections. *Pediat. Infect. Dis. J.*, **6**, 664–7.

Barthez-Carpentier, M. A., Rozenberg, F., Dussaix, E., Lebon, P., Goudeau, A., Billard, C. et al. (1995). Relapse of herpes simplex encephalitis. *J. Child Neurol.*, **10**, 363–8.

Benedetti, J., Corey, L. & Ashley, R.(1994). Recurrence rates in genital herpes after symptomatic first episode infection. *Ann. Int. Med.*, **121**, 847–54.

Binkin, N. J. & Koplan, J. P. (1989). The high cost and low efficacy of weekly cultures for pregnant women with recurrent genital herpes: a reappraisal. *Med. Decis. Making*, **9**, 225–30.

Boggess, K. A., Watts, D. H., Hobson, A. C., Ashley, R. L, Brown, Z. A. & Corey, L. (1997). Herpes simplex virus type 2: detection by culture and polymerase chain reaction and relationship to genital symptoms and cervical antibody status during the third trimester of pregnancy. *Am. J. Obstet. & Gynecol.*, **176**, 443–51.

Boucher, F. D., Yasukawa, L. L., Bronzan, R. N., Hensleigh, P. A., Arvin, A. M. & Prober, C. G. (1990). A prospective evaluation of primary genital herpes simplex virus type 2 infections acquired during pregnancy. *Pediat. Infect. Dis. J.*, **9**, 499–504.

Brocklehurst, P., Charney, O. & Ross, E. (1995). The management of recurrent genital herpes in pregnancy: a postal survey of obstetric practice. *Br. J. Obstet. Gynecol.*, **101**, 791–7.

Brocklehurst, P., Kinghorn, G., Carney, O., Helsen, K., Ross, E., Ellis, E., Shen, R., Cowan, F. & Mindel, A. (1998). A randomised placebo controlled trial of suppressive acyclovir in late pregnancy in women with recurrent genital herpes infection. *Br. J. Obstet. Gynaecol.*, **105**, 275–80.

Brown, Z.A., Benedetti, J., Ashley, R., Burchett, S., Selke, S., Berry, S., Vontver, L.A. & Corey, L. (1991). Neonatal herpes simplex virus infection in relation to asymptomatic maternal infection at the time of labor. *N. Engl. J. Med.*, **324**, 1247–52.

Brown, Z. A., Benedetti, J. K., Watts, D. H., Selke, S., Berry, S., Ashley, R. L. & Corey, L. (1995). A comparison between detailed and simple histories in the diagnosis of genital herpes complicating pregnancy. *Am. J. Obstet. Gynecol.*, **172**, 1299–303.

Brown, Z. A., Benedetti, J., Selke, A., Ashley, R., Watts, D. H. & Corey, L. (1996). Asymptomatic maternal sheding of herpes simplex virus at the onset of labor: relationship to preterm labor. *Obstet. & Gynecol.*, **87**, 483–8.

Brown, Z. A., Selke, S., Zeh, J., Kopelman, J., Maslow, A., Ashley, R. L., Watts, D. H., Berry, S., Herd, M. & Corey, L. (1997). The acquisition of herpes simplex virus during pregnancy. *N. Engl. J. Med.*, **337**, 509–15.

Brown, Z. (1998). Genital herpes complicating pregnancy. *Dermatol. Clin.*, **16**, 805–10.

Bryson, Y., Dillon, M., Bernstein, D. I., Radolf, J., Zakowski, P. & Garratty, E. (1993). Risk of acquisition of genital herpes simplex virus type 2 in sex partners of persons with genital herpes: a prospective couple study. *J. Infect. Dis.*, **167**, 942–6.

Buchman, T. G., Roizman, B., Adams G. & Stover, B. H. (1978). Restriction endonuclease fingerprinting of herpes simplex DNA: a novel epidemiological tool applied to nosocomial outbreak. *J. Infect. Dis.*, **138**, 488–98.

Buchman, T. G., Roizman, B. & Nahmias, A. (1979). Demonstration of exogenous reinfection with herpes simplex virus type-2 by restriction enzyme digestion. *J. Infect. Dis.*, **140**, 295–304.

Cone, R. W., Hobson, A. C., Brown, Z., Ashley, R., Berry, S., Winter, C. & Corey, L. (1994). Frequent detection of genital herpes simplex virus DNA by polymerase chain reaction among pregnant women. *J. A. M. A.*, **272**, 792–6.

Corey, L. & Spear P.G. (1986a). Infections with herpes simplex viruses I. *N. Engl. J. Med.*, **314**, 686–91.

Corey, L. & Spear P. G. (1986b). Infections with herpes simplex viruses II. *N. Engl. J. Med.*, **314**, 749–57.

Corey, L. (1988). First episode, recurrent and asymptomatic herpes simplex infections. *J. Am. Acad. Dermatol.*, **18**, 169–72.

Corey, L., Whitley, R. J., Stone, E. F. & Mohan, K. (1988). Difference between herpes simplex virus type 1 and type 2 neonatal encephalitis in neurological outcome. Lancet, **i**, 1–4.

Cowan, I. M., Johnson, A. M., Ashley, R., Corey, L. & Mindel, A. (1996). Relationship between antibodies to herpes simplex virus (HSV) and symptoms of HSV infection. *J. Infect. Dis.*, **174**, 470–5.

Diamond, C., Mohan, K., Hobson, A., Frenkel, L. & Corey, L. (1999). Viremia in neonatal herpes simplex virus infections. *Pediat. Infect. Dis. J.*, **18**, 487–9.

Enders, G., Risse, B., Zauke, M. & Knotek, F. (1999). Seroprevalence study of herpes simplex virus type 2 among pregnant women in Germany using a type-specific enzyme immunoassay.

Eur. J. Clin. Microbiol. Infect. Dis., **17**, 870–2.

Englund, J.A., Courtney, V., Fletcher, P. & Balfour, H.H. (1991). Acyclovir therapy in neonates. *J. Pediatrics,* **119**, 129–35.

Fonnest, G., De La Fuente Fonnest, I. & Weber, T. (1997). Neonatal herpes in Denmark 1977–1991. *Acta Obstet. Gynecol. Scand.,* **76**, 355–8.

Forsgren, M. (1990). Genital herpes simple virus infection and incidence of neonatal disease in Sweden. *Scand. J. Infect. Dis.* Suppl. **69**, 37–41.

Forsgren, M., Skoog, E., Jeansson, S., Olofsson, S. & Giesecke, J. (1994). Prevalence of antibodies to herpes simplex virus in pregnant women in Stockholm in 1969, 1983 and 1989: implications for STD epidemiology. *Int. J. STD AIDS,* **5**, 113–16.

Frenkel, L. M., Brown, Z. A., Bryson, Y. J., Corey, L., Unadkat, J. D., Hensleigh, P. A. Arvin, A. M., Prober, C. G. & Connor, J. D. (1991). Pharmacokinetics of acyclovir in the term human pregnancy and neonate. *Am. J. Obstet. Gynecol.,* **164**, 569–76.

Frenkel, L. M., Garratty, E. M., Shen, J. P., Wheeler, N., Clark, O. & Bryson, Y. J. (1993). Clinical reactivation of herpes simplex virus type 2 infection in seropositive pregnant women with no history of genital herpes. *Ann. Int. Med.,* **118**, 414–18.

Haddad, J., Langer, B., Astruc, D., Messer, J. & Lokiec, F. (1993). Oral acyclovir and recurrent genital herpes during late pregnancy. *Obstet.Gynecol.,* **82,** 102–4.

Hagadorn, J. I., Bogin, F. J. & Rasmussen, C. A. (1996). Vesicular neonatal rash at the site of vacuum application. *Obstet. Gynecol.,* **87**, 879.

Hensleigh, P. A., Andrews, W. W., Brown, Z., Greenspoon, J., Yasukawa, L. & Prober, C.G. (1997). Genital herpes during pregnancy: inability to distinguish primary and recurrent infections clinically. *Obstet. Gynecol.,* **89**, 891–5.

Kimberlin, D. W., Lakeman, F. D., Arvin, A. M., Prober, C. G., Corey, L., Powell, D. A., Burchett, S. K., Jacobs, R. F., Starr, S. E. & Whitley, R. J. (1996a). Application of the polymerase chain reaction to the diagnosis and management of neonatal herpes simplex virus disease. *J. Infect. Dis.,* **174**, 1162–7.

Kimberlin, D., Powell, D., Gruber, W., Diaz, P., Arvin, A., Kumar M. et al., (1996b). Administration of oral acyclovir suppressive therapy after neonatal herpes simplex virus disease limited to the skin, eyes and mouth: results of a phase I/II trial. *Pediat. Infect. Dis. J.,* **15**, 247–54.

Kimberlin, D.F., Weller, S., Whitley, R. J., Andrews, W. W., Hauth, J. C., Lakeman, F. & Miller, G. (1998). Pharmacokinetics of oral valacyclovir and acyclovir in late pregnancy. *Am. J. Obstet. Gynecol.,* **179**, 846–51.

Kimura, H., Aso, K., Kiyotaka, K., Hanada, N., Shibata, M. & Morishima, T. (1991a). Relapse of herpes simplex encephalitis in children. *Pediatrics,* **89**, 891–4.

Kimura, H., Futamura, M., Kito, H., Ando, T., Goto, M., Kuzushima, K. et al. (1991b). Detection of viral DNA in neonatal herpes simplex virus infections: frequent and prolonged presence in serum and cerebrospinal fluid. *J. Infect. Dis.,* **164**, 289–93.

Koskiniemi, M., Happonen, J. M., Jarvenpaa , A. L., Pettay, O. & Vaheri, A. (1989). Neonatal herpes simplex virus infection: a report of 43 patients. *Pediat. Infect. Dis. J.,* **8**, 30–5.

Koutsky, L. A., Stevens, C. E., Holmes, K. K., Ashley, R. L., Kiviat, N. B., Critchlow, C. W. & Corey, L. (1992). Underdiagnosis of genital herpes b·y current clinical and viral-isolation procedures. *N. Engl. J. Med.*, **326**, 1533–9.

Kulhanjian, J.A., Soroush V., Au, D.S., Bronzan, R. N., Yasukawa, L. L., Weylman, L. E., Arvin, A.M. & Prober, C. G. (1992). Identification of women at unsuspected risk of primary infection with herpes simplex virus type 2 during pregnancy. *N. Engl. J. Med.*, **326**, 916–20.

Lakeman, A. D., Nahmias, A. J. & Whitley, R. J. (1986). Analysis of DNA from recurrent genital herpes simplex virus isolates by restriction endonuclease digestion. *J. Sexually Transm. Dis.*, **13**, 61–6.

Lanouette, J. M., Duquette, D. A., Jacques, S. M., Qureshi, F., Johnson, M. P. & Berry, S. M. (1996). Prenatal diagnosis of fetal herpes simplex infection. *Fetal Diagn. Ther.*, **11**, 414–16.

Löwhagen, G-B., Jansen, E., Nordenfelt, E. & Lycke, E. (1990). Epidemiology of genital herpes infections in Sweden. *Acta Derm. Venereol.*, **70**, 330–4.

Malm, G. & Forsgren, M. (1999). Neonatal herpes simplex virus infections: HSV-DNA in cerebrospinal fluid and serum. *Arch. Dis. Child.*, **81**, F24–9.

Malm, G., Forsgren, M., el Azazi, M. & Persson, A. (1991). A follow-up study of children with neonatal herpes simplex virus infections with particular regard to late nervous disturbances. *Acta Paediat. Scand.*, **80**, 226–34.

Malm, G., Berg, U. & Forsgren, M. (1995). Neonatal herpes simplex: clinical picture and outcome in relation to type of maternal infection. *Acta Paediat.*, **84**, 256–60.

Mertz, G. J., Benedetti, J., Ashley, R., Selke, S. A. & Corey, L. (1992). Risk factors for the sexual transmission of genital herpes. *Ann. Int. Med.*, **116**, 197–202.

Mertz, G. J., Loveless, M. O., Levin, M. J., Kraus, S. J., Fowler, S. L., Goade, D. & Tyring, S. K. (1997a). Valaciclovir versus aciclovir in patient initiated treatment of recurrent genital herpes: a randomised, double blind clinical trial. International Valaciclovir HSV Study Group. *Genitourin. Med.*, **73**, 110–16.

Mertz, G. J., Loveless, M. O., Levin, M. J., Kraus, S. J., Fowler, S. L., Goade, D. & Tyring, S. K. (1997b). Oral famciclovir for suppression of recurrent genital herpes simplex virus infection in women. A multicenter, double-blind, placebocontrolled trial. Collaborative Famciclovir Genital Herpes Research Group. *Arch. Int. Med.*, **157**, 343–9.

Mizrahi, E. M. & Tharp, B. R. (1985). A characteristic EEG pattern in neonatal herpes encephalitis. *Neurology*, **32**, 1215–20.

Nahmias, A. J., Keyserling, H. G. & Kerick, G. M. (1983). Herpes simplex. In *Infectious Diseases of the Fetus and Newborn Infant*, ed. J. S. Remington & J. O. Klein, pp. 636–78. Philadelphia: W.B. Saunders Company.

Nahmias, A., Lee, F. K. & Beckman-Nahmias, S. (1990). Seroepidemiological and sociological patterns of herpes simplex virus infection in the world. *Scand. J. Infect. Dis. Suppl.*, **69**, 19–36.

Peng, J., Krause, P. J. & Kresch, M. (1993). Neonatal herpes simplex virus infection after cesarean section with intact amniotic membranes. *J. Am. Med. Assoc.*, **270**, 77–82.

Prober, C. G., Sullender, W. M., Yasukawa, L. L., Au, D. S., Yeager, A. S. & Arvin, A. M. (1987). Low risk of herpes simplex infections in neonates exposed to the virus at the time of delivery to mothers with recurrent genital herpes simplex infections. *N. Engl. J. Med.*, **316**, 240–4.

Randolph, A. G., Washington, A. E. & Prober, C. G. (1993). Cesarean delivery for women presenting with genital herpes lesions. Efficacy, risks, and costs. *J. Perinatol.*, **16**, 397–9.

Randolph, A. G., Hartshom, R. M. & Washington, A. E. (1996). Acyclovir prophylaxis in late pregnancy to prevent neonatal herpes: a cost-effectiveness analysis. *Obstet. Gynecol.*, **88**, 603–10.

Sakaoka H., Aamori, T., Gouro, T. & Kumamoto, Y. (1995). Demonstration of either endogenous recurrence or exogenous reinfection by restriction endonuclease cleavage analysis of herpes simplex virus from patients with recrudescent genital herpes. *J. Med. Virol.*, 387–96.

Scott L. L . (1999). Prevention of perinatal herpes: prophylactic antiviral therapy? *Clin. Obstet. Gynecol.*, **42**, 134–48.

Smith, R. J., Cowan, F. M. & Munday, F. (1998). The management of herpes simplex virus infection in pregnancy. *Br. J. Obstet. Gynecol.*, **105**, 255–60.

Stray-Pedersen, B. (1990). Acyclovir in late pregnancy to prevent neonatal herpes simplex. *Lancet*, **336**, 756.

Sugimoto, T., Woo, M., & Okazaki, H., Nishida, N., Hara, T., Yasuhara, A., Kasahara, M. & Kobayashi, Y. (1985). Computed tomography in young children with herpes simplex virus encephalitis. *Pediat. Radiol.*, **15**, 372–6.

Tookey, P. & Peckham, C. S. (1996). Neonatal herpes simplex virus infection in the British Isles. *Paediatr. Perinat. Epidemiol.*, **10**, 432–42.

Van der Meijden, W. I. & Dumas, A. M. (1987). Consensus preventie van herpes neonatorum. *Nederl. Tijdschr. Geneeskd.*, **131**, 2030–4.

Van Everdingen, J. J., Peeters, M. F. & ten Have, P. (1993). Neonatal herpes policy in The Netherlands. Five years after a consensus conference. *J. Perinat. Med.*, **21**, 371–5.

Wald, A., Zeh, J., Selke, S., Ashley, R.L. & Corey, L. (1995). Virologic characteristics of sub-clinical and symptomatic genital herpes infections. *N. Engl. J. Med.*, **333**, 770–5.

Wald, A., Zeh, J., Barnum, G., Davis, L. G. & Corey, L. (1996). Suppression of subclinical shedding of herpes simplex virus type 2 with acyclovir. *Ann. Intern. Med.*, **124**, 8–15.

Wald, A., Corey, L., Cone, R., Hobson, A., Davis, G. & Zeh, J. (1997). Frequent genital herpes simplex virus 2 shedding in immunocompetent women. Effect of acyclovir treatment. *J. Clin. Investig.*, **99**, 1092–7.

Whitley, R. J. (1995). Herpes simplex virus infections of the central nervous system: therapeutic and diagnostic considerations. Review. *Clin. Infect. Dis. J.*, **20**, 414–20.

Whitley, R. J. & Arvin, A. M. (1995). Herpes simplex virus infections. In *Infectious Diseases of the Fetus and Newborn Infant*, 4th edn, ed. J. S. Remington & J. O. Klein, pp. 354–74. Philadelphia: W. B. Saunders Company.

Whitley, R., Arvin, A., Prober, C., Burchett, S., Corey, L., Powell, D. et al. (1991a). A controlled trial comparing vidarabine with acyclovir in neonatal herpes simplex virus infection. Infectious Diseases Collaborative Antiviral Study Group. *N. Engl. J. Med.*, **324** , 444–9.

Whitley, R., Arvin, A., Prober, C., Corey, L., Burchett, S., Plotkin, S. et al. (1991b). Predictors of morbidity and mortality in neonates with herpes simplex virus infections. *N. Engl. J. Med.*, **324**, 450–4.

Yeager, A. S. & Arvin, A. M. (1984). Reasons for the absence of a history of recurrent genital infections in mothers of neonates infected with herpes simplex virus. *Pediatrics*, **73**, 188–93.

Young, E. J., Chafizadeh, E., Oliveira, V. L. & Genta, R. M. (1996). Disseminated herpes virus infection during pregnancy. *Clin. Infect. Dis.*, **22**, 51–8.

10

Vertical transmission of hepatitis viruses

Laurent Mandelbrot and Marie-Louise Newell

Introduction

Hepatitis is a general term for inflammation of the liver due to a variety of causes, of which viruses are the most common, but which can also include toxic and auto-immune disorders. The consequences of liver disease in pregnancy, including maternal and fetal outcome, are beyond the scope of this chapter, which focuses on vertical transmission. Acute hepatitis in the mother must be distinguished from other types of liver disease, either unique to pregnancy, such as cholestasis of pregnancy, acute fatty liver of pregnancy and preeclampsia / HELLP syndrome, or pre-existing liver disease, such as cholelithiasis. Although a number of viruses, including herpes simplex and cytomegalovirus, can cause hepatitis, viral hepatitis refers to infections caused by the hepatitis viruses.

Six distinct hepatitis viruses are known: A, B, C, D, E and G, which are not easily distinguished on clinical grounds. Hepatitis A and E are transmitted by the faecal–oral route, and are not commonly transmitted vertically. However, they can cause either asymptomatic infection or fulminating acute hepatitis, notably for HEV in pregnant women. HBV, HCV, HDV and HGV are bloodborne agents, which can lead to chronic carriage, and subsequently to mother-to-child transmission. The clinical significance of HGV remains undetermined, and HDV is dependent upon co-infection with HBV for replication. Hence, HBV and HCV are the most important. They have similar epidemiological and clinical features, and in both infections, asymptomatic carrier mothers can be identified only if serologic testing is performed. Yet there are also important differences. HBV has been known for decades, has a high risk of mother-to-child transmission, with potentially serious long-term consequences for the child, but which can be effectively prevented with immune prophylaxis. HCV was discovered more recently, has a lower risk of mother-to-child transmission, with consequences for the child which are poorly understood at present, and no prophylaxis against mother-to-child HCV transmission is yet available.

Hepatitis B virus infection

Hippocrates provided one of the earliest descriptions of epidemic jaundice more than 2000 years ago, but the first recorded outbreak of jaundice that clearly fits the epidemiology of hepatitis B occurred in Bremen, Germany in 1883 after the vaccination of shipyard workers against smallpox with a vaccine manufactured from human lymph (Greenberg, 1993). Hepatitis B is an important infection in the community and remains a major problem for public health. Each year, about 1 million people die from the acute and chronic sequelae of HBV infection, making it one of the major causes of morbidity and mortality worldwide. HBV causes a spectrum of liver diseases, including acute and chronic hepatitis and cirrhosis, and is one of the few known viral causes of cancer (Zuckerman et al., 1997). Primary liver cancer is among the ten most common cancers in the world, and HBV is second only to tobacco smoking as an identified cause of death from cancer.

Hepatitis B virus

Hepatitis B virus (HBV) is a small enveloped DNA virus, belonging to the family of hepadna viruses (Blumberg, 1995). The structure of the virus includes a double-stranded DNA, surrounded by the hepatitis B core antigen (HBcAg) and the hepatitis Be antigen (HBeAg), which is derived from the core component. The viral envelope carries the surface antigen (HBsAg). The pathological effect of HBV is caused by the attack of the host immune system on the hepatocytes containing HBcAg and probably other viral antigens on their surface rather than by a direct effect of the virus on liver cells (Blumberg, 1995).

The natural history of hepatitis B covers a wide spectrum. There is a long incubation period lasting 6 weeks to several months, on average 10 weeks. In adults and children beyond the age of 3 years, acute infection usually has non-specific clinical manifestations including fatigue and nausea, but jaundice or kernicterus are absent in the majority of cases, and the hepatitis can be asymptomatic. Fulminant liver failure occurs in less than 1% of acute infections. Following acute infection, some individuals develop chronic infection, defined as lack of clearance of the virus beyond 6 months. The immune mechanisms involved are complex, and may lead to either active chronic hepatitis or persistent chronic hepatitis, or carrier state. This distinction is important for clinical management, but in epidemiological studies, the term carrier state includes all types of chronic HBsAg detection, and is therefore usually but not always asymptomatic. Among carriers of HBV, those in whom HBeAg is detected often have some degree of active chronic hepatitis and are the most infectious, whereas those with antibody to HBeAg (anti-HBe) are generally of low infectivity.

The outcome of HBV infection is largely dependent on age at acquisition and the reaction of the immune system (McMahon et al., 1985). If the number of HBV-infected hepatocytes is still small at the time when an efficient immune defence is initiated, the infection is self-limited and remains without symptoms (Grob, 1998). Perinatally infected children are most likely to become chronic carriers, whereas over 90% of individuals infected as adults clear the virus.

Several therapies have been tested in hepatitis B, including alpha interferon, lamivudine, famciclovir, and alpha-interferon combined with lamivudine. The best results were observed in cases of acute hepatitis with active viral replication lasting beyond 6 weeks, preventing progression to chronic hepatitis. For individuals, as well as in terms of public health, the most effective measures against hepatitis B are not therapy, but prevention.

Diagnosis of HBV infection

The diagnosis of hepatitis B infection depends on the identification of specific serological markers. HBsAg is the first marker of infection to occur after infection, occurring within weeks, and persisting for several weeks to months. Its presence reflects infectivity but cannot distinguish acute from chronic infection. The disappearance of HBsAg is usually followed two to six weeks later by detection of antibody against surface antigen (anti-HBs). This indicates recovery from infection and persistent immunity which protects against re-infection. Anti-HBs is produced without other markers of HBV infection after successful vaccination. HBcAg is found only in the liver, and is not detectable in blood. Anti-HBc antibody is usually the first antibody to appear following clinical illness (first IgM then IgG). The presence of anti-HBc indicates either current or past HBV infection. The HBeAg appears after HBsAg and disappears before HBsAg. Its presence is indicative of active viral replication and it is thus a marker of infectivity. Anti-HBe antibody appears following the disappearance of HBeAg and persists for many years. HBV DNA in serum is the most sensitive index of viral replication and can be found in sera of patients with acute or chronic infection. High levels are usually present in the serum of chronic HBeAg positive carriers. HBV DNA usually disappears before, or simultaneously with, anti-HBe seroconversion.

Continued presence of HBsAg for more than 6 months indicates a chronic carrier state. As mentioned above, chronic hepatitis is usually asymptomatic, and liver enzymes may be elevated or normal. Markers of active viral replication include high titres of HBsAg, the presence of HBeAg and HBV DNA in the serum, and the presence of HBcAg, HBeAg and HBV DNA in the liver. However, active viral replication may occur without expression of HBe antigen. A variety of screening tests are available for the detection of HBsAg, the most popular being ELISAs, which have a high sensitivity. Commercial ELISA kits are available for the detection of HBeAg and antibody, HB core antibodies, as well as HBsAg and

Table 10.1. Modes of transmission of HBV

Percutaneous
Contact with blood or blood products
Contaminated needles or syringes, instruments, etc.
Injecting drug use
Surgery
Tattooing, piercing

Mother-to-child
Intrauterine (rare)
Perinatal
Postnatal

Intimate or sexual contact

---

antibody. Pregnant women are first screened for HBsAg and, if positive, tested for HBe antigen and antibody to determine infectivity and for anti-core IgM antibody to differentiate recent acute infection from the carrier state.

Modes of acquisition of HBV infection

HBV is present in certain body fluids of individuals with acute infection as well as in those of chronic carriers, who act as the main reservoir for infection. The risk of transmission of HBV is ten times more frequent than for hepatitis C, and 100 times more than HIV-1. HBV is transmitted through infected blood or blood products, including through sharing of needles and syringes in injecting drug use and inoculation injury in health care workers (Table 10.1). The efficiency of transmission through contaminated blood transfusion is assumed to be 90%, and through needlestick injuries between 7 and 30%. In areas where blood is not routinely screened and where surgical instruments are not adequately sterilized, contamination through these routes remains a risk.

HBV is present in semen and vaginal secretions and acquisition of infection through sexual contact is a major route of infection in low prevalence countries. Chronic carriers may not be aware that they can transmit the infection to their sexual partners. The risk increases with the number of sexual partners, number of years of sexual activity and the presence of other sexually transmitted diseases (Wright, 1975; Szmuness et al., 1975). Although low levels of HBV have been identified in many body fluids, such as sweat, tears, urine and faeces, these are not considered to play a role in transmission. Saliva has been implicated in transmission through biting; kissing and sharing cups are not considered likely to lead to infection.

Mother-to-child transmission is one of the most important factors contributing to the continued high prevalence of HBV in many parts of the world. Carrier status in childhood not only results in liver disease in later life, but it also produces a reservoir of chronic carriers which facilitates intra-familial, child-to-child, and community transmission and perpetuates the cycle of perinatal transmission (Davis et al., 1989).

HBV Prevalence

In 1996 more than a third of the world's population, 2 billion people, were estimated to have serological evidence of HBV infection, with more than 350 million people (or about 5% of the world's population) estimated to be chronically infected with the HBV (Kane et al., 1993). The prevalence of chronic HBV infection in women of childbearing age varies greatly between countries and between populations within a country. To reflect this variation three areas of endemicity are commonly identified: high, low and intermediate.

In countries in Southeast Asia, China and Africa, parts of the Middle-East, the central Asian republics and some countries of Eastern Europe, prevalence of infection is high, with 70–80% of adults having serological evidence of past HBV infection and 8–20% of pregnant women being chronic symptomless carriers of HBV. In intermediate prevalence countries, such as Japan, Eastern Europe, Russia and the Mediterrean countries, 20–30% of women have evidence of past infection, and 2–7% are carriers. In Northern and Western Europe and North America the prevalence is low, and fewer than 10% of adults have experienced HBV infection and less than 1% of pregnant women are chronic carriers of the virus (Denis et al., 1994; Mortimer & Miller 1997; Royal College of Physicians, 1996; Krugman, 1988). Prevalence and incidence of HBV infection vary across Europe, and in general the level increases from north to south and from west to east.

In low prevalence areas adults usually acquire infection through sexual contact or from injecting drug use and perinatal infection is uncommon. However, it is important to bear in mind that immigrants in low prevalence countries have similar HBV carrier rates to those women in their country of origin (Denis et al., 1994; McMenamin, 1996; Dwyer & McIntyre, 1996), and such groups may thus need to be targeted for intervention.

Rates and determinants of vertical HBV transmission

Infants at risk of HBV infection are those born to mothers who are chronic, usually asymptomatic, HBsAg-positive carriers. Acute hepatitis in pregnancy is an uncommon event. Transmission following acute HBV infection during the first trimester of pregnancy is rare, unless the mother develops persistent infection. The risk is about 6% in the second trimester and rises significantly to 67% if infection is acquired in the third trimester of pregnancy (Beasley, 1982). The risk of mother-to-child transmission of HBV is strongly related to the infectivity of maternal blood (Burk et al., 1994; Lee et al., 1988). Infection rates are highest in infants exposed to HBsAg positive women who are also HBeAg positive (Stevens et al., 1975; Beasley, 1982). Nearly 90% of infants born to mothers who are HBeAg positive become infected compared with 40% of infants of HBeAg-negative/HBe antibody-negative mothers. For the small number of carrier mothers with HBe antibody, the risk of vertical transmission is much lower, 10–20%, and does not lead to chronic HBV infection in those children who are infected.

The differences in HBeAg positivity in part account for the wide variation in transmission rates in different populations. Rates are particularly high in Southeast Asia, where 35–50% of HBsAg-positive pregnant women are HBeAg positive, and as a result perinatal transmission is the major route of acquisition of infection. Africa and the Middle East are areas of high endemicity of HBV, but the prevalence of HBeAg among adults is low, with 10–20% of HBsAg-positive pregnant women being HBeAg positive. In these countries, perinatal transmission is less common, but infection is acquired rapidly among young children within families, and 80–90% of children are infected by the age of 10 years. In countries with a low overall prevalence of HBV infection, most people remain uninfected, and nearly all infection is acquired by adults.

Presence of HBeAg is a surrogate marker for high viral load, which is itself the major determinant of transmission risk. Among HBeAg-positive mothers, non-transmitters were more likely than transmitters to have low titres of HBeAg (Ip et al., 1989). Quantification of serum HBV DNA is a direct marker of viral load, which appears to be a strong predictor of transmission risk, particularly among HBeAg-positive mothers. In a cohort of 773 HBsAg-positive Taiwanese women and their infants, the odds of vertical transmission were strongly associated with HBV DNA viral load in HBeAg-positive, but not in HBeAg negative women (Burk et al., 1994). In a multivariate analysis, the risk of vertical transmission associated with the presence of HBeAg was similar to the effect of high viral load, but the risk of persistence of infection in the infant was far greater in infected infants of mothers with high viral load than of mothers with HBeAg. This would suggest that both viral load and HBeAg exert an independent effect on the risk of vertical transmission, and that the association with viral load is stronger than the association with presence of HBeAg.

Timing of vertical HBV transmission

Transmission can occur in utero, but this accounts for only a small proportion (about 5%) of vertically acquired infection. Early in utero infection occurs very rarely or not at all, and there is no embryopathy or fetopathy. Even in the case of acute maternal hepatitis in the first half of pregnancy there is no evidence of transmission occurring at that time. The virus does not readily cross the placenta and cases of intrauterine infection are probably due to leakage of maternal blood into the fetal circulation late in pregnancy (Lee et al., 1978; Lin et al., 1987). In utero infection can be affirmed when HBsAg and HBV DNA are present at significantly higher titres than in the mother, appear within 2 weeks or persist over a week in peripheral blood samples from the neonate. Cord blood should not be used, as there is potential for contamination with maternal blood, and positive results can be due to microtransfusions during delivery. HBeAg crosses the placenta, and is therefore not a diagnostic criterion, and anti-HBc IgM is not produced by congenitally infected infants. It is possible that in utero transmission is underestimated, because of a prolonged incubation period which mistakenly leads to the assumption of intra-partum acquisition of infection. The incidence of in utero infection is increased when the mother has high levels of HBe antigen, serum HBV DNA, and PBMC infection (Brossard, 1992).

The majority of infections are acquired at the time of birth, which is suggested by the seroconversion profile in infants and the remarkable efficacy of immuno-prophylaxis at birth. However, the routes of intrapartum HBV transmission are difficult to determine. In a study from Taiwan (Chen et al., 1998), the presence of HBsAg in the neonatal gastric aspirate was associated with the risk of trans-mission. This could be interpreted as evidence for exposure to infected vaginal secretions or maternal blood via the oral route, although presence of virus in the gastric aspirate may also be a marker for high maternal viral load, and does not in itself indicate whether transmission occurred through the ascending route, via swallowing during the birth process, or transplacentally. There is clear evidence that parenteral exposure occurs because of microtransfusions at the time of delivery (Lin et al., 1996). Interestingly, there is selection of a single variant of HBV during mother-to-child transmission (Friedt et al., 1999).

Whether the risk is higher in infants delivered vaginally than in those delivered by caesarean section is not well established, although this was reported in one study (Lee et al., 1988). Breastfeeding does not seem to be associated with an increased risk of mother-to-child transmission, but conclusive evidence to sup-port this is lacking, because of the introduction of interventions before appropri-ate epidemiological studies were carried out (Beasley et al., 1975). Any effect of vaginal delivery or breastfeeding is likely to be minimal when the infant is protected by immunoglobulin and vaccine.

Even when infection is not acquired during the perinatal period, children of HBV-infected mothers remain at risk of acquiring chronic HBV infection by person-to-person (horizontal) transmission during the first 5 years of life (Advis-ory Committee Immunization Practices, 1991).

Outcome in children

Most infected infants develop an asymptomatic carrier state. The age of acquisition of HBV is inversely related to the risk of chronic infection. While infection during infancy and early childhood is usually asymptomatic, it frequently progresses to the chronic carriage state. On the other hand, due to the immaturity of the immune response, fulminant hepatitis never occurs before the age of 3 months. Persistent HBsAg carriage occurs in 70–90% of neonates and declines to less than 10% when infection is acquired after 6 years of age. The likelihood of chronic HBV infection in the child is related to the mother's viral load and immune status. Infants born to HBeAg-positive mothers are not only likely to be infected, but also to become carriers. The risk is lower in babies born to HBeAg-negative mothers. Those born to mothers with anti-HBe antibodies have a low risk of being infected and do not become chronic carriers, but may develop acute hepatitis at about 3 months of age.

Children with chronic HBV infection are at risk of developing chronic active hepatitis, liver cirrhosis and primary hepatocellular carcinoma (Beasley, 1982). Although the cause and effect relation of HBV to hepatocellular carcinoma is as yet unproven, there is a strong association between chronic HBV infection and the development of liver cancer in both children and adults. In Taiwan (Chang et al., 1997), virtually all children with hepatocellular carcinoma are HBsAg positive, as compared with 70–80% of adults with the disease. Integration of the HBV genome into the host genome of hepatocelllar carcinoma has been reported in children (Chang et al., 1991). In addition to the impact on their own health, chronically HBV infected children also constitute a reservoir of virus for infection of others. Interferon has been used in the treatment of chronic hepatitis B in children, with variable response rates (Vajro et al., 1998). Interferon therapy appeared to be less effective in case of vertical, as compared to postnatal, acquisition of infection.

Prevention of HBV infection and carriage in exposed infants

In the late 1970s, the discovery of HBsAg and the development of assays to measure HBs-specific antibody led to the recognition that anti-HBs antibody provides lifelong protection against reinfection with HBV (Greenberg, 1993). Subsequently it was shown that the serum of an HBsAg positive patient, heated to inactivate infectious virus, would serve as an immunogen to produce anti-HBs (Krugman, 1988). HBIG is prepared from the blood of donors who are negative for HBsAg and whose plasma contains a high titre of anti-HBs antibody. The human plasma from which HBIG is prepared is screened for antibodies to HIV and hepatitis C virus (HCV); in addition, the process used to prepare HBIG inactivates and eliminates HIV and HCV from the final product (Advisory Committee Immunization Practices, 1991).

The efficacy of passive immunization of neonates exposed to HBV was demonstrated in a trial performed in Taiwan (Beasley et al., 1981). In this trial, 71% of the children receiving multiple injections of hepatitis B immune globulin (HBIG) did not become chronic carriers. However, one of its major limitations is that the strategy becomes ineffective if HBIG is not given immediately at birth. The chimpanzee model showed that the efficacy of HBIG disappears if it is given more than 4 hours after birth (Iwarson, 1989), and this is consistent with clinical data. The other major limitations of passive immunization are that it must be repeated monthly, and offers no protection against the risk of postnatal transmission. Therefore passive immunization should not be used alone for the prevention of mother-to-child transmission, but in association with vaccination.

Active-passive immunization of the neonate born to an HBsAg-positive mother is the most successful example of postexposure prophylaxis. Two aspects of HBV infection account for this remarkable efficacy, its long incubation period and the predominance of exposure of the fetus/neonate around the time of delivery. The beneficial impact of vaccination programmes became evident in less than a decade. For instance, in Taiwan a nationwide HBV vaccination programme was implemented in 1984, and the incidence of hepatocellular carcinoma in children declined substantially, from 0.52 per 100 000 for those born between 1974 and 1984 to 0.13 per 100 000 for those born between 1984 and 1986 (Chang et al., 1997). Immunization of neonates also reduces the reservoir of virus, decreasing the incidence of horizontal transmission.

Active HBV vaccination provides long-term protection against HBV infection. In addition to its use as pre-exposure prophylaxis, rapid and energetic vaccination is effective as postexposure prophylaxis, as is the case in rabies, when it is started early enough. The first HBV vaccine was developed in 1976 in France, and safe and effective vaccines have been available since the early 1980s. Initial vaccines were derived from plasma from HBV infected healthy donors, but the cost and insecurity about the supply of human serum stimulated the development of recombinant vaccines. The recombinant vaccines are produced by using HBsAg synthesized by *Saccharomyces cerevisiae* (common baker's yeast) or CHO cell lines, into which a plasmid containing the gene for HBsAg has been inserted. Purified HBsAg is obtained by lysing the yeast cells and separating HBsAg from the yeast components by biochemical and biophysial techniques. HBV vaccine is packaged to contain 10–40 microgram of HBsAg protein per millilitre after adsorption to aluminum hydroxide (0.5 mg/ml); thimerosal (1:20 000 concentration) is added as a preservative (Salisbury & Begg, 1996).

In a study in Hong Kong, different vaccination regimens were evaluated as well as the additional effect of immunoglobulin administration (Wong et al., 1984). Vaccination alone reduced mother-to-child transmission by about two-thirds.

Table 10.2. HBV immunoprophylaxis

	HB vaccine	HBIG
Mother HBsAg positive and HBeAg positive	yes	yes[a]
Mother HBsAg positive without e markers (or where they have not been determined)	yes	yes
Mother with acute HBV during pregnancy	yes	yes[a]
Mother HBsAg positive and anti-HBe positive	yes	no

HBIG is given as rapidly as possible at birth (in the delivery ward) . The first dose of vaccine is given at the same time. Both are injected intramuscularly in an anteriolateral thigh, but at different sites. The second dose of vaccine should be given at 1 month, and the third at 6 or 12 months. (An alternative schedule would be birth, 1, 2 and 12 months.) [a] The usual dosage of HBIG is 100 IU (1 ml); although some programmes recommend a 200 IU dose, to be repeated at 1 month when the mother is HBeAg-positive, had acute hepatitis in the 3rd trimester, or a high level of serum HBV DNA. The recommended dosages of HB vaccine for infants born to HBeAg-positive mothers are 5 µg (Merck) or 10 µg (SmithKline). Follow-up should include, if possible, testing for HBsAg and anti-HBs antibody titre at 4 months. Universal vaccination of all neonates is recommended in several countries.

Transmission from HBe antigen-positive mothers occurred in 21% with vaccination alone, vs. 73.2% in controls. Combination with a single or multiple injections of HBIG led to transmission rates of 6.8% and 2.9%, respectively. Vaccination together with the administration of HBIG was significantly more effective than vaccination alone. The safety and effectiveness of recombinant vaccines has been documented in several well-conducted trials and studies (Sangfelt et al., 1995; Lemon & Thomas, 1997). In settings where HBIG is not available, vaccination alone offers a substantial benefit. Vaccination alone is most effective when the maternal viral load is low, and least effective when the viral load is high, as measured by HBe antigen titer or HBV DNA quantification. Therefore, vaccination without HBIG is an effective measure in regions such as the Sahel.

Prophylaxis of an exposed infant must start shortly after birth *in the delivery room* before antigenaemia has developed, usually with a combination of hepatitis B immunoglobulin and hepatitis B vaccine (Sangfelt et al., 1995) (Table 10.2). Vaccine and HBIG (100 IU) are injected intramuscularly at two different sites. Neonates born to women who are HBsAg and HBeAg positive should receive both HBIG and HBV vaccine, as should those born to HBsAg positive mothers whose HBeAg status has not been assessed or who had active hepatitis during pregnancy. Only those neonates whose mothers are known to have anti-HBe antibodies do not require the HBIG but should receive the vaccine. Optimal protection is achieved by giving immunoglobulin immediately after birth together with a three-dose schedule of acellular vaccine, in the first 6 months, starting at birth (Table 10.2). Several different vaccination schedules are currently used, as there is no evidence to suggest superior efficacy for one of these. The classical schedule is 0–1–2–12 months, but an 0–1–6 months' schedule is also widely used. The dosage of vaccines vary from 2.5 to 30 μg. Some authors have recommended a more intensive prevention in neonates whose mothers are HBeAg-positive or HBV DNA positive, with an HBIG dose of 200 IU repeated at one month.

Acquisition of HBV infection after birth

Horizontal transmission of HBV during the first 5 years of life occurs frequently in populations in which HBV infection is endemic, with HBsAg positive children being an effective source of infection.. The risk of chronic infection after horizontal transmission is age dependent, ranging from 30% to 60% for children 1–5 years of age (McMahon et al., 1985). Neonatal vaccination has been shown to offer long-term protection, even though anti-HBs levels may become low or decline below detectable levels (Fortuin et al., 1993; Whittle et al., 1995; Lee et al., 1995). This is of particular importance because infants born to HBsAg-positive mothers remain at risk of being infected postnatally in the absence of vaccination. Current studies suggest a good retention of immunological memory over 5–12 years, and suggest that there is no need for routine booster vaccination in children who received the full schedule at birth for at least 5 years, possibly longer (Lemon & Thomas, 1997; Fortuin et al., 1993; Whittle et al., 1995, Poovorawan et al., 1997). Passive immunization with specific immunoglobulin does not affect the development of active immunity in response to vaccine.

Frequency and reasons for failed prophylaxis

The main reason prophylaxis fails is probably because it is not performed, delayed, suboptimally dosed, or incomplete. For instance, in the USA, between a quarter (MMWR, 1997) and a half (Pierce et al., 1999) of the infants born to HBsAg-positive mothers were not receiving both vaccine and hepatitis B immune globulin as recommended. However, even when active–passive immunoprophylaxis is correctly carried out, a small proportion of infants are nonetheless infected. These infections may be due to in utero infection, high maternal viral load, or poor response to vaccine by the infant.

Because in utero transmission is estimated to occur in about 5% of cases, it may account for the majority of prophylactic failures (Brossard, 1992). However, because the incubation period is long, vaccination at birth may still be effective postexposure prophylaxis weeks after the time of exposure. It has been suggested that a high maternal viral load increases the risk of prophylactic failure (Ngui et al., 1998), although this has not been confirmed (Chang et al., 1996). Because high viral load is associated with an increased risk of in utero transmission, it is difficult to determine whether it has an independent effect on breakthrough infection. Many programs recommend the use of higher as well as repeated doses of HBIG in infants born to mothers with high titre HBeAg and/or HBV DNA (Brossard, 1992).

Approximately 5% of neonates do not respond to vaccination. This may be due to the host's inability to mount an antibody response, or insufficient dosage or immunogenicity of the vaccine preparation. In recent years, attention has been given to escape mutant virus as a cause for failed immunoprophylaxis (Hsu et al., 1997; Chong-Jin et al., 1999; Matsumoto et al., 1997). Surface gene (S) mutants emerge or are selected under the immune pressure generated by the host or by the administration of vaccine and HBIG. In a British study (Ngui et al., 1997), mother–infant sequence mismatches in the HBV S gene were found in only 2 of 17 infants infected, despite full active–passive immunopropylaxis. The frequency of potential vaccine escape mutants is low, and there are minor variants in the mother (Ngui et al., 1997).

Other factors have been suggested to play a role in immunization failure. HBV genome was detected at birth in the peripheral blood mononuclear cells of a high proportion of children who did not respond to HB vaccine (Lazizi et al., 1997). This was interpreted to indicate that in utero exposure to HBsAg induced a specific immune tolerance, which may be transient or prolonged, leading to failure of vaccination in these infants. In another study, low anti-HBc antibody titres in the mother (and the infant) were strongly related to failure of prophylaxis, suggesting that anti-HBc may play a positive role in modulating vertical transmission (Chang et al., 1996).

Amniocentesis

Invasive needling procedures carry the potential risk of transmitting blood-borne infectious agents (see hepatitis C). Leakage of blood through the placenta may occur, in particular during chorionic villi sampling, or when the needle crosses the placenta, and direct parenteral exposure may occur during fetal blood sampling. Follow-up of large cohorts would be required to evaluate whether or not amniocentesis actually increases the risk of HBV infection in the child. In a small retrospective study (Grosheide et al., 1994), no evidence of increased transmission was found, and in a study from Taiwan (Ko et al., 1994), the failure rates of immunoprophylaxis were the same in 32 infants who had an amniocentesis as in other infants born to HBsAg-positive mothers. In the subgroup with HBeAg-positive mothers, amniocentesis was associated with a higher failure rate (30% vs. 14%), although the difference did not reach statistical significance. Because data are lacking, there is no consensus for clinical management, and no basis to contraindicate invasive procedures in HBsAg-positive pregnant women. When performing amniocentesis, the transplacental route should be avoided whenever possible. In case of percutaneous fetal blood sampling, HBIG (50 IU/kg estimated fetal weight) may be injected intravenously before withdrawing the needle (Brossard, 1992).

Prevention strategies
Antenatal testing

Optimal intervention to prevent mother-to-child transmission requires knowledge of maternal serostatus. In order for infants born to HBsAg-positive mothers to receive immunoglobulin and the first vaccine dose immediately after birth, antenatal testing policies are of clear benefit. Whether testing should be systematically offered, or only to women with risk factors varies according to the seroprevalence in the antenatal population, as well as economic and cultural considerations. In many countries, testing is offered at the first prenatal visit, although in France, where testing for HBs antigen has been mandatory since 1992, it is done in the sixth month of pregnancy. In the Netherlands, a programme for first trimester HBsAg screening was launched in 1989, and by 1992 84% of women were screened. In North Carolina, 92% of pregnant women were screened for HBs following a policy of universal screening. Selective screening appears less effective, even in low-prevalence areas, because hepatitis B is not limited to identifiable risk groups, and because preventing mother-to-child transmission is of great importance on an individual as well as a public health level, there is a strong basis for universal screening.

The most cost-effective screening is the detection of HBs antigen. To the extent that resources are available, all women who test positive for HBs antigen should be tested for HBe antigen, and if negative for anti-HBe antibody and HBV DNA. In addition to this work-up, the objective of which is to optimize prevention of vertical transmission, women should be offered liver function tests and appropriate long-term follow-up for their own health.

Expanded prevention programmes

Ultimately, the most effective prevention of mother-to-child HBV transmission is the prevention of hepatitis B in the general population. This prevention includes blood safety programs, universal precautions in healthcare facilities, risk reduction programmes for intravenous drug users, STD control including condoms in high risk groups, and vaccination. Integrating HBV vaccine into childhood vaccination programmes in populations with high rates of childhood infection has been shown to interrupt HBV transmission (Advisory Committee Immunization Practices, 1991). Over 75 countries have adopted a national policy of immunizing all infants with hepatitis B vaccine, most of which are in Eastern and Southeast Asia, the Pacific Basin, and the Middle East.

In Western industrialized countries, where the prevalence is lower, immuniz-ation policies are either universal, or targeted at risk groups. These include, of course, neonates born to HBV-infected mothers, but also healthcare workers (Joint Working Party of the Hospital Infection Study Group, 1992), children in close daily living contact such as day care centres and special schools or collective residential facilities (Salisbury & Begg, 1996), drug users, and sexual partners of HBV-infected persons. All healthcare workers, including labour ward staff, should be vaccinated against hepatitis B, and universal precautions for the prevention of transmission of blood borne virus infection should be strictly adhered to (Joint Working Party of the Hospital Infection Study Group, 1992; Advisory Committee on Dangerous Pathogens, 1995).

Universal childhood HB vaccination has been adopted in several countries, including France, where HB vaccine is part of the recommended immunization calendar starting at 2–4 months. The American Academy of Pediatrics recom-mends HB vaccination of all neonates at birth, but with a higher vaccine dosage and HBIG when the mother is HbsAg-positive. Recently, there has been concern that hepatitis vaccination may increase the incidence of multiple sclerosis in certain persons. Although this has not been confirmed in large-scale surveys, it has led to a controversy in Europe over the policies of mass vaccination. In the UK, antenatal screening of all pregnant women for HBV is recommended, but there is no universal childhood vacccination programme in place.

A programme of universal hepatitis B vaccination in infancy was implemented in Israel in 1992, where all infants are vaccinated at birth and at 1 and 6 months of age. Contrary to the American programme, this was conducted without HBIG, and without HBsAg screening during pregnancy. This strategy has been reported to be effective, even among subgroups with high HBsAg prevalence (Zamir et al., 1999).

In areas with high prevalence and restricted resources, such mass vaccination of all infants, as early as possible after birth, may be the most cost-effective strategy. The approach is sub-optimal in Asia, where vertical transmission accounts for most infections, and therefore active–passive immunization immediately at birth is advised whenever possible. In parts of Africa where both vertical and early postnatal mother-to-child transmission are of importance, universal vaccination in infancy has been shown to be effective. For instance, in a Gambian study (Fortuin et al., 1993), the vaccine was 84% effective against infection and 94% effective against chronic carriage at 3–4 years follow-up.

The recommended three intramuscular doses of HBV vaccine induces a protective antibody response (anti-HBs greater than 10 milli-international units per ml) in over 95% of infants, children and adolescents and over 90% of healthy adults (Sangfelt et al., 1995; Salisbury & Begg, 1996; Lemon & Thomas, 1997). HBV vaccine should be administered in the deltoid muscle of adults or children or in the anterolateral thigh muscle of neonates and infants; the immunogenicity of the vaccine for adults is substantially lower when injections are administered in the buttock. When infants receive hepatitis B vaccine at the same time as other vaccines, separate sites in the anterolateral thigh are recommended (Salisbury & Begg, 1996). HBV vaccine is generally well tolerated and the most common adverse reactions are soreness and redness at the injection site (Salisbury & Begg, 1996; Lemon & Thomas, 1997). It has been shown that concurrently administered vaccines do not interfere with the immunological response to hepatitis B vaccine, and that hepatitis B vaccine does not interfere with the other childhood vaccines. Attention is now focused on the development of combined vaccines (Lemon & Thomas, 1997).

Conclusion

Hepatitis B is a major public health problem worldwide, with significant public health consequences even in Europe where the prevalence is low, and where most childhood infections are acquired from mother-to-child transmission. Most perinatal or early infant HBV infection results from infection at delivery rather than in utero, and prophylaxis must start immediately after birth before anti-genaemia has developed. The risk of mother-to-infant transmission of HBV is related to the infectivity of maternal blood, which is high when HBeAg is present, and low in the presence of anti-HBe antibody. Universal HBsAg testing in pregnancy allows for the rapid and effective active–passive immunoprophylaxis starting at birth, with an efficacy of over 90% in preventing carriage of HBV in the child. Over the last two decades, hepatitis B prevention in neonates has been shown to have a major impact on the incidence of chronic liver disease, cirrhosis and hepatocarcinoma, as well as limiting the horizontal and vertical spread of HBV in new generations. Making this prevention available worldwide is a major challenge.

Hepatitis C virus infection

Hepatitis C virus (HCV) is a single stranded, positive sense RNA virus of approximately 9500 bases, identified in 1989 as the major causal agent of non-A non-B hepatitis (Choo et al., 1989). At least six genotypes and more than 80 subtypes have been described, which can be detected with serological and HCV RNA tests. The distribution of subtypes varies according to geographic location and route of infection (Consensus Panel, 1999). Positivity of antibody tests does not denote protection against the virus, but rather prior or current infection with the virus.

Acute HCV infection is asymptomatic in over two-thirds of cases, but leads to chronic hepatitis C in up to 70% of cases. Most patients with chronic hepatitis C remain asymptomatic for many years, however there are high rates of long-term morbidity and mortality, as a consequence of destruction of hepatocytes by the host's immune system. It has been estimated that approximately 35% of HCV infected people progress to cirrhosis after 20 years, and 20–25% develop hepatocellular carcinoma 30 years after acquiring HCV infection (Resnick & Koff, 1993; Di Bisceglie et al., 1991). Chronic HCV infection has also been associated with a large array of autoimmune manifestations, including mixed cryoglubulinemia, rheumatic disorders, diabetes, and thyroiditis, and possibly with an increased frequency of B-cell lymphoma.

Although progress has been made in recent years, in the majority of patients existing therapies do not result in long-term clearance of hepatitis C. The first established therapy for chronic hepatitis C is alpha-interferon 2; however, only 10–20% of patients show a sustained response with persistent disappearance of detectable viraemia and normalization of ALT levels. A low pretreatment serum HCV RNA level, HCV genotype non-1a and non-1b, and mild liver damage are the main independent predictors of a sustained treatment response. Tolerance is variable; the most common side effect is a flu-like syndrome, but haematological toxicity is the most frequent cause of interruption of therapy. Combination therapy of interferon and ribavirin has been shown to be more effective than interferon alone, and is now the standard of care (Consensus Panel, 1999). However, ribavirin is teratogenic and mutagenic and cannot be used in pregnancy. No vaccine has yet been developed against HCV.

Prevalence of HCV

Hepatitis C is a major public health problem worldwide. Prevalence rates among unselected pregnant women in Western Europe are about 1%. Highest prevalence (sometimes greater than 10%) has been reported from parts of the Middle East, sub-Saharan Africa and Japan (Kiyosawa et al., 1994; El Gohary et al., 1995; Louis et al., 1994). Some studies from Europe have reported higher rates of ELISA positivity among women from sub-Saharan Africa than among native Europeans or immigrants from other countries (Marcellin et al., 1993; Aussel et al., 1991). However, Roudot-Thoroval et al. (1993) found that higher prevalence among immigrant women recorded at initial ELISA testing virtually disappeared after supplementary testing, suggesting that in these women there was a high frequency of false positive ELISA results. Not all women who are HCV seropositive are also HCV RNA viraemic, and there is little evidence for a role of raised ALT levels in predicting the presence of HCV infection (Tanzi et al., 1995; Wahl et al., 1994; Lin et al., 1993).

HCV diagnostic tests

The first serological test, detecting anti-C100 antibodies, was developed after the identification of HCV in 1989, but lacked sensitivity and specificity. Second- and third-generation ELISA and recombinant immunoblot assays have sensitivities of 90–95%. However, in low prevalence populations, the false positive rate is in the order of 10 to 20%. Thus, for screening pregnant women or children born to HCV-positive mothers, positive ELISA tests require a confirmation immunoblot test, such as RIBA III, on a second blood sample.

HCV RNA becomes positive 2 weeks after infection, and is persistently detectable in about two thirds of patients with HCV antibodies. Commercial assays available include Amplicor (Roche, Basel), and branched DNA (Quantiplex, Chiron). Detection limits of the first generation tests are 700 copies/ml and 200 000 copies/ml, respectively. Second generation tests are now available, with lower detection limits (down to 100 copies/ml). Thus, the definition of negative viraemia differs according to the test used, and furthermore there are considerable sources of error and variation in plasma RNA testing. The RT PCR and bDNA tests also allow for quantification of viraemia, i.e. plasma HCV RNA levels, however the limits of detection of these tests are higher than for qualitative tests.

Mother-to-child transmission of HCV infection

There is clear evidence to suggest mother-to-child transmission exists (Weiner et al., 1993; Inoue et al., 1992; Gish et al., 1996; Lin et al., 1994; Ohto et al., 1994). Analysis of phylogenic trees revealed transmission through two (Inoue et al., 1992) and even three generations (Tahara et al., 1996). In the study by Ohto et al., three infants showing genomic sequences of HCV nearly identical to those of their mothers were followed prospectively from birth, documenting vertical transmission (Ohto et al., 1994).

Diagnosis of HCV infection in children born to seropositive mothers

A variety of diagnostic criteria have been used, based on HCV RNA detection and/or serology. The diagnosis of HCV infection in exposed children cannot be based on antibody testing before 18 months of age. HCV antibodies can be detected in most infants born to HCV-infected mothers for a period of several months, due to the passive transfer of maternal IgG. These usually disappear within the first year of life, although, when maternal antibody titre is particularly elevated, such as in women co-infected with HIV-1, passively acquired maternal anti-HCV antibodies may persist longer (Resti et al., 1998). Antibody response may be delayed in some infected children, leading to cases of transient seronegativity during the period in which maternal antibodies are no longer detected and the infant is not yet producing antibodies. Such cases of delayed seroconversion (Katayama et al., 1998) appear to be rare, and have been reported mostly in HIV-1 co-infected infants (Granovsky et al., 1998). Because of these variations both in the disappearance of maternal antibodies and in the production of antibodies by the child serological testing alone is unable to distinguish vertical transmission from potential cases of postnatal horizontal transmission.

Transaminase levels are not useful for diagnosis, as they may be normal in infected children, or transiently elevated in uninfected children (Wejstal et al., 1990; Nagata et al., 1992, 1994). In practice, diagnosis of whether the child is infected or not should be based at least on HCV RNA performed after 3 months of age, and preferably between 6 months and 1 year, confirmed by serostatus at 18 months. Reverse-transcriptase polymerase chain reaction (PCR) to detect HCV RNA in serum or plasma samples is a highly sensitive assay allowing for an early diagnosis of infection in perinatally exposed infants (Thomas et al., 1997), although much variation exists in the reliability of these tests between laboratories. In clinical practice at least two positive PCR results in separate samples are required to confirm the diagnosis of infection. Cord blood samples must not be used, as there is a high rate of false-positive results (Uehara et al., 1993; Reinus et al., 1992; Silverman et al., 1993). These may be due to transfer of HCV through the placenta up through the third stage of labour, without necessarily leading to infection of the child, or to contamination of the sample with maternal blood. On the other hand, HCV RNA can offer false-negative results, especially if it is performed too early or too late.

Several studies have reported transitory viraemia among seroreverting children (Paccagnini et al., 1995; Zanetti et al., 1995; Tovo et al., 1997; Mazza et al., 1998). These observations may be due to false positive PCR findings, as no case was documented by more than one positive peripheral blood sample and sequence homology between samples in the mother and child. However, it can be hypothesized that some children contracted the infection, but definitively cleared the virus without seroconverting. Further research on these children could contribute to identifying the underlying mechanisms responsible for virus control and the immunological target for a future vaccine.

Mother-to-child HCV transmission rates

Among the numerous studies published, crude transmission rates have varied from 0 to 100%. Many of the discrepancies can be explained by methodological weaknesses, such as small populations, lack of appropriate follow-up, and differences in criteria for the diagnosis of HCV infection in exposed infants (Thomas et al., 1998). However, most of the difference is likely to be due to differences in the populations under study. The role of some putative risk factors (see below) has not yet been clarified, but two factors are clearly important: maternal HIV

Table 10.3. Mother-to-child transmission rates from HIV negative, HCV seropositive, viraemic mothers (restricted to studies with more than 20 infants, with more than 6 months of follow-up)

Reference	Infants exposed	Infants infected	MCT (%)
Chang, 1996	20	3	15.0
Croxson et al., 1997	30	2	6.6
Fischler et al., 1996	38	0	0
Giacchino et al., 1996	45	4	8.8
Granovsky et al., 1998	25	2	8
Kumar & Shahul, 1998	65	3	4.6
Lam et al., 1993	38	4	10.5
La Torre et al., 1998	56	2	3.6
Matsubara et al., 1995	21	3	14.3
Mazza et al., 1998	43	2	4.7
Moriya et al., 1995	87	2	2.3
Nagata et al., 1994	20	1	5
Ohto et al., 1994	31	3	9.7
Polywka et al., 1997	62[a]	4	6.7
Resti et al., 1998	275	13	4.7
Spencer et al., 1997	63	6	9.5
Wejstal et al., 1990	21	1	4.8
Zanetti et al., 1998	176	8	4.6

[a] only children with > 6 months follow-up included.

infection status and HCV viraemia (Fischler et al., 1996; Thomas et al., 1998). Transmission from non-viraemic mothers appears to be rare (Novati et al., 1992; DeVoid et al., 1993; Thomas et al., 1998; Granovsky et al., 1998).

When considering only HCV RNA-positive, viraemic, mothers and distinguishing those who were co-infected with HIV, a more consistent pattern appears (Table 10.3). Among 38 studies, published between 1992 and 1999, a total of 94 cases of transmission were reported from 1345 viraemic, HIV-negative mothers, giving a crude transmission rate of 7%, similar to the rates found in two large Italian cohorts (Resti et al., 1998; Zanetti et al., 1998). When excluding the smallest studies, with fewer than 20 mother–infant pairs, 66 of 1137 infants (5.8%) born to HIV-negative, HCV viraemic mothers were found to be infected. Although transmission rates ranged from 0 to 14.3%, the 95% confidence intervals for nearly all of the studies were consistent with that of the largest study (Resti et al., 1998), which was 2 to 7%.

Table 10.4. Mother-to-child transmission rates from HIV-1 co-infected, HCV seropositive, viraemic (PCR+) mothers (restricted to studies with follow-up of 20 or more mother–infant pairs for more than 6 months)

Reference	Infants exposed	Infants infected	MCT (%)
Granovsky et al., 1998	47	4	9
Nigro[a]	23	2	8.7
Mazza et al., 1998	20	4	20
Papaevangelou et al., 1998	31	4	12.9
Thomas et al., (WITS[b]), 1998	140	13	9.3
Tovo et al., 1997[c]	165	25	15.1
Zanetti et al., 1998	32	9	28.1

[a] Mother's PCR unknown. Includes only HIV+ children.
[b] No maternal PCR.
[c] Women and infants transmission study.

Among women with HIV co-infection, estimates of transmission rates vary from 0 (Reinus et al., 1992; Fischler et al., 1996) to 44% (Maccabruni et al., 1993). However, several of the studies only included small numbers, or have been updated in more recent multicentre cohorts (Gamboa et al., 1994; Thomas et al., 1998). When seven publications with 20 or more mother–infant pairs are considered, and known overlaps excluded, transmission rates ranged from 8.7 to 28.1%, and a total of 61 of 458 exposed infants (13.1%) were found to be HCV-infected (Table 10.4). These results are consistent with the rates observed in the two largest studies to date (Tovo et al., 1997; Thomas et al., 1998), which were 9.3% and 15.1%, respectively.

Factors related to HCV transmission risk

A number of factors have been investigated, which could potentially be related to the risk of mother-to-child transmission. Apart from maternal viral load and HIV co-infection, these include immunosuppression, viral subtype, maternal characteristics, obstetrical factors, breastfeeding and HCV–antibody complexing. The cohort studies published to date have lacked power to investigate all potential risk factors, owing to the small numbers of infected women and the low transmission rate. Although some of the putative risk factors are probably interrelated, the small overall numbers have precluded multivariate analysis of risk factors. It is to be expected that, as for other blood-transmitted viruses, the higher the viral burden, the higher the risk of transmission. The available evidence is consistent with the hypothesis that maternal viral load is the most important factor determining

Table 10.5. Viral load and vertical HCV transmission

Reference	Method	Transmitters		Non-transmitters	
		N	RNA eq/ml	N	RNA eq/ml
Aizaki et al., 1996	RT–PCR	1	10^6	8	Median $10^{5.5}$
Fugisawa (in Thomas S. et al., 1998)	RT–PCR	5	10^6–10^7	17	10^4–10^9
Garland et al., 1998	RT–PCR	3	5×10^5	42	1.2×10^4
Giacchino et al., 1996	bDNA	4 ?	Mean 5.76 meq $\times 10^6$	25	1.11 meq $\times 10^6$
Granovsky et al., 1998	Mostly bDNA	7	3.7×10^6	66	4.2×10^6
Kudo et al., 1995	bDNA	6	Median 1.2×10^6	6	2.2×10^6
La Torre et al., 1998	RT–PCR	2	2×10^4 and 4×10^5	17	4×10^3–1×10^6
Lin et al., 1995	Competitive RT-PCR	1	10^{10}	7	5×10^5–5×10^6
Manzini et al., 1995	Limited dilution	1	ND	27	10^3–10^4–$> 10^4$
Matsubara et al., 1995	Limited dilution	3	Mean $10^{5.3}$	16	Mean $10^{4.4}$
Mazza et al., 1998	PCR differential hybridization assay	5	Median$10^{7.2}$	36	Median$10^{7.35}$
Moriya et al., 1995	bDNA	4	8.6×10^6–9.6×10^7	46	$< 2 \times 10^5$–5.6×10^7
Nagata et al., 1992	bDNA	1	10^7	1	$< 10^7$
Ohto et al., 1994	Limited dilution	7	Mean $10^{6.5}$	33	Mean 104.4
Papaevangelou et al., 1998	bDNA	5	Median $< 3.5 \times 10^5$	40	Median 4.1×10^5
Pipan et al., 1996	bDNA	0	–	13	6.5×10^5–4.6×10^6
Resti et al., 1998	RT–PCR	13	3.8×10^5	258	2.4×10^5
Spencer et al., 1997	RT–PCR	6	Median 8.9×10^5	46	Median 3.9×10^5
Thomas D. L. et al., 1998	RT–PCR	13	2×10^6	142	3.5×10^5
Zanetti et al., 1998	bDNA	8	Median 10^7	10	Median 6.7×10^6

infectivity (Nagata et al., 1992; Lin et al., 1994; Ohto et al., 1994; Matsubara et al., 1995; Moriya et al., 1995; Giacchino et al., 1996; Zanetti et al., 1998). As discussed above, transmission by HCV RNA negative mothers is rare. In a few studies (Kudo et al., 1997; Granovsky et al., 1998; La Torre et al., 1998), there was no difference in the median and/or distribution of viral loads between transmitting and non-transmitting mothers. In the largest study with an HIV-negative population (Resti et al., 1998), no difference was found in RNA load between transmitters and non-transmitters, and there was remarkable overlap in the distribution of values $(0.02$ to $56) \times 10^5$ copies/ml, vs. $(0.01$ to $92.7) \times 10^5$, respectively.

The data summarized in Table 10.5 suggest that there is no threshold value of viral load below which transmission does not occur. In a widely cited publication from Japan (Ohto et al., 1994), no case of transmission occurred from mothers with viraemias below 10^6/ml (using a limited dilution test). However, more recent studies failed to detect a threshold (Thomas et al., 1998; Papaevangelou et al., 1998). In the study by Resti (Resti et al., 1998), transmission occurred with a viral load as low as 2×10^3 copies/ml (using RT–PCR). It should, however, be stressed that the level of viraemia may change markedly over the course of pregnancy (Kumar & Shahul, 1998), and few of the studies reported serial determinations at standardized time points, such as delivery.

As discussed above, rates of vertical transmission appear to be approximately two to three times higher from mothers with HIV co-infection, compared to HIV-negative mothers (Zuccotti et al., 1995; Maccabruni et al., 1995; Paccagnini et al., 1995; Tovo et al., 1997; Thomas et al., 1998; Granovsky et al., 1998; Papaevangelou et al., 1998; Zanetti et al., 1998). Although HIV co-infection is the foremost known risk factor for vertical HCV transmission, the reasons are poorly understood. It is interesting to note that HCV co-infection has also been reported to be a risk factor for vertical HIV transmission, and both HCV and HIV cohort studies show unexpectedly high proportions of infants infected with both HIV and HCV. HIV-infected infants were more likely than HIV-uninfected infants to be infected with HCV (Zanetti et al., 1995; Tovo et al., 1997; Thomas et al., 1998; Papaevangelou et al., 1998). These findings point to common risk factors for vertical transmission of both viruses.

Theoretically, any immunodeficiency condition in the mother, leading to an enhanced viral load, could result in an increased risk of HCV transmission to the offspring. HIV-induced immunosuppression may play a role in increasing levels of HCV viraemia. One study reported lower CD4 counts among HIV coinfected mothers who transmitted HCV infection (Kumar & Shahul, 1998), but this was not the case in another (Papaevangelou et al., 1998). Coinfection with HIV may result in increased levels of HCV viraemia. Two studies investigated levels of HCV viraemia according to maternal HIV serostatus, one of which reported significantly higher viraemia levels among 18 HIV co-infected mothers compared to 10 HIV negative mothers (Kumar & Shahul, 1998), whereas the other (using a semi-quantitative assay) found no significant association between maternal HIV sero-status and viraemia levels in 27 non-transmitting mothers (Manzini et al., 1995). In the WITS study (Thomas et al., 1998), maternal HCV RNA levels were higher in cases where the child was coinfected with HCV and HIV. In the study by Granovsky et al., (1998), there was a trend towards increasing HCV transmission with increasing maternal HIV-1 viral load and/or low CD4 counts, however it did not approach statistical significance due to the relatively small population studied.

Most women with HCV antibodies, including those with detectable plasma HCV RNA, are clinically asymptomatic. Although data on maternal liver enzyme levels were lacking in most perinatal cohort studies, it is likely that few of the women had advanced liver damage. Furthermore, there is a trend towards transient normalization of liver enzyme levels during pregnancy. It has been suggested (Xiong et al., 1998) that transmission may be increased in women with elevated liver enzymes. Such a relation may theoretically be due to higher levels of circulating HCV in patients with advanced disease, as well as to shifts in the host's immune response. However, other larger studies (Zanetti et al., 1998) did not observe a significant difference in transmission according to whether the mother had, or did not have, chronic liver disease or elevated transaminase levels.

A higher risk of transmission may occur, due to the presence of high levels of viraemia and the absence of antibodies during primary infection. There are few data on seroconversion during pregnancy, and furthermore there is clear potential for selection bias towards women with symptomatic acute hepatitis. Two cases of vertical transmission were reported in mothers who were infected during the third trimester, and another two cases of acute hepatitis C in the third trimester without vertical transmission have been reported (Gurakan et al., 1994; Zuckerman et al., 1997).

The clinical course of chronic HCV infection has been reported to vary according to the subtype, but it is not clear whether subtypes are also related to transmissibility. The distribution of HCV subtypes has been found to differ between populations. It is not clear whether this is due to a 'founder effect' or to differences in transmission via different routes for different subtypes. Subtypes 1a and 1b are those most commonly observed in Western Europe and North America, and appear to respond less well to therapy than other subtypes (Consensus Panel, 1999). Transmission of various subtypes has been reported, including 1a, 1b, 2a and 3a, and more rarely 6a, 2a/2c and 4c/4d. The subtype detected in the infant was nearly always detected in the mother. However, only one subtype was transmitted, even from mothers with more than one subtype present. There is some suggestion that selection may occur (Kudo et al., 1997; Mazza, 1998; Thomas, 1998; Granovsky, 1998; Spencer, 1997; La Torre, 1998). It is not possible to conclude at present whether some subtypes are more transmissible, or whether the distribution of subtypes among infected children simply reflects the prevalence of each subtype among the mothers studied.

The role of maternal immune response has been suggested particularly in studies of women co-infected with HIV (see above). In one study (Mazza et al., 1998), a significant relationship was found between the absence of reactivity to C100 on RIBA and transmission risk. A more solid line of evidence suggests that the maternal immune response plays an important role in preventing transmission of the virus (Weiner et al., 1993; Kudo et al., 1997; Ni et al., 1997). In these studies, a unique HCV variant was transmitted in each case by mothers with multiple variants. Interestingly, the variant which was transmitted was not dominant in the mother, suggesting that selection occurred. Kudo et al. (1997) found that the virus had higher densities in non-transmitters than transmitters, and because densities of the virus are believed to increase in reaction to humoral response, concluded that this selection process was due to the maternal immune response.

Timing of vertical HCV transmission

When vertical transmission takes place remains unclear. There is sufficient evidence to suggest that both in utero and intrapartum transmission can occur, but their relative contributions are difficult to establish. HCV RNA has been found immediately after birth in venepuncture samples of some infected children (Giacchino et al., 1996; Resti et al., 1998), which would indicate that in utero infection had occurred. However, in some of them HCV RNA was detected only at birth and not subsequently, and this was interpreted as possible clearance of infection, a false-positive finding or maternal contamination. In other investigations, infected children were PCR negative at birth and became positive only a few weeks later, suggesting peripartum transmission (Tovo et al., 1997; Mazza et al., 1998; Papaevangelou et al., 1998).

Obstetric factors and transmission

Because there is circumstantial evidence suggesting that peripartum transmission can occur, it may be expected that the circumstances of labour and delivery would have an impact on transmission. Because elective caesarean section involves less microtransfusions, it can have a protective effect against transmission of blood-borne viruses such as HCV. HCV has also been detected in the cervicovaginal secretions of infected mothers (Kurauchi et al., 1993). Whether direct contact in the birth canal and/or ascending route transmission of HCV can also occur during vaginal delivery or emergency caesarean section is not known. Existing studies have lacked power to investigate the relation between mode of delivery and vertical HCV transmission, and are unable to distinguish between elective and emergent caesarean sections. In four studies (Paccagnini et al., 1995; Chang, 1996; Tovo et al., 1997; Granovsky et al., 1998), lower transmission rates were observed in case of caesarean versus vaginal delivery, although this did not reach statistical significance. It is interesting to note that these studies were all composed of a majority of HIV- co-infected women, and that the trend towards lower transmission with caesarean section was observed only in the co-infected subgroups (Zanetti et al., 1998). In the largest studies, no difference in transmission was observed according to mode of delivery (Thomas, 1998; Resti, 1998; Papaevangelou, 1998; La Torre, 1998; Zanetti, 1998).

The only other obstetrical factor investigated is duration of rupture of membranes. It was significantly longer among infected than uninfected children in one

Table 10.6. The presence of HCV RNA in breastmilk

Reference	Number of women	Number of RNA +milk/colostrum
Aizaki et al., 1996	5	1
Croxson et al., 1997	30	5
Garland et al., 1998	12	0
Gish et al., 1996	1	0
Grayson et al., 1995	17	0
Gurakan et al., 1994	1	1
Kage et al., 1997	11	0
Kumar & Shahul, 1998	65	65[a]
Kurauchi et al., 1993	12	0
Lin et al., 1995	15	6
Ogasawara et al., 1993	10	0
Polywka et al., 1997	34	0
Spencer et al., 1997	38	0
Straus et al., 1993	2	0
Uehara et al., 1993	7	2
Zimmerman et al., 1995	10	2

[a] Colostrum supernatant and precipitate.

study (Spencer et al., 1997). In the WITS cohort, which showed a relation between membrane rupture and vertical transmission of HIV, no relation was found between membrane rupture and transmission of HCV (Thomas et al., 1998).

Effect of breastfeeding on HCV transmission

Excretion of HCV in breast milk has been described, but the prevalence, variability over time and correlates of excretion have not been evaluated. No case of excretion in milk has been reported in women who were HCV antibody positive, but RNA negative. In the studies which tested colostrum and/or breast milk for HCV RNA, the proportion of samples with detectable virus varied widely (Table 10.6). However, each of these studies comprised small numbers of mother–infant pairs, and had many methodological differences, such as number of samples, time of sampling, and type of sample (colostrum or milk, homogenate, supernatant or pellet).

No study has observed a significantly increased rate of transmission to breastfed infants (Table 10.6 and (Polywka et al., 1997; Spencer et al., 1997)), but the statistical power of these observational studies was insufficient to rule out transmission through breastfeeding. Very few women co-infected with HIV breastfed their child because of the known risk of HIV transmission; therefore the relation between breastfeeding and transmission of HCV can be evaluated only among women who were not co-infected. This further decreased the number of infected children evaluated. In addition, many infants were breastfed for short periods. Ohto et al. found that infected infants were breastfed for longer than non-infected infants (6.6 ± 3.6 months vs. 2.0 ± 2.9 months), but this difference did not reach statistical significance, and there was no difference in the transmission rate itself according to feeding practice (Ohto et al., 1994).

A relatively unequivocal case of late postnatal transmission was reported in a Japanese study (Uehara et al., 1993), in an infant who was HCV RNA negative at birth and at 6 months, but had a positive result at 10 months. This child had been continuously breastfed, and HIV RNA was detected in the mother's milk. In another study (Kumar & Shahul, 1998), the authors suspected breastfeeding as the cause of three cases of transmission. The three infants were reported to have become both clinically ill and HCV RNA positive for the first time by 5–6 months of age. All three of these infants' mothers had developed clinical symptoms in the 3 months following delivery, and showed an increase in HCV RNA of over three log copies/ml both in blood and milk. In the same study, another 62 infants who were breastfed for a mean duration of 8 months, including two whose mothers also developed clinical symptoms in the postpartum period, were not infected, despite detection of HCV RNA in the colostrum of all their mothers. Similarly, in the study by Lin et al. (1995), four infants whose mothers had HCV RNA detected in colostral supernatants (10^2 to 10^4 copies/ml) were breastfed for a mean duration of 2 months and were not infected.

Two additional large retrospective studies (Meisel et al., 1995; Power et al., 1995) offer further evidence that postnatal mother-to-child transmission is rare. These studies of children born to women infected via contaminated anti-D immunoglobulin were excluded from the above analyses due to lack of prospective follow-up and uncertainty about maternal HCV serostatus before delivery. None the less, many of the children were thought to have been breastfed during the period of primary infection in the mothers, yet few were infected at any point in time. The most recent consensus (Consensus Panel, 1999) is not to discourage HCV-infected women from breastfeeding.

Natural history of HCV infection in children

The natural history of HCV infection in children is ill defined, and there are only anecdotal reports in vertically infected children (Tovo & Newell, 1999). Data available seem to indicate a persistence rate comparable to that of adults, in the order of 60–80%. These figures are likely to be an underestimate, because the majority of studies considered disappearance of circulating HCV RNA and normalization of ALT levels as evidence of resolved infection. However, repeatedly negative PCRs for HCV RNA in serum and normal ALT levels do not necessarily implicate clearance of infection, because the virus may persist in the liver or peripheral blood mononuclear cells of subjects with undetectable viraemia (Tovo & Newell, 1999). Of 33 children infected by transfusion who were followed for 3 years, spontaneous biochemical remission and disappearance of HCV RNA lasting for more than 1 year occurred in 4 (8.3%) cases, in one of whom HCV RNA was still detectable in the liver and eventually reappeared in the serum.

Information regarding the histologic features of chronic hepatitis C (CHC) in children is scarce. The histological characteristics of adult CHC, such as lymphoid aggregate, bile duct epithelial damage, and steatosis have also been reported in children. However, there have been few long-term prospective follow-up studies, and most of the data come from infants presenting with clinical signs of hepatitis. Furthermore, most of the infants followed up were infected postnatally through contaminated blood products, and there is little long-term follow-up of vertically infected children. The available data suggest that disease progression is slower in children, with appearance of symptoms and signs of CHC in young adulthood only.

In a study of 109 Japanese children, most had normal liver biopsies or minimal fibrosis, and none had progressed to full-blown cirrhosis during a follow-up of 4–14 years (Tovo & Newell, 1999). Among 80 European children who underwent liver biopsy, only one child had cirrhosis and all the others had normal biopsies or mild to moderate fibrosis. In this study, the presence of fibrosis was associated with duration of disease. Signs of fibrosis were more frequently found in a series of 40 North American children, 78% of whom had signs of portal fibrosis, including bridging fibrosis with architectural distortion (22%) and cirrhosis (8%); the necroinflammatory activity was generally mild, even in children with advanced stage of fibrosis. Comparing 24 paediatric and 32 adult patients with a similar duration of CHC (mean 11.4 and 11.9 years, respectively), the mildest forms of liver damage were significantly more frequent in the former. ALT levels and viral load were also lower in children.

Limited information is available on histological pictures of vertically infected children. A case of fulminant hepatitis leading to death at 5 months was reported in a perinatally infected child (Kong & Chung, 1994). Most studies suggest mild or moderate liver insult, with higher degree of abnormalities being detected in older patients (Tovo & Newell, 1999). It is generally assumed that liver injury is not primarily due to the direct cytopathic effect of HCV, but rather to the host immune response against the virus. The slower disease course in children could be accounted for by the hyporeactivity of the immune system in the first years of life.

Children with chronic liver disease are exposed to a risk of hepatocellular carcinoma, however they may be expected not to develop these disorders until adolescence and young adulthood. An increased risk, as described in adults, of developing B-cell non-Hodgkin's lymphoma is an additional cause for concern. Because tissue autoantibodies have been found in up to two-thirds of HCV infected children, it is also likely that children with chronic hepatitis C may eventually develop, after a long latency period, autoimmune manifestations which are seen in infected adults.

The experience with IFN treatment in children is limited and based on uncontrolled trials only. The most recent studies have shown sustained responses in about one third of children one year after treatment (Tovo & Newell, 1999), with an incidence of side effects similar to that reported in adults. However, the objective of therapy is to avoid relapses in the long term. This is particularly true for children. Combined therapy with IFN and oral ribavirin holds considerable promise, but no data are available as yet in children.

Conclusions

After adopting standardized diagnostic criteria, originally widely divergent estimates of the rate of vertical transmission of HCV have narrowed down to the order of 5% in most unselected HIV negative pregnant populations. Transmission was more than twofold more frequent from HIV co-infected mothers, and was largely restricted to women with demonstrable HCV viraemia during pregnancy or delivery. Findings from a limited number of studies suggest that transmission risk increases with increasing maternal viral load, but fail to identify a threshold below which transmission never occurs. There is no definitive evidence to prove the existence of other potential risk factors for HCV transmission, such as viral genotype, mode of acquisition of infection by the mother, degree of liver disease or mode of delivery. There is at present no convincing evidence that breastfeeding increases the risk of mother-to-child transmission.

Concern about the public health importance of HCV infection has led to discussion of antenatal screening for HCV infection. Much information is now available for decision-makers: the prevalence of HCV infection among pregnant women, the risk of vertical transmission of HCV, the natural history of HCV infection in vertically infected infants, and the effectiveness of drugs used to treat established infections in women and children. One rationale for offering HCV testing to pregnant women is to offer them an opportunity to seek follow-up and care for themselves. However, pregnancy is not necessarily the most appropriate time to make this diagnosis. In Italy, where the prevalence of HCV infection in pregnancy is about 1%, HCV testing is offered, free of charge, to all pregnant women. In France and in the UK, on the other hand, with similarly high prevalences, antenatal testing for HCV is not routine, nor has it been recommended by the

American Academy of Pediatrics. On the other hand, selective screening in pregnancy based on perceived high-risk groups alone fails to detect many infected women, because a substantial proportion have no risk factors indicating HCV exposure.

As long as no intervention has been proven effective to reduce the risk of mother-to-child transmission, the case for universal antenatal testing will remain open for debate. As mentioned above, neither caesarean section nor formula feeding can be recommended at present, and there has been no study of prophylactic therapy during pregnancy. Alpha interferon could potentially be considered in order to decrease maternal viral load. Although it has been shown not to cross the human placenta, the high incidence of side effects is likely to limit its tolerance in pregnant women. The reproductive toxicity profile of ribavirin precludes its use in pregnancy. Clinical studies have been advocated using hyperimmune anti-HCV immunoglobulins, by analogy with the prevention of hepatitis B transmission. Priority must be given in the next years towards research for the prevention of mother-to-child HCV transmission.

HCV infection also raises a number of safety issues in the perinatal setting. For instance, although transmission through breastfeeding has not been documented, the possible excretion of HCV in milk has led a number of milk banks to require antibody testing of donors. When assisted reproductive technology is required for an HCV-infected woman, the risk of nosocomial infection must be considered. HCV screening is recommended and IVF should be performed only if the laboratory is properly equipped for virological security.

Knowledge of their HCV status may be useful to women who are planning a pregnancy. If the presence of HCV antibodies is confirmed, testing for liver enzymes and HCV RNA should be performed first. If HCV RNA is not detected, the risk of transmission to the child is negligible. If HCV RNA is detected, risk factors for transmission can be estimated by HIV testing and a quantitative HCV RNA assay. Women infected with HCV should be provided with specialized follow-up and care, including counselling to avoid hepatotoxic substances such as alcohol and certain medications, with monitoring of liver enzymes and liver biopsy when indicated. The benefit of interferon alpha or interferon and ribavirine therapy has been demonstrated only for people with high Knodell scores on biopsy. It is likely that HCV RNA positive women should benefit from combination therapy before starting pregnancy, in order to reduce viral load. However, reproduction is discouraged for both men and women within 6 months of completion of ribavirin therapy, because of its potential toxicity to germ cells.

Other hepatitis viruses

Hepatitis A and hepatitis E

Hepatitis A and hepatitis E, both of which are transmitted faeco-orally, may be transmitted vertically, but they are mostly of concern because of the risk of fulminant hepatitis, which may be increased among pregnant women in developing countries. Hepatitis A virus has rarely been implicated in congenital infections (Leikin et al., 1996). An isolated case of congenital infection was reported following maternal hepatitis A at 13 weeks' gestation (McDuffie & Bader, 1999). Ultrasonographic examinations revealed fetal ascites (20 weeks) and meconium peritonitis (33 weeks), and a perforated distal ileum was diagnosed after birth. Elevated levels of hepatitis A immunoglobulin G persisted in the infant 6 months after delivery.

Hepatitis E (HEV) is a small RNA virus. Like hepatitis A, it is transmitted oro-faecally, is endemic in parts of all developing countries, and causes acute viral hepatitis. The course of the disease is usually benign with production of protective antibodies, and little risk of chronic infection and cirrhosis. However, in pregnant women, HEV is associated with a high rate of fulminant hepatitis (Hamid et al., 1996; Hussaini et al., 1997), which is often fatal in developing countries. Immune serum globulins have not been found to be effective for prevention (Arankalle et al., 1998), but there is promise for a vaccine in the near future. At present, only a clean water supply will reduce the number of cases in areas where the virus is endemic. Vertical transmission of HEV has been observed, but is thought to be unusual. In a study from India (Khuroo et al., 1995), six of eight babies born to mothers infected with hepatitis E during the third trimester had evidence of hepatitis E infection, and two of them died within 24 hours. However, the incidence of vertical transmission, and the clinical course of congenital HEV infection remain to be determined.

Hepatitis D

The hepatitis D (HDV) or delta virus is a small RNA virus. Because it uses the envelope of HBV, infection with HDV occurs only in subjects infected with HBV. It is estimated that 5–20% of chronic HBs antigen positive subjects are co-infected with HDV. A few cases of mother-to-child tranmission of HDV have been reported (Ramia & Bahakim, 1988; Zanetti et al., 1982; Huang et al., 1999). Hepatitis B immunoblogulin and vaccination of all neonates born to HBs antigen-positive mothers appear to also prevent transmission of HDV.

Hepatitis G

Hepatitis G virus (HGV), also named GB virus type C (GBV-C), was identified in 1995. Although its epidemiology ressembles non-A non-B hepatitis, available data indicate that it does not lead to either acute or chronic liver disease. The presence of HGV RNA is about 1–2% in blood donors in the USA and Europe, and is higher in populations at risk for blood-borne viruses (Lefrere et al., 1999). Presence of HGV RNA denotes carriage of the virus, and presence of anti-E2 antibodies denotes recovery. In immunocompetent individuals, the prevalence of anti-E2 antibody is about twice that of HGV RNA, which suggests the frequency of recovery from HGV infection (Lefrere et al., 1999).

Mother-to-child transmission of HGV has been documented by genetic homology between the virus present in the mother and the child (Fischler et al., 1997). It occurs frequently, in the order of one-third to two-thirds (Fischler et al., 1997; Inaba 1997; De Martino 1998; Lin et al., 1998; Zanetti et al., 1998; Menendez et al., 1999). It is thought that most cases of transmission occur perinatally, however postnatal horizontal transmission may account for some cases of HGV in children born to HGV RNA-positive mothers (Menendez et al., 1999). The determinants of mother-to-child transmission have not yet been investigated in large prospective cohorts. In a study from Taiwan (Lin et al., 1998), high maternal viraemia was associated with frequent transmission. In this study, no child born by elective caesarean section was infected, but the size of the study (25 infants followed) was not large enough to offer any definitive conclusion. Several studies have shown that infected children may either have a positive or an initially negative HGV RNA at birth, suggesting that both in utero and intrapartum transmission can occur.

Whether or not congenital HGV infection may have consequences is unknown at present, as there is no long-term follow-up available. In adults, there is no evidence for an association between HGV and impaired liver function. This has led some authors (Lefrere et al., 1999) to suggest that the virus should be renamed, as it does not cause liver damage. At present, there has been no report of liver damage in any child infected with HGV.

REFERENCES

HBV

Advisory Committee Immunization Practices. (1991). Hepatitis B virus, a comprehensive strategy for eliminating transmission in the United States through universal childhood vaccination. *M.M.W.R.*, **40**, 1–19.

Advisory Committee on Dangerous Pathogens. (1995). *Protection Against Blood-borne Infections in the Workplace*, pp. ii–53. London: HMSO.

Beasley, R. P. (1982). Hepatitis B virus as the etiologic agent in hepatocellular carcinoma. Epidemiologic considerations. *Hepatology*, **2**, 21S–6S.

Beasley, R. P., Stevens, C. E., Shiao, I-S. & Meng, H-C. (1975). Evidence against breast-feeding as a mechanism for vertical transmission of hepatitis B. *Lancet*, **ii**, 740–1.

Beasley, R. P., Hwang, L. Y., Lin, C. C., Stevens, C.E., Wang, K. Y., Sun, T. S., Hsieh, F. J. & Szmuness, W. (1981). Hepatitis B immunoglobulin (HBIG) efficacy in the interruption of perinatal transmission of hepatitis B virus carrier state. *Lancet*, **ii**, 388–93.

Blumberg, B. S. (1995). Complex interactions of hepatitis B virus with its host and environment. *J. R. Coll. Physicians*, **29**, 31–40.

Brossard, Y. (1992). Transmission périnatale de l'hépatite B, prévention. In *Virus et Grossesses*, ed. M. Azoulay & J. F. Delfraissy, pp. 245–77. Paris: INSERM.

Burk, R. D., Hwang, L., Ho, G. Y. F., Shafritz, D. A. & Beasley, R. P. (1994). Outcome of perinatal hepatitis B virus exposure is dependent on maternal virus load. *J. Infect. Dis.*, **170**, 1418–23.

Chang, M. H., Chen, C. J., Lai, M. S., Hsu, H. M., Wu, T-C., Kong, M-S., Shau, W. Y., Chen, D. S. & Taiwan Childhood Hepatoma Study Group. (1997). Universal hepatitis B vaccination in Taiwan and the incidence of hepatocellular carcinoma in children. *N. Engl. J. Med.*, **336**, 1855–89.

Chang, M. H., Hsu, H. Y., Huang, L. M., Lee, P. I., Lin, H.H. & Lee, C. Y. (1996). The role of transplacental hepatatis B core antibody in the mother-to-infant transmission of hepatitis B virus. *J. Hepatol.*, **24**, 674–9.

Chang, M. H., Chen, P. J., Chen, Y.J. Lai, M. Y, Hsu, H. C., Lian, D. C., Liu, Y. G. & Chen, D. S. (1991). Hepatitis B virus integration in hepatitis B virus-related hepatocellular carcinoma in childhood. *Hepatology*, **13**, 316–20.

Chen, W. H., Yin, C. S., Chang, Y. K., Yan, J. S. & Chu, M. L. (1998). Neonatal gastric aspirates as a predictor of perinatal hepatitis B virus infections. *Int. J. Gynaecol. Obstet.*, **60**, 15–21.

Chong-Jin, O., Wei Ning, C., Shiuan, K. & Gek Keow, L. (1999). Identification of hepatitis B surface antigen variants with alterations outside the 'a' determinant in immunized Singapore infants. *J. Infect. Dis.*, **179**, 259–63.

Davis, G. L., Weber, D. J. & Lemon, S. M. (1989). Horizontal transmission of hepatitis B virus. *Lancet*, **i**, 889–93.

Denis, F., Tabaste, J. L. & Ranger, S. (1994). Prévalence de l'AgHBs chez près de 21500 femmes enceintes. Enquête de douze CHU français. *Pathol. Biol.*, **42**, 533–8.

Dwyer, M. J. & McIntyre, P. G. (1996). Antenatal screening for hepatitis B surface antigen, an appraisal of its value in a low prevalence area. *Epidemiol. Infect.*, **117**, 121–31.

Fortuin, M., Chotard, J., Jack, A. D., Maine, N. P., Mendy, M., Hall, A. J., Inskip, H. M., George, M. O. & Whittle, H. C. (1993). Efficacy of hepatitis B vaccine in the Gambian expanded programme on immunisation. *Lancet*, **341**, 1129–31.

Friedt, M., Gerner, P., Lausch, E., Trubel, H., Zabel, B. & Wirth, S. (1999). Mutations in the basic core promotor and the precore region of hepatitis B virus and their selection in children with fulminant and chronic hepatitis B. *Hepatology*, **29**, 1252–8.

Greenberg, D. P. (1993). Pediatric experience with recombinant hepatitis B vaccines and relevant safety and immunogenicity studies. *Pediatr. Infect. Dis. J.*, **12**, 438–45.

Grob, P. (1998). Hepatitis B, virus, pathogenesis and treatment. *Vaccine*, **16**, S11–S16.

Grosheide, P. M., Quartero, H. W., Schalm, S. W., Heijtink, R. A. & Christiaens, G. C. (1994). Early invasive prenatal diagnosis in HBsAg-positive women. *Prenat. Diagn.*, **14**, 553–8.

Hsu, H. Y., Chang, M. H., Ni, Y. H., Lin, H. H., Wang, S. M. & Chen, D. S. (1997). Surface gene mutants of heptatits B virus in infants who develop acute or chronic infections despite immunoprophylaxis. *Hepatology*, **26**, 786–91.

Ip, H. M. H., Lelie, P. N., Wong, V. C. M., Kuhns, M. C. & Reesink, H. W. (1989). Prevention of hepatitis B virus carrier state in infants according to maternal serum levels of HBV DNA. *Lancet*, **ii**, 406–9.

Iwarson, S. (1989). Post-exposure prophylaxis for hepatitis B, active or passive? *Lancet*, **ii**, 146–8.

Joint Working Party of the Hospital Infection Study Group. (1992). Risks to surgeons and patients from HIV and hepatitis, guidelines on precautions and management of exposure to blood or body fluids. *B.M.J.*, **305**, 1337–43.

Kane, M. A., Clements, J. & Hu, D. (1993). Hepatitis B. In *Disease Control Priorities in Developing Countries. A World Bank Book*, ed. D. T. Jamison, D. T., W. H. Mosley, A. R. Measham & J. Bobadilla, pp. 321–30. New York: Oxford University Press.

Ko, T. M., Tseng, L. H., Chang, M. H., Chen, D. S., Hsieh, F. J., Chuang, S. M. & Lee, T. Y. (1994). Amniocentesis in mothers who are hepatitis B virus carriers does not expose the infant to an increased risk of hepatitis B virus infection. *Arch. Gynecol. Obstet.*, **255**, 25–30.

Krugman, S. (1988). Hepatitis B virus and the neonate. *Ann. NY Acad. Sci.*, **549**, 129–34.

Lazizi, Y., Badur, S., Perk, Y., Ilter, O. & Pillot, J. (1997). Selective unresposiveness to HBsAg vaccine in newborns related with an in utero passage of hepatitis B virus DNA. *Vaccine*, **15**, 1095–100.

Lee, A., Ip, H. & Wong, V. (1978) Mechanisms of maternal fetal transmission of hepatitis B virus. *J. Infect. Dis.*, **138**, 668–71.

Lee, S. D., Lo, K. J., Tsai, Y. T., Wu, J. C., Wu, T. C., Yang, Z. L. & Ng, H. T. (1988). Role of caesarean section in prevention of mother-infant transmission of hepatitis B virus. *Lancet*, **ii**, 833–4.

Lee, P. I., Lee, C. Y., Huang, L. M. & Chang, M. H. (1995). Long-term efficacy of recombinant hepatitis B vaccine and risk of natural infection in infants born of mothers with hepatitis e antigen. *J. Pediatr.*, **126**, 716–21.

Lemon, S. M. & Thomas, D. L. (1997). Vaccines to prevent viral hepatitis. *N. Engl. J. Med.*, **336**, 196–204.

Lin, H. H., Lee, T. H., Chen, D. S., Sung, J. L., Ohto, H., Etoh, T., Kawana, T. & Mizuno, M. (1987). Transplacental leakage of HBeAg-positive maternal blood as the most likely route in causing intrauterine infection with hepatitis B virus. *J. Pediatr.*, **111**, 877–81.

Lin, H. H., Kao, J. H., Hsu, H. Y., Mizokami, M., Hirano, K. & Chen, D. S. (1996). Least microtransfusion from mother to fetus in elective cesarean delivery. *Obstet. Gynecol.*, **87**, 244–8.

McMahon, B. J., Alward, W. L. M., Hall, D. B., Heyward, W. L., Bender, T. R., Francis, D. P. & Maynard, J. E. (1985). Acute hepatitis B virus infection, relation of age to the clinical expression of disease and subsequent development of the carrier state. *J. Infect. Dis.*, **151**, 599–603.

McMenamin, J. (1996). Hepatitis B in the UK, who is at risk, who succumbs? Role of screening. In *Prevention of Hepatitis B., in the Newborn, Children and Adolescents*, ed. A. Zuckerman, pp. 1–7, London: Royal College of Physicians.

Matsumoto, T., Nakata, K., Hamasaki, K., Daikokuku, M., Nakao, K., Yamashita, Y., Shirahama, S. & Kato, Y. (1997). Efficacy of immunization of high-risk infants against hepatitis B virus evaluated by polymerase chain reaction. *J. Med. Virol.*, **53**, 255–60.

Mortimer P. & Miller E. (1997). Commentary: antenatal screening and targeting should be sufficient in some countries. *B. M. J.*, **314**, 1036–7.

Ngui, S. L., O'Connell, S., Eglin, R. P., Heptonstall, J. & Teo, C. G. (1997). Low detection rate and maternal provenance of hepatitis B virus S., gene mutants in cases of failed postnatal immunoprophylaxis in England and Wales. *J. Infect. Dis.*, **176**, 1360–5.

Ngui, S. L., Andrews, N. J., Underhill, G. S., Heptonstall, J. & Teo, C. G. (1998). Failed postnatal immunoprophylaxis for hepatitis B characteristics of maternal hepatitis B virus as risk factors. *Clin. Infect. Dis.*, **27**, 100–6.

Pierce, R. L., Smith, S., Rowe-West, B. & Sterritt, B. (1999). Hepatitis B maternal screening, infant vaccination, and infant prophylaxis practices in North Carolina. *Arch. Pediatr. Adolesc. Med.*, **153**, 619–23.

Poovorawan, Y., Sanpavat, S., Chumdermpadetsuk, S. & Safary, A. (1997). Long-term hepatitis B vaccine in infants born to hepatitis Be antigen positive mothers. *Arch. Dis. Child.*, **77**, F47–51.

Royal College of Physicians. (1996). *Prevention of Hepatitis B in the Newborn, Children and Adolescents*, ed. A., Zuckerman, pp. 1–113. London: Royal College of Physicians of London.

Salisbury, D. M., & Begg, N. T. (1996). *Immunisation Against Infectious Disease*, pp. 1–290. London: HSMO.

Sangfelt, P., Reichard, O., Lidman, K., von Sydow, M. & Forsgren, M. (1995). Prevention of hepatitis B by immunization of the newborn infant – a long term follow-up study in Stockholm, Sweden. *Scand. J. Infect. Dis.*, **27**, 3–7.

Stevens, C. E., Beasley, R. P., Tsui, J. & Lee, W. L., (1975). Vertical transmission of hepatitis B antigen in Taiwan. *N. Engl. J. Med.*, **292**, 771–4.

Szmuness, W., Much, M. I., Prince, I., Hoofnagle, J. M., Cherubin, C. E., Harley, E. J. & Block, G. H. (1975). On the role of sexual behaviour in the spread of hepatitis B infection. *Ann. Int. Med.*, **83**, 489–95.

Vajro, P., Migliaro, F. & Fontanella, O. G. (1998). Interferon, a meta-analysis of published studies in pediatric chronic hepatitis B. *Acta Gastroenterol. Belg.*, **61**, 219–23.

Whittle, H. C., Maine, N. P., Pilkington, J., Mendy, M., Fortuin, M., Bunn, J., Allison, L., Howard, C. & Hall, A. J. (1995). Long-term efficacy of continuing hepatitis B vaccination in infancy in two Gambian villages. *Lancet*, **345**, 1089–92.

Wong, V. C. W., Ip, H., Reesink, H. W., Lelie, P. N., Reerink-Brongers, E. E., Yeung, C. Y. & Ma, H. K. (1984). Prevention of the HBsAg carrier state in newborn infants of mothers who are chronic carriers of HBsAg and HBeAg by administration of hepatitis B vaccine and hepatitis B immunoglobulin. *Lancet*, **i**, 921–6.

Wright, R. A., (1975). Hepatitis B., and the HBsAg carrier. An outbreak related to sexual contact. *J.A.M.A.*, **232**, 717–21.

Zamir, C., Dagan, R., Zamir, D., Rishpon, S., Fraser, D., Rimon, N. & Ben Porath, E. (1999). Evaluation of screening for hepatitis B surface antigen during pregnancy in a population with a high prevalence of hepatitis B surface antigen-positive/hepatitis Be antigen-negative carriers. *Pediatr. Infect. Dis. J.*, **18**, 262–6.

Zuckerman, A. (1997). Prevention of primary liver cancer by immunisation. *N. Engl. J. Med.*, **336**, 1906–7.

HCV

Aizaki, H., Saito, A., Kuzakawa, I., Ashiwara, Y., Nagamori, S., Toda, G., Suzuki, T., Ishii, K., Matsuura, Y. & Miyamura, T. (1996). Mother-to-child transmission of a hepatitis C virus variant with an insertional mutation in its hypervariable region. *J. Hepatol.*, **25**, 608–13.

Aussel, L., Denis, F., Ranger, S., Martin, Ph., Caillaud, M., Alain, J., Baudet, J. & Tabaste, J. L. (1991). Prevalence of antibodies to the hepatitis C virus in pregnant foreign residents in France. *Path. Biol. Paris*, **39**, 991–6.

Chang, M. H., (1996). Mother-to-infant transmission of hepatitis C virus. *Clin. Invest. Med.*, **19**, 368–72.

Choo, Q-L., Kuo, G., Weiner, A. J., Overby, L. R., Bradley, D. W. & Houghton, M. (1989). Isolation of a cDNA clone derived from a blood-borne non-A non-B viral hepatitis genome. *Science*, **244**, 359–62.

Consensus Panel. (1999). EASL International Consensus Conference on Hepatitis C – Consensus statement. *J. Hepatol.*, **30**, 956–61.

Croxson, M., Couper, A., Voss, L., Groves, D. & Gunn, T. (1997), Vertical transmission of hepatitis C virus in New Zealand. *N. Z. Med. J.*, **110**, 165–7.

DeVoid, D. E., Minkoff, H., Goedert, J., Biswas, R. & Di Bisceglie, A. M. (1993). Perinatal transmission of hepatitis C [Abstract]. *Hepatology*, **18**, 229A.

Di Bisceglie, A. M., Goodman, Z. D., Ishak, K. G., Hoofnagle, J. H., Melpolder, J. J. & Alter, H. J. (1991). Long-term clinical and histopathological follow-up of chronic posttransfusion hepatitis. *Hepatology*, **14**, 969–74.

El Gohary, A., Hassan, A., Nooman, Z., Lavanchy, D., Mayerat, C., El Ayat, A., Fawaz, N., Gobran, F, Ahmed, M., Kawano, F. et al. (1995). High prevalence of hepatitis C virus among urban and rural population groups in Egypt. *Acta Tropica*, **59**, 155–61.

Fischler, B., Lindh, G., Lindgren, S., Forsgren, M., Von Sydow, M., Sangfelt, P., Alaeus, A., Harland, L., Enockson, E. & Nemeth, A. (1996) Vertical transmission of hepatitis C virus infection. *Scand. J. Infect. Dis.*, **28**, 353–6.

Gamboa, R., Castro, R. G., Flores, R. G., Maciel, C. A. S. & Leyva, G. B. (1994). Seroprevalence of antibodies against hepatitis C virus among the obstetrical population at the new Hospital Civil de Guadalajara (in Spanish). *Gin. Obstet. Mex.*, **62**, 399–402.

Garland, S. M., Tabrizi, S., Robinson, P., Hughes, C., Markman, L., Devenish, W. & Kliman, L. (1998). Hepatitis C – role of perinatal transmission. *Aust. N. Z. J. Obstet. Gynaecol.*, **38**, 424–7.

Giacchino, R., Tasso, L., Timitilli, A., Cristina, E., Picciotto, A., Sinelli, N., Gotta, C., Giambartolomei, G. & Moscatelli, P. (1996). Vertical transmission of HCV infection from HIV seronegative mothers can occur. Usefulness of viremia detection. [Abstract]. *IX Triennial International Symposium on Viral Hepatitis and Liver Disease (Rome)*, 168.

Gish, R. G., Cox, K. L., Mizokami M., Ohno, T. & Lau, J. Y. N. (1996). Vertical transmisson of hepatitis C. *J. Pediatr. Gastroenterol. Nutr.*, **22**, 118–9.

Granovsky, M. O., Minkoff, H. L., Tess, B. H., Waters, D., Hatzakis, A., DeVoid, D. E., Landesman, S. H., Rubinstein, A., Di Bisceglie, A. M. & Goedert, J. J. (1998). Hepatitis C virus infection in the mothers and infants cohort study. *Pediatrics*, **102**, 355–9.

Grayson, M. L., Branitt, K. M., Bowden, D. S. & Turnidge, J. D. (1995). Breastfeeding and the risk of vertical transmission of hepatitis C virus. *Med. J. Aust.*, **163**, 107.

Gurakan, B., Oran, O. & Yigit, S. (1994). Vertical transmission of hepatitis C virus. *N. Engl. J. Med.*, **331**, 399

Inoue, Y., Takeuchi, K., Chou, W-H., Unayama, T., Takahashi, K., Saito, I. & Miyamura, T. (1992). Silent mother-to-child transmission of hepatitis C virus through two generations determined by comparative nucleotide sequence analysis of the viral cDNA. *J. Infect. Dis.*, **166**, 1425–8.

Kage, M., Ogasawara, S., Kosai, K. I., Nakashima, E., Shimamatsu, K., Kimura, A., Fujisawa, T., Matsukuma, Y., Ito, Y., Kondo, S., Kawano, K. & Sata M. (1997). Hepatitis C virus RNA present in saliva but absent in breast milk of the hepatitis C carrier mother. *J. Gastroenterol. Hepatol.*, **12**, 518–21.

Katayama, Y., Tajiri, H., Tada, K., Okada, S., Tong, W. Y., Ishido, S. & Hotta, H. (1998). Follow up study of hypervariable region sequences of the hepatitis C virus (HCV) genome in an infant with delayed anti-HCV antibody response. *Microbiol. Immunol.*, **42**, 75–9.

Kiyosawa, K., Tanaka, E., Sodeyama, T., Yoshizawa, K., Yabu, K., Furuta, K., Imai, H., Nakano, Y, Usuda, S., Uemura, K. et al. (1994). Transmission of hepatitis C in an isolated area in Japan: community-acquired infection. *Gastroenterology*, **106**, 1596–602.

Kong, M-S. & Chung, J-L. (1994). Fatal hepatitis C in an infant born to a hepatitis C positive mother. *J. Pediatr. Gastroenterol. Nutr.*, **19**, 460–3.

Kudo, T., Morishima, T., Shibata, M., Miwata, H., Matsushima, M., & Tsuzuki, K., (1995). Low humoral responses to hepatitis C virus among pediatric renal transplant recipients. *Acta Paediatr.*, **84**, 677–82.

Kudo, T., Yanase, Y., Oshiro, M., Yamamoto, M., Morita, M., Shibata, M. & Morishima, T. (1997). Analysis of mother-to-infant transmission of hepatitis C virus, quasispecies nature and buoyant densities of maternal virus populations. *J. Med. Virol.*, **51**, 225–30.

Kumar, R. M. & Shahul, S. (1998). Role of breastfeeding in transmission of hepatitis C virus to infants of HCV-infected mothers. *J. Hepatol.*, **29**, 191–7.

Kurauchi, O., Furai, T., Itakura, A., Ishiko, H., Sugiyama, M., Ohno, Y., Ando, H., Tanamura, A., Ishida, T., Nawa, A. et al. (1993). Studies on transmission of hepatitis C virus from mother-to-child in the perinatal period. *Arch. Gynecol. Obstet.*, **253**, 121–6.

Lam, J. P., McOmish, F., Burns, S. M., Yap, P. L., Mok, J. Y. & Simmonds, P. (1993). Infrequent vertical transmission of hepatitis C virus. *J. Infect. Dis.*, **167**, 572–6

La Torre, A., Biadaioli, R., Capobianco, T., Colao, M. G., Monti, M., Pulli, F., Visiolo, C. B., Zignego, A-L. & Rubaltelli, F. (1998). Vertical transmission of HCV. *Acta Obstet. Gynecol. Scand.*, **77**, 889–92.

Lin, H-H., Kao J-H., Leu J-H., Young Y-C., Lee T-Y., Chen P-J. & Chen D-S. (1993). Comparison of three different immunoassays and PCR for the detection of hepatitis C virus infection in pregnant women in Taiwan. *Vox Sang*, **65**, 117–21.

Lin, H-H., Kao, J-H., Hsu, H-Y., Ni, Y-H., Yeh, S-H., Hwang, L-H., Chang, M-H., Hwang, P-J., Chen, P-J. & Chen, D-S. (1994). Possible role of high-titer maternal viremia in perinatal transmission of hepatitis C virus. *J. Infect. Dis.*, **169**, 638–41.

Lin, H-H., Kao, J-H., Hsu, H-Y., Ni, Y-H., Chang, M-H., Huang, S-C., Hwang, L-H., Chen, P-J. & Chen, D-S. (1995). Absence of infection in breast-fed infants born to hepatitis C virus-infected mothers. *J. Pediatr.*, **126**, 589–91.

Louis, F. J., Maubert, B., Le Hesran, J-Y., Kemmegne, J., Delaporte, E. & Louis, J-P. (1994). High prevalence of anti-hepatitis C virus antibodies in Cameroon rural forest area. *Trans. R., Soc. Trop. Med. Hyg.*, **88**, 53–4.

Maccabruni, A., Caselli, D., Mondelli, M., Degioanni, M. & Cerino, A. (1993). Vertical transmission of hepatitis C virus and HIV. *AIDS*, **7**, 1024–5.

Maccabruni, A., Bossi, G., Caselli, D., Cividini, A., Silini, E. & Mondelli, M. U. (1995). High efficiency of vertical transmission of hepatitis C virus among babies born to human immunodeficiency virus-negative women. *Pediatr. Infect. Dis. J.*, **14**, 921–2.

Manzini, P. M., Saracco, G., Cerchier, A., Riva, C., Musso, A., Ricotti, E., Palomba, E., Scolfaro, C., Verme, G., Bonino, F. et al. (1995). Human immunodeficiency virus infection as risk factor for mother-to-child hepatitis C virus transmission: persistence of anti-hepatitis C virus in children is associated with mother's anti-hepatitis C virus immunoblotting pattern. *Hepatology*, **21**, 328–32.

Marcellin, P., Bernuau, J., Martinot-Peignoux, M., Larzul, D., Xu, L-Z., Tran, S., Bezeaud, A, Guimont, M-C., Levardon, M., Aumont, P. et al. (1993). Prevalence of hepatitis C virus infection in asymptomatic anti-HIV1 negative pregnant women and their children. *Digest. Dis. Sci.*, **38**, 2151–5.

Matsubara, T., Sumazaki, R. & Takita, H. (1995). Mother-to-infant transmission of hepatitis C virus, a prospective study. *Eur. J. Pediatr.*, **154**, 973–8.

Mazza, C., Ravaggi, A., Rodella, A., Padula, D., Duse, M., Lomini, M., Puoti, M., Rossini, A., Cariani, E. & Study Group for Vertical Transmission (1998). Prospective study of mother-to-infant transmission of hepatitis C virus (HCV) infection. *J. Med. Virol.*, **54**, 12–19.

Meisel, H., Reip, A., Faltus, B., Lu, M., Porst, H., Weise, M., Roggendorf, M. & Kruger D. V. (1995). Transmission of hepatitis C virus to children and husbands by women infected with contaminated anti-D immunoglobulin. *Lancet*, **345,** 1209–11.

Moriya, T., Ohno, N., Mohri, H., Katayama, K., Sasaki, F. & Yoshizawa, H. (1995). Study of perinatal HCV transmission – expression and persistence of HCV RNA in infants' peripheral blood. [Abstract]. *Int. Hepatol. Commun.*, **3**(Suppl.), S54.

Nagata I., Shiraki, K., Tanimoto, K., Harada, Y., Tanaka, Y. & Okada, T. (1992). Mother-to-infant transmisson of hepatitis C virus. *J. Pediatr.*, **120**, 432–4.

Nagata, I., Iizuka, T., Harada, Y., Okada, T., Matsuda, R., Tanaka, Y., Tanimoto, K. & Shiraki, K. (1994). Prospective study of mother-to-infant transmission of hepatitis C virus. In *Viral Hepatitis and Liver Disease, Proceedings of the International Symposium on Viral Hepatitis and Liver Disease, Tokyo, Japan*, ed. K. Nishioka, H. Suzuki, S. Mishiro & T. Oda, pp. 468–70. Baltimore: Williams and Wilkins.

Ni, Y-H., Chang, M. H., Chen, P-J., Lin, H. H. & Hsu, H-Y. (1997). Evolution of hepatitis C virus quasispecies in mothers and infants infected through mother-to-infant transmission. *J. Hepatol.*, **26**, 967–74.

Nigro, G., D'Orio, F., Catania, S., Badolato, M. C., Livadiotti, S., Bernardi, S. & D'Argenio, P. (1997). Mother to infant transmission of coinfection by human immunodeficiency virus and hepatitis C virus, prevalence and clinical manifestations. *Arch. Virol.*, **142**, 453–7.

Novati, R., Thiers, V., D'Arminio Monforte, A., Maisonneuve, P., Principi, N., Conti, M., Larrarin, A. & Brechot, C. (1992). Mother-to-child transmission of hepatitis C virus detected by nested polymerase chain reaction. *J. Infect. Dis.*, **165**, 720–3.

Ogawawara, S., Kage, M., Kosai, K., Shimamatsu, K. & Kojiro, M. (1993). Hepatitis C virus RNA in saliva and breastmilk of hepatitis C carrier mothers. *Lancet*, **341**, 561.

Ohto, H., Okamoto, H. & Mishiro, S. (1994). Vertical transmission of hepatitis C virus. *N. Engl. J. Med.*, **331**, 400

Paccagnini, S., Principi N., Massironi E., Tanzi E., Romano L., Muggliasca, M. L., Ragni, M. C. & Salvaggio, L. (1995). Perinatal transmission and manifestation of hepatitis C virus infection in a high risk population. *Pediatr. Infect. Dis. J.*, **14**, 195–9.

Papaevangelou, V., Pollack, H., Rochford, G., Kokka, R., Hou, Z., Chernoff, D., Hanna, B., Krasinski, K. & Borkowsky, W. (1998). Increased transmission of vertical hepatitis C virus (HCV) infection to human immunodeficiency virus (HIV)-infected infants of HIV- and HCV-coinfected women. *J. Infect. Dis.*, **178**, 1047–52.

Pipan, C., Amici, S., Astori, G., Ceci, G. P. & Botta, G. A. (1996). Vertical transmission of hepatitis C virus in low-risk pregnant women. *Eur. J. Clin. Microbiol. Infect. Dis.*, **15**, 116–20.

Polywka, S., Feucht, H. & Laufs, R. (1997). Hepatitis C virus infection in pregnancy and the risk of mother-to-child transmission. *Eur. J. Clin. Microbiol. Infect. Dis.*, **16**, 121–4.

Power, J. P., Davidson, F., O'Riordan, J., Simmonds, P., Yap, P. L. & Lawlor, E. (1995). Hepatitis C infection from anti-D immunoglobulin. *Lancet*, **346**, 372–3.

Reinus, J. F., Leiken, E. L., Alter, H. J., Cheng, L., Shindo, M., Jett, B., Piazza, S. & Shih, J.W-K. (1992). Failure to detect vertical transmission of hepatitis C virus. *Ann. Intern. Med.*, **117**, 881–6.

Resnick, R. H. & Koff, R. (1993). Hepatitis C-related hepatocellular carcinoma. Prevalence and significance. *Arch. Intern. Med.*, **153**, 1672–7.

Resti, M., Azzari, C., Mannelli, F., Moriondo, M., Novembre, E., de Martino, M., Vierucci, A. & Tuscany Study Group on Hepatitis C Virus Infection in Children (1998). Mother to child transmission of hepatitis C virus, prospective study of risk factors and timing of infection in children born to women seronegative for HIV-1. *B. M. J.*, **317**, 437–41.

Roudot-Thoraval, F., Pawlotsky, J-M., Deforges, L., Girollet, P-P. & Dhumeaux, D. (1993). Anti-HCV seroprevalence in pregnant women in France. *Gut*, **34**(2 Suppl), S55–6.

Silverman, N. S., Jenkin, B. K., Wu, C., McGillen, P. & Knee, G. (1993). Hepatitis C virus in pregnancy. Seroprevalence and risk factors for infection. *Am. J. Obstet. Gynecol.*, 169, 583–7.

Spencer, J. D., Latt, N., Beeby, P. J., Collins, E., Saunders, J. B., McCaughan, G. W. & Cossart Y. E. (1997). Transmission of hepatitis C virus to infants of human immunodeficiency virus-negative intravenous drug-using mothers, rate of infection and assessment of risk factors for transmission. *J. Viral Hepat.*, **4**, 395–409.

Strauss, R. M., Nolte, F. S. & Boyer, T. D. (1993). Is human breast milk a source of hepatitis C virus? *Hepatology*, **18**, 802A.

Tahara, T., Toyoda, S., Mukaide, M., Hikiji, K., Ohba, K-I. & Mizokami, M. (1996). Vertical transmission of hepatitis C through three generations. *Lancet*, **347**, 409.

Tanzi, M. L., Verrotti, C., Volpicelli, A., Cavatorta, E., Bracchi, U., Tagger, A., Ribero, M., Benaglia, G., Grignaffini, A., Tagliavini, M. et al. (1995). Risk factors and prevalence of HCV antibodies in pregnant women and in their babies. *Int. J. Gynaecol. Obstet.*, **2**, 66–72.

Thomas, D. L., Villano, S. A., Riester, K., Hershow, R., Mofenson, L., Landesman, S., Hollinger, F. B., Davenny, K., Riley, L., Diaz, C. et al. (1998). Perinatal transmission of hepatitis C virus from human immunodeficiency virus type 1-infected mothers. *J. Infect. Dis.*, **177**, 1480–8.

Thomas, S. L., Newell, M-L., Peckham, C., Ades, A. E. & Hall, A. J. (1997). Use of polymerase chain reaction and antibody tests in the diagnosis of vertically transmitted hepatitis C infection. *Eur. J. Clin. Microbiol. Infect. Dis.*, **16**, 711–19.

Thomas, S. L., Newell, M-L., Peckham, C. S., Ades, A. E. & Hall, A. J. (1998). A review of hepatitis C virus (HCV) vertical transmission, risks of transmission to infants born to mothers with and without HCV viraemia or human immunodeficiency virus infection. *Int. J. Epidemiol.*, **27**, 108–17.

Tovo, P-A. & Newell, M-L. (1999). Hepatitis C in children. *Curr. Opin. Infect. Dis.*, **12**, 245–50.

Tovo, P-A., Palomba, E., Ferraris, G., Principi, N., Ruga, E., Dallacasa, P., Maccabruni, A. & Italian Study Group for HCV Infection in Children (1997). Increased risk of maternal–infant hepatitis C virus transmission for women coinfected with human immunodeficiency virus type 1. *Clin. Infect. Dis.*, **25**, 1121–4.

Uehara, S., Abe, Y., Saito, T., Yoshida, Y., Wagatsuma, S., Okamura, K., Yajima, A. & Mandai, M. (1993). The incidence of vertical transmission of hepatitis C virus. *Tohoku J. Exp. Med.*, **171**, 195–202.

Wahl, M., Hermonsson, S., Leman, J., Lindholm, A., Wejstal, R. & Norkrans, G. (1994). Prevalence of antibodies against hepatitis B and C virus among pregnant women and female blood donors in Sweden. *Serodiagn. Immunother. Infect. Dis.*, **6**, 127–9.

Weiner, A. J., Thaler, M. M., Crawford, K., Ching, K., Kansopon, J., Chein, D. Y., Hall, J.E., Hu, F. & Houghton, M. (1993). A unique, predominant hepatitis C virus variant found in an infant born to a mother with multiple variants. *J. Virol.*, **67**, 4365–8.

Wejstal, R., Hermodsson, S., Iwarson, S. & Norkrans, G. (1990). Mother to infant transmission of hepatitis C virus infection. *J. Med. Virol.*, **30**, 178–80.

Xiong, SK., Okajima, Y., Ishikawa, K., Watanabe, H. & Inaba, N. (1998). Vertical transmission of hepatitis C virus, risk factors and infantile prognosis. *J. Obstet. Gynaecol. Res.*, **24**, 57–61.

Zanetti, A. R., Tanzi, E., Principi, N., Pizzocolo, G., Caccamo, M. L., D'Amico, E., Cambie, G., Vecchi, L. & the Lombardy Study Group on Vertical HCV Transmission (1995). Mother-to-infant transmission of hepatitis C virus. *Lancet*, **345**, 289–91.

Zanetti, A. R., Tanzi, E., Romano, L., Zuin, G., Minola, E., Vecchi, L. & Principi, N. (1998). A prospective study on mother-to-infant transmission of hepatitis C virus. *Intervirology*, **41**, 208–12.

Zimmerman, E., Perucchini, D., Fauchere, J. C., Jolier-Jemelka, H. Geyer, M., Huch, R. & Huch, A. (1995). Hepatitis C virus in breast milk. *Lancet*, **345**, 928.

Zuccotti, G. V., Ribero, M. L., Giovannini, M., Fasola, M., Riva, E., Portera, G., Biasucci, G., Decarlis, S., Profeta, M. L. & Tagger, A. (1995). Effect of hepatitis C genotype on mother-to-infant transmission of virus. *J., Pediatr*, **127**, 278–80.

Zuckerman, M. A., Aitken, C., Whitby, K., Deaville, R., Sanders, E., Glynn, M. J., Swain, C. P. & Garson, J. A. (1997). Acute hepatitis C viral infection during pregnancy, failure of mother-to-infant transmission. *J. Med. Virol.*, **52**, 161–3.

Other hepatitis viruses

Arankalle, V. A., Chadha, M. S., Dama, B. M., Tsarev, S. A., Purcell, R. H. & Banerjee, K. (1998). Role of immune serum globulins in pregnant women during an epidemic of hepatitis E. *J. Viral Hepat.*, **5**, 199–204

De Martino, M. Azari, C., Resti, M. Moriondo, M., Rossi, M. E., Galli, L. & Vierucci, A. (1998). Hepatitis G virus infection in human immunodeficiency virus type 1 – infected mothers and their children. *J. Infect. Dis.*, **178**, 862–5.

Fischler, B., Lara, C., Chen, M., Sönnerborg, A., Nemeth, A. & Sällberg. M. (1997). Genetic evidence for mother-to-infant transmission of hepatitis G virus. *J. Infect. Dis.*, **176**, 281–5.

Hamid, S. S., Jafri, S., Khan, H., Shah, H., Abbas, Z. & Fields, H. (1996). Fulminant hepatic failure in pregnant women, acute fatty liver or acute viral hepatitis? *J. Hepatol.*, **25**, 20–7.

Huang, Y. H., Wu, J. C., Lu, S. N., Chiang, T. Y., Chang, F. Y. & Lee, S. D. (1999). Phylogenetic analysis to document a common source of hepatitis D virus infection in a mother and her child. *Chung Hua I. Hsueh Tsa Chih (Taipei)*, **62**, 28–32.

Hussaini, S. H., Skidmore, S. J., Richardson, P., Sherratt, L. M., Cooper, B. T. & O'Grady, J. G. (1997). Severe hepatitis E infection during pregnancy. *J. Viral Hepat*, **4**, 51–4.

Inaba, N., Okajima, Y., Kang, X. S., Ishikawa, K. & Fukasawa, I. (1997). Maternal–infant transmission of hepatitis G virus. *Am. J. Obstet. Gynecol.*, **177**, 1537–8.

Khuroo, M. S., Kamili, S. & Jameel, S. (1995). Vertical transmission of hepatitis E virus. *Lancet*, **345**, 1025–6.

Lefrere, J. J., Roudot-Thoraval, F., Morand-Joubert, L., Brossard, Y., Parnet-Mathieu, F., Mariotti, M., Agis, F., Rouet, G., Lerable, J., Lefevre, G., Girot, R. & Loiseau, P. (1999). Prevalence of GB., virus type C/hepatitis G virus RNA., and of anti-E2 in individuals at high or low risk for blood-borne or sexually transmitted viruses, evidence of sexual and parenteral transmission. *Transfusion*, **39**, 83–94.

Leikin, E., Lysikiewicz. A., Garry, D. & Tejani, N. (1996). Intrauterine transmission of hepatitis A virus. *Obstet. Gynecol.*, **88**, 690–91.

Lin, H. H., Kao, J. H., Yeh, K. Y., Liu, D. P., Chang, M. H., Chen, P. J. & Chen, D. S. (1998). Mother-to-infant transmission of GB virus C/hepatitis G virus, the role of high-titered maternal viremia and mode of delivery. *J. Infect. Dis.*, **177**, 1202–6.

McDuffie, R. S., Jr & Bader, T. (1999). Fetal meconium peritonitis after maternal hepatitis A. *Am. J. Obstet. Gynecol.*, **180**, 1031–2.

Menendez, C., Sanchez-Tapias, J. M., Alonso, P. L., Gimenez-Barcons, M., Kahigwa, E., Aponte, J. J., Mshinda, H., Navia, M. M., Jimenez de Anta, M. T., Rodes, J. & Saiz, J. C. (1999). Molecular evidence of mother-to-infant transmission of hepatitis G virus among women without known risk factors for parenteral infections. *J. Clin. Microbiol.*, **37**, 2333–6.

Ramia, S. & Bahakim, H. (1988). Perinatal transmission of hepatitis B virus-associated hepatitis D virus. *Ann. Inst. Pasteur/Virol.*, **139**, 285–90.

Zanetti, A. R., Feroni, P., Magliano, E. M., Pirovano, P., Lavarini, C., Massaro, A. L., Gavinelli, R., Fabris, C. & Rizetto, M. (1982). Perinatal transmission of the hepatitis B virus and of the HBV-associated delta agent from mothers to offspring in northern Italy. *J. Med. Virol.*, **9**, 139–48.

Zanetti, A. R., Tanzi, E., Romano, L., Principi, N., Zuin, G., Minola, E., Zapparoli, B., Palmieri, M., Marini, A., Ghisotti, D., Friedman, P., Hunt, J. & Laffler, T. (1998). Multicenter trial on mother-to-infant transmission of GBV-C virus. The Lombardy Study Group on Vertical/Perinatal Hepatitis Viruses Transmission. *J. Med. Virol.*, **54**, 107–12.

that HPV infections of the genital tract in the male partner is an STD (Barrasso et al., 1987; Schiffman, 1992). The prevalence of anogenital warts in both partners of sexual couples has been reported to be greater than 90%, and more than 60% of exposed contact develop clinical or subclinical lesions (Barrett et al., 1954; Oriel, 1971; Schneider et al., 1988; Maymon et al., 1994). However, in other studies the concordance of HPV types between sexual partners has been surprisingly low. Typed by *in situ* hybridization (ISH), both partners were HPV-positive in 66 (24%) cases, but HPV types were identical in only 15 of these couples (Hippeläinen et al., 1994).

Support for a non-sexual route comes from studies on HPV DNA detection in genital samples of virginal women, with HPV DNA present in 12–20% of women (Ley et al., 1991; Pao et al., 1993; Wheeler et al., 1993). These findings are substantiated by a growing number of case reports (Valente et al., 1991; Yell et al., 1993; Craigo et al., 1995).

Horizontal transmission

The increased incidence of cutaneous warts in children older than 5 years is believed to be due to exposure during physical education during the first years at school (Schiffman, 1994). It has also been suggested that non-sexual transmission of genital HPV infection may occur through close contact during bathing or by bath towels or other shared objects (Rock et al., 1986; Gibson et al., 1990; Obalek et al., 1990; Padel et al., 1990; Pacheco et al., 1991; Handley et al., 1993). However, this is not confirmed in all studies (Puranen et al., 1996a).

Fomite transmission has also been postulated, based on the detection of HPV DNA in gynaecological settings (McCance et al., 1986; Ferenczy et al., 1989; Lou et al., 1991) and in the CO_2-laser fume while treating the HPV lesions (Garden et al., 1988; Ferenczy et al., 1990; Kashima et al., 1991). However, laser surgeons are not found to be at an increased risk of acquiring warts compared to the general population (Gloster & Roenigk, 1995).

Vertical transmission

HPV infections and pregnancy

Genital HPV types contain mediatory hormone responsive elements such as positive transcription regulatory signals of glucocorticoid hormones, like progesterone. Their activity may play a particularly important role in the biology of genital HPV infections. For example, expression of viral functions may fluctuate with the temporal hormonal status of the host (Fuchs & Pfister, 1994). A marked variation in detectability of HPV DNA by Southern blot hybridization (SBH) in cervical smears during pregnancy with an increase from the first to third trimester, and a sharp decline post-partum has been reported in some (Rando et al., 1989;

Schneider et al., 1987; Czegledy et al., 1989; Soares et al., 1990), but not all studies (de Roda Husman et al., 1995a).

Abramson et al. (1987) studied the effect of pregnancy on the course of laryngeal papillomatosis in 10 women. Four women had active lesions just prior to pregnancy, and in three of these, growth was substantially increased with progression of pregnancy. After delivery, the severity of the disease markedly decreased. Pregnancy resulted in activation of latent laryngeal papillomatosis in one of the remaining six patients. In one report, laryngeal papillomatosis recurred during pregnancy after 21 years of remission and led to the death of the pregnant woman (Helmrich et al, 1992).

Transmission of HPV from an infected mother to her infant

Despite the overwhelming evidence in favour of the sexual route as the main mode of HPV transmission in sexually active age groups, there is also convincing evidence to suggest that HPV is not exclusively an STD. Like other viral infections, HPVs can be vertically transmitted from an infected mother to her newborn baby. In 1956, Hajek wrote: 'Multiple laryngeal papillomata are found in small children and adolescents. They are not hereditary, but in 20% of cases can be found at birth'. In the same article, he reported probably the first recorded case of a suspected transmission of a viral wart from the mother to her child at birth (Hajek, 1956).

Laryngeal papillomas

Since then, a number of studies have shown the relation between the juvenile onset recurrent respiratory papillomatosis (JO–RRP) and maternal genital condylomata (Cook et al., 1973; Strong et al., 1976; Quick et al., 1980; Hallden & Majmudar, 1986; Abramson et al, 1987; Alebrico et al., 1995). Among 109 cases of JO-RRP, only one child had been delivered by caesarean section (Shah et al., 1986). HPV DNA was found in 11 of 23 nasopharyngeal aspirates of infants born by vaginal delivery to the mothers with genital HPV infection (Sedlacek et al., 1989), whereas both children born by caesarean section were HPV DNA-negative. Amniotic fluid samples after rupture of the membranes were obtained from 13 patients, 2 of which were positive for HPV DNA (Sedlacek et al., 1989).

Compared to controls, children with JO-RRP are more often first-born, delivered vaginally and born to a teenage mother, whereas adults with AO-RRP report more life-time sexual partners and a higher frequency of oral sex (Kashima et al., 1992). A maternal history of genital condyloma at the time of delivery or during pregnancy is reported for 54%–67% of children with RRP (Cook et al., 1973; Quick et al., 1980; Hallden & Majmudar, 1986). It has been estimated that caesarean delivery is associated with a nearly five-fold decrease in the risk of

JO–RRP, first order births with a nearly two-fold increase; and maternal age less than 20 years with a more than doubling of risk (Shah et al., 1998).

Evidence for vertical transmission of HPV

A large number of studies have shown a relation between maternal genital HPV infection and HPV DNA detection in the oral, nasopharyngeal or genital mucosa of neonates. Fredericks et al., sampled cervical cells from 11 women 6 weeks postpartum and took buccal scrapes of their babies for analysis of HPV DNA by PCR with an identical HPV type detected in eight mother–child pairs (Fredericks et al., 1993). Pakarian et al. (1994) detected HPV DNA in cervical swabs of 20 out of 31 pregnant women between 20th and 38th weeks of pregnancy and buccal and genital swaps of 12 of 32 infants at birth. Ten mother–infant pairs demonstrated concordant HPV types at six weeks, HPV DNA persisted in eight infants. Of the eight mothers who transmitted HPV infection to their infants, four with a previous history of abnormal smears and two with previous genital warts had significantly higher viral load than those who did not (Kaye et al., 1994).

Cason et al. (1995) found four positive nasopharyngeal aspirates from the babies born to 15 mothers with HPV DNA positive cervical swabs. HPV DNA persisted at least for 6 weeks in 80% and 6 months in 65% of these infants. Concordant variants or prototypic sequences were detected in 9 out of 13 mother/infant samples (Kaye et al., 1996). Alberico et al. (1996) collected endocervical biopsies during the first and/or second trimester of pregnancy and/or at the onset of labour, and oropharyngeal secretions from their infants, in 32 mother–infant pairs. The concordance of HPV DNA positivity between the mothers and their infants was nearly 60%.

In a larger study cervical scrapes of 105 mothers and nasopharyngeal aspirate fluids (NPAFs) of their infants at the time of delivery were analysed (Puranen et al., 1996b). Both maternal and neonatal samples were positive for the same type of HPV in 29 mother–infant pairs. Interestingly, five infants born by caesarean section were HPV DNA positive for the same HPV type as their mother; overall concordance between HPV types in mother and newborn was 69%. HPV DNA was found in 30 of 78 infants delivered vaginally and in 9 of 26 infants delivered by caesarean section. HPV DNA remained detectable up to 3 years in 16 children, but in the other 15 it was no longer detectable at 2–4 days. Similar results were reported by Tseng et al. (1998) who assessed the presence of HPV 16 and 18 DNA sequences by PCR in genital swabs of 301 pregnant women and buccal swabs of their infants. The overall frequency of HPV 16/18 DNA among the pregnant women was 23% (68/301). At birth 18 of 35 vaginally delivered infants and 9 of 33 infants delivered by caesarean section were HPV positive (Tseng et al., 1998). These findings confirm those of Shah et al. (1998) and suggest that vaginally

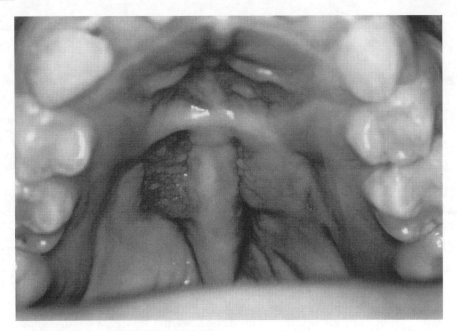

Figure 11.1   Oral papilloma in a child with HPV infection.

delivered infants are at higher risk than those delivered by cesarean section.

Whereas most studies report a high rate of transmission of HPV in infants born to HPV infected mothers, in some detection rates have been much lower, which may have been due to less sensitive laboratory techniques (Smith et al., 1995; Monk et al., 1994). Watts et al. (1998) reported a low perinatal transmission rate for HPV in 151 infants. Koch et al. (1997) reported a low prevalence of oral or anogenital HPV infection in randomly selected Danish children aged 0 to 17 years. This study population represents a randomly selected cohort, and the prevalence of HPV DNA is also expected to be significantly lower than among the children born to HPV infected mothers.

St. Louis et al. (1993) assessed the frequency of HPV infection in cervico-vaginal lavage specimens of 52 HIV-infected women and their children at the time of delivery. Oropharyngeal and perineal specimens from 21 HIV-seropositive and 60 HIV-seronegative 3-year-old children of these mothers were also collected. Detection of HPV in the mother was strongly associated with HIV; ten children had HPV DNA but detection of HPV in children was not associated with the mothers' HPV or HIV status or with the child's own HIV status. In 98 children aged 0 to 12 years, born to mothers included in a prospective cohort study for genital HPV infection (Puranen et al., 1996b), HPV DNA was found in 31 oral scrapings. At the time of delivery, five mothers had genital HPV infection with the same virus type as found in her child. In addition 11 mothers had a genital HPV infection with the same virus type as the child a few months before or after delivery. One child had an oral papilloma in which HPV 16 DNA was detected which type was also present in her mother's genital tract at the time of delivery (Fig. 11.1). These results suggest that vertically transmitted HPV infection can persist for years (Puranen et al., 1996b).

Transmission in utero

In utero transmission of HPV has been seriously considered only recently. Intrauterine HPV transmission can occur via blood, ascending infection or through sperm at the time of conception. Haematogenous HPV transmission has been considered unlikely, because HPV is known to multiply locally at the site of entry on the skin or mucous membranes, and there has been no convincing evidence of disseminated HPV viraemia (Mounts & Shah, 1984). In some studies, however, HPV DNA has been found in peripheral blood leukocytes (Tseng et al., 1992; Kedzia et al., 1992; Pao et al., 1991; Jalal et al., 1992; Hönig et al., 1995).

The results of one study refer to ascendent HPV transmission in utero. Favre et al. (1998) detected HPV DNA in the amniotic fluid and placental biopsies. The child was born by caesarean section and the amniotic fluid specimen was taken prior to the rupture of membranes. HPV 3, 5, 8, 24 and 36 were detected in the amniotic fluid and placental specimens as well as in the skin lesions of the mother suffering from epidermodysplasia verruciformis. No viral sequences were detected in peripheral blood mononuclear cells collected 2 years and 6 months before the caesarean section, suggesting ascendent HPV infection via the birth canal.

Some reports suggest sperm as a vector for HPV delivery in utero (Chan et al., 1995, 1996; Lai et al., 1996). HPV DNA and RNA have been detected in seminal plasma and sperm cells suggesting that HPV can infect human sperm cells and certain HPV genes are expressed actively in infected sperm cells. The infected sperm cells conceivably can behave as vectors or carriers for the transmission of HPV (Lai et al., 1996).

Further support for intrauterine acquisition of infection is provided by reports of congenital condylomata (Tang et al., 1978) after caesarean section without premature rupture of the membranes (Rogo & Nyansera, 1989). HPV DNA has been found in amniotic fluid from women with cervical HPV lesions by some (Armbruster-Moraes et al., 1994), but not all researchers (Maxwell et al., 1998). Pao et al. (1995) found HPV DNA in hydatiform moles and in placental choriocarcinomas. Recently, Hermonat et al. (1997) found HPV infection more prevalent in 25 spontaneous abortion specimens than in 15 samples from elective abortions and identified syncytiotrophoblasts as the predominant cellular target of HPV (Hermonat et al., 1998).

In conclusion, vertical transmission of HPV infection does occur, but the relative contribution of intrauterine, intrapartum and postpartum routes is not yet quantified or fully understood. Study populations have mostly been quite small and detection methods for HPV DNA have not been equally sensitive. The estimated rates of transmission from mother-to-child range from 4–87%, but, because of the small size of most studies and the inconsistently sensitive HPV DNA tests used, no accurate rates can be calculated.

Diagnosis of perinatally transmitted HPV infections

Like most DNA viruses, HPVs may induce clinical, subclinical and latent infections. The terms subclinical and latent HPV infections are commonly misused concepts ascribed to different issues by different authors (Syrjänen, 1989a), and criteria for these three categories have only recently been outlined (Syrjänen, 1990, 1992, 1995). Clinical infection should be readily apparent by colposcopy, cytology and histology. In subclinical infection, HPV DNA is found with DNA hybridization or PCR amplification methods with minor epithelial changes seen with colposcopy after acetic acid application, in PAP-smears or in biopsy. Latent infection is not detectable on colposcopy, cytology or histology, but HPV DNA should be demonstrated in clinically and histologically normal epithelium. Confusion has been created, e.g. the use of the term subclinical infection as a synonym to flat condyloma (Roman & Fife, 1989; Meisels et al., 1983). Genital HPV infections can run an extremely fluctuating course, with transition from subclinical or latent infection to clinical infection.

Gross appearance and colposcopy

On gross appearance, HPV-induced lesions are either exophytic, inverted (endophytic) or flat (Meisels & Fortin, 1976). Exophytic lesion can be either papillary or verrucous, flat and inverted lesions are usually not seen with the naked eye. The colour varies from that of the adjacent normal skin or mucosa to red or white, depending on vascularization and keratinization of the lesion (Syrjänen et al., 1987). Application of 3–5% acetic acid, usually combined with colposcopy, has been used to detect flat and subclinical HPV lesions in the anogenital tract of both women and men (Gross, 1987; Cone et al., 1991; Costa et al., 1992). The exact mechanism whereby the epithelium changes its colour to white after acetic acid application is not fully understood. It is important to realize, however, that this reaction is not specific for HPV infection. Acetowhite staining may also be seen in cases of chronic inflammation, epithelial thickening or minor abrasions (Schneider et al., 1988; Griffiths et al., 1991).

Cytology and histology

Cytology is an important tool in screening a variety of abnormal changes in the uterine cervix. Clinical and subclinical HPV infections induce typical cytological changes in the epithelial cells. These changes are referred to as koilocytosis, characterized by perinuclear vacuolization, pyknosis-, enlargement- and hyperchromasia of the nucleus, and double- or multiple nuclei (Koss, 1987). In HPV-derived lesions, squamous cells with enlarged, dark, pyknotic nuclei without koilocytosis may also be seen, called 'dyskeratinocytes' (Koss, 1987).

On light microscopic examination, exophytic HPV lesions have a distinct morphology. The epithelium is thickened with acanthosis, hyperkeratosis and papillomatosis. Rete pegs show thickening and elongation. The surface of the epithelium frequently shows hyperorto- or hyperparakeratosis (Purola & Savia, 1977). In benign HPV lesions, cell maturation is discernible in all cell layers, koilocytes being present just above the parabasal layer or higher. Nuclear pleomorphism and nuclear enlargement are minimal or absent and mitoses are normal. In intraepithelial neoplasia, on the other hand, atypical cell maturation is seen, and koilocytes are found in the upper 1/3 of the epithelium, sometimes with a haphazardous, focal distribution. Nuclear pleomorphism, enlargement and abnormal mitoses are typically present (Syrjänen, 1989b).

Immunohistochemistry and DNA hybridization techniques

Before DNA hybridization and PCR, the detection of viral structural proteins (viral antigens) in biopsies with poly- or monoclonal antibodies was used in HPV diagnosis. With immunohistochemistry (IHC), however, only productive infections where structural proteins are expressed, can be detected. Latent and other non-replicating infections or cases where HPV DNA is integrated into the host genome cannot be detected by IHC (Maitland et al., 1987; Syrjänen, 1989b). Due to this serious limitation, DNA techniques have entirely replaced IHC in HPV diagnosis.

Nucleic acid hybridization techniques are based on the ability of specific small nucleotide sequence, the probe, to form a hybrid with the complementary sequence in the denatured target DNA molecule. Hybridization may be performed to the DNA isolated from the sample and attached to the filter (dot blot, SBH, reverse blot and sandwich hybridizations), or directly to the tissue sections or cytological samples (ISH and filter *in situ* [FISH] hybridization) (Maitland et al., 1987; Syrjänen, 1990). In the hybrid capture method, DNA is hybridized with RNA probe and the hybrids are detected with antibodies to RNA–DNA hybrids and chemiluminescent reaction, e.g. HCII (Digene)(Cox et al., 1995).

Polymerase chain reaction (PCR), single-strand conformation polymorphism (SSCP) and DNA sequencing

In HPV diagnosis, the PCR primers can be designed to detect a specific viral type or multiple different types at the same time. Different HPV types have highly conserved regions of nucleotides within their genomes. The consensus primers which detect several different HPV types are designed to flank the most conserved parts of HPV genome (Gregoire et al., 1989; Manos et al., 1989; Snijders et al., 1990; Contorni & Leoncini, 1993; de Roda Husman et al., 1995b). Recently, PCR amplification has also been applied directly on the tissue sections, subjected to ISH. Theoretically, this *in situ* PCR would substantially increase the power of the conventional ISH method in detecting HPV-infected cells with simultaneous histological localization (Haase et al., 1990; Nuovo et al., 1991a, b). This novel application of PCR still needs further development, however, before becoming suitable for routine use.

The SSCP method is based on the principle that under non-denaturating conditions, single-stranded DNA molecules form unique secondary structures depending on their primary nucleotide sequences. Secondary structures (conformers) result in diverse band patterns from the DNA fragments examined (Kurvinen et al., 1995; Zehbe et al., 1996). Combined use of PCR amplification and SSCP analysis has provided a rapid and powerful tool for HPV diagnosis and typing (Zehbe et al., 1996).

The linking of PCR amplification, direct sequencing and computer data bank analysis provides a new approach in the detection of different HPVs and has several advantages over existing methodology. These advantages include increased precision in the rapid characterization of known HPVs, detection of mutations, and identification of new HPV types (Rady et al., 1993). Data on sequence variations are mandatory while attempting to identify routes of virus transmission (Ho et al., 1993).

Serology

For most viruses, evidence of infection is based on the detection of serum antibodies which react with viral proteins. HPV cannot be grown in cell cultures and in most clinical samples virions are rarely present. Antibodies have been difficult to develop because of the lack of suitable antigen targets and the development of serological assays has lagged behind DNA testing (Galloway & Jenison, 1990; Galloway, 1992). Bacterially expressed fusion proteins, synthetic peptides, HPV 11 propagated in a xenograft system (Galloway, 1992), and virus-like particles (Kirnbauer et al., 1992, 1993) are now used as antigen targets in ELISA (enzyme-linked immunosorbent assays) and Western blotting (Galloway, 1992). Because of the lack of suitable antigen targets for antibody production, data on humoral immune responses in HPV infection are only now emerging (Stanley et al., 1995).

The advantages of the serological assays over HPV DNA detection tests include the potential of serology to detect past HPV infections among people who no longer have measurable viral DNA, thus providing insight into the risk factors for HPV persistence and disease progression (Palefsky, 1995). While performing HPV DNA detection tests, sampling errors are always a problem. Serological assays should provide a more accurate measurement of a previous or current exposure to HPVs (Galloway, 1992). Serological tests are also needed in planning and controlling of the planned vaccination programmes.

Management of perinatal HPV infections

Vertically transmitted HPV can cause a true infection in the upper aero-digestive tract or genital region of the child. Theoretically, the time of acquiring HPV infection is crucial: if infection is acquired when lymphocytes are developing tolerance to own tissues of the body, it would be possible that lymphocytes also become tolerant to HPV. Immunological mechanisms would then fail to recognize HPVs as foreign antigens. It is also possible that infection acquired at a time when the child's own immunological response is not fully developed may act like vaccination towards infections encountered later in life. Another unsolved issue is the latency period of HPV infection. Is vertically transmitted HPV infection able to remain latent for years or decades and cause disease after a long period of latency? The HPV genome has been reported to persist in cell cultures in vitro without any signs of virus growth in cell morphology for 4 to 11 months after infection (Lancaster & Meinke, 1975; La Porta & Taichman, 1982). Activation or reactivation of latent HPV infection after 21 (Helmrich et al., 1992), 33 (Bergström, 1982) and even 79 years (Yell et al., 1993) has been suggested.

Management of the child and the family
Genital HPV infections

Controversy remains regarding the manner in which children acquire anogenital warts (Fig. 11.2). It has been suggested that lesions are transmitted to the child by one (or more) of four dominant means: perinatal infection, digital inoculation or autoinoculation, fomite and casual social contact, and sexual abuse (Gutman et al., 1993). The issue of genital warts in children originating from sexual abuse was raised in the 1980s, when vulvar condylomata in young children, previously considered extremely rare, were reported with increasing frequency (Stumpf, 1980). Anogenital lesions recognized within the first year after birth are considered to be perinatally acquired (Gutman et al., 1993). To confirm or exclude sexual abuse, a wide range of information must be obtained: age-appropriate diagnostic disclosure interviews of the child by skilled personnel, a forensic medical examination and an evaluation for other STDs, an assessment of the adequacy of supervision of the child, prior events relating to abuse, behavioral indicators of

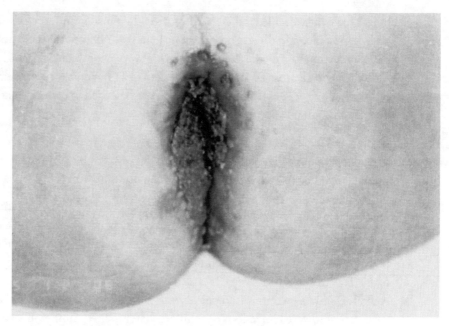

Figure 11.2   Anal warts in an HPV-infected child. (Picture courtesy of Dr Olli Ruuskanen.)

abuse, and a review of medical records for events indicating possible abuse or neglect (Gutman et al., 1993). Also oral abuse, during which secretions from the assailant come into contact with the child's oral cavity, is a common type of sexual abuse particularly in younger children. Therefore examinations should include an inspection of the oral mucosa (Gutman et al., 1993). In addition, HPV typing is important in determining whether the infection is derived from mucosal or cutaneous transmission (Padel et al., 1990).

Recurrent respiratory papillomatosis (RRP)

Laryngeal papillomas, the most common benign tumours of the larynx in infants and children, account for substantial morbidity in affected children (Cohen et al., 1980). Laryngeal papillomas have a bimodal age distribution with the first peak in children before 4 years of age and a second in adults between 20 and 30 years of age (Abramson et al., 1987; Kashima & Mounts, 1987; Hartley et al., 1994). According to the age of onset, laryngeal papillomatosis (LP) or recurrent respiratory papillomatosis (RRP) have been classified as juvenile-onset (JO) and adult-onset (AO) disease. The incidence of JO-RRP is estimated to be 0.2–0.8/100 000 and the prevalence 0.8/100 000 in a Danish population at risk (Mounts & Shah, 1984; Christensen et al., 1985; Bomholt, 1988; Lindeberg et al., 1989; Lindeberg & Elbrønd, 1991). The incidence of JO-RRP seems to be considerably higher in the USA, up to 4.3/100 000 (Derkay, 1995). Assuming that 25% of pregnant women have genital HPV infection, of which 2–5% are clinically overt, it has been estimated that the number of births at risk for HPV infection in USA is between 72 000 and 180 000 (Shah et al., 1986). However, the prevalence of genital condylomata in women of child-bearing age far exceeds the reported number of new cases of JO-RRP. Thus, the risk of a newborn contracting a laryngeal lesion as a result of viral transmission from an HPV-infected mother must be relatively low; according to the best estimates, in the order of 1:80 to 1:1.500 (Shah et al., 1986).

Clinical symptoms usually start with a changing voice or hoarseness with subsequent respiratory distress and stridor (Cohen et al., 1980; Hirschfield & Steinberg, 1989). Laryngeal papillomas are usually located on the vocal cords and epiglottis or subglottis but can involve the entire larynx as well as the tracheobronchial tree and even the lungs (Christensen et al., 1985; Hirschfield & Steinberg, 1989). The lesions may be single or multiple. The need for surgical removal is greater in children than in adults, and also malignant conversion appears to be more common in the JO than in AO disease (Mounts & Shah, 1984).

The most notable characteristics of laryngeal papillomas is their tendency to recur even after radical surgical removal. Operations may be required at annual intervals or sometimes as frequently as every 2 weeks (Mounts & Shah, 1984; Kashima & Mounts, 1987). Another characteristic of laryngeal papillomas is their tendency to regress spontaneously. Remission can be temporary or for the lifetime of the patient (Bergström, 1982; Abramson et al., 1987). Spontaneous remissions have been described at puberty, and recurrence or increase in the severity of disease during pregnancy (Kashima & Mounts, 1987; Hirschfield & Steinberg, 1989).

Malignant conversion of RRP has been ascribed to irradiation, smoking and alcohol consumption (Lindeberg et al., 1989; Lindeberg & Elbrønd, 1991). Among 113 patients with laryngeal papillomatosis, Lindeberg and Elbrønd (1991) showed a 16-fold higher risk of respiratory tract carcinoma in irradiated patients as compared to non-irradiated patients. However, there are reports on malignant conversion of laryngeal papillomas in the absence of these co-factors (Cohen et al., 1980; Simma et al., 1993). Although no exact incidence figures for malignant conversion of RRP are available, Yoder and Batsakis (1980) estimated that RRP is followed by laryngeal carcinoma in 2–3% of cases.

Prevention of HPV transmission

Antenatal screening

A caesarean section delivery may reduce the risk of HPV transmission, and the option of caesarean delivery should be discussed with a mother who has condyloma at the time of delivery (Shah et al., 1998). Although HPV DNA has been shown in human semen (Ostrow et al., 1986; Inoue et al., 1992; Astori et al., 1995) and in sperm (Chan et al., 1994), HPV transmission via sperm in utero must be confirmed before screening programmes for sperm can be started. The role of breast milk in HPV transmission or the possible protective value of breast milk in the form of HPV antibodies is not known. Currently, antenatal screening for HPV infections at a population level is not feasible. Any measures to prevent the development of HPV infection in the newborn are linked with adequate treatment of the disease in the mother.

Treatment of the mother

Women who have HPV lesions without CIN require only careful follow-up without treatment because the majority of such lesions resolve spontaneously (Syrjänen et al., 1992). It is not known whether such HPV induced lesions should be treated to prevent transmission of HPV infection either sexually or vertically. When HPV induced lesions are treated during pregnancy, surgical methods are safe for the mother and her infant (Ferenczy, 1984; Matsunaga et al., 1987; Schwartz et al., 1988). Surgical methods in the treatment of HPV induced lesions include excision, electrodiathermy, cryotherapy, CO_2-laser vaporization and conization (cold knife conization, laser conization) as well as large loop excision of the transformation zone (LLETZ). During pregnancy, conization and LLETZ are avoided if not necessary for the prompt eradication of high-grade CIN. The success rates of any surgical treatment of HPV induced lesions is generally excellent. Surgical treatment significantly affects the clinical course of genital HPV infections but does not guarantee total clearance of the virus (Yliskoski et al., 1989, 1991).

Antiviral agents used in the treatment of HPV lesions include podophyllotoxin (podofilox) and podophyllin, concentrated tricloroacetic acid (TCA), 5-fluorouracil and interferons. Podophyllin and podophyllotoxin (podofilox) are antimitotic agents, which are absorbed systematically. Therefore, both are contra-indicated during pregnancy (Beutner, 1987). 5-fluorouracil is a pyrimidine antagonist, acts through inhibition of DNA and RNA synthesis and has an anti-proliferative effect (Krebs, 1991). Like podophyllin and podophyllotoxin, 5-fluorouracil is contraindicated during pregnancy. Unlike podophyllin and 5-fluorouracil, TCA has not been shown to be teratogenic and is not contra-indicated during pregnancy (Schwartz et al., 1988). The success rates of chemotherapeutic treatment of HPV lesions reported in the literature vary considerably (Cowsert, 1994; Phelps & Alexander, 1995).

Although some studies show good response rates for interferon treatment of HPV lesions, current data are not consistent. Interferon therapy has a high frequency of adverse effects and high costs, therefore it is currently less often used

(Cowsert, 1994). The effect of interferon therapy on pregnancy and fetus is not known. Interferon therapy should not be used during pregnancy, unless the benefits for the mother are clearly justified over the possible harm for the fetus. A new approach for the treatment of LP with intralesional injections of cidofovir [(S)-1-(3-hydroxy-2-phosphonylmethoxypropyl) cytosine] has recently been published (Snoeck et al., 1998). This new chemotherapeutic is well tolerated and so far, no significant side effects have been noted.

Prophylactic vaccination

A vaccine to prevent genital HPV infections, especially those types associated with malignancy, would significantly reduce morbidity and mortality from cervical and other genital tract cancers (Fife, 1998). However, HPV vaccine development is hampered by several problems. The immune response to natural HPV infection is incompletely understood and there is uncertainty about which viral antigen(s) should be included in a candidate vaccine. It is clear that immunization of several animal species with the L1 major capsid protein (usually in the form of virus-like particles) induces production of anti-HPV antibodies that are neutralizing in several assay systems. However, it is not clear if neutralizing antibody will be present in the genital tract in sufficient quantities to block infection. A second problem is the lack of a reliable serological assay for HPV. This is a major problem for clinical trials in which the identification of susceptible individuals, and incident infections, usually relies on a serological diagnosis. There is also interest in the development of a vaccine that is used to treat individuals who are already infected, a therapeutic vaccine (Fife, 1998).

It is likely that a therapeutic vaccine will need to target different or additional antigens to those in a prophylactic vaccine (Fife, 1998). The design of such vaccines has evolved from an understanding of the nature of HPV infections and their consequences, together with an evaluation of the efficacy of different approaches to vaccination in animal models. These studies have resulted in several different vaccine preparations which are currently undergoing Phase I and II clinical trials. The justification for the widespread implementation of prophylactic HPV vaccines will depend on the outcome of larger scale studies of vaccine efficacy that take into account the epidemiology of HPV infections and associated disease. Although the effectiveness of these vaccines cannot be evaluated in such small studies, they constitute an important step toward the development of therapeutic uterine cervix cancer vaccines (Duggan-Keen et al., 1998; Gariglio et al., 1998). In planning prophylactic vaccination programmes, it is essential to know the true frequency of vertical transmission of HPV infection. Most patients experience the clinically apparent HPV infection in the early adulthood, but in fact, HPV infection may have been acquired far earlier.

Other preventive measures

A high standard of hygiene and adequate cleaning of contaminated articles is important in controling HPV transmission. HPVs have capsids consisting only of protein. Because of the lack of a lipid envelope, HPVs are resistant to lipid solvents such as ether, chloroform or sodium deoxycholate that destroy enveloped viruses. Formaldehyde, dilute hydrochloric acid and sodium hypochlorite will disinfect HPV-contaminated articles (White, 1994). The use of a 2% glutaraldehyde bath for the sterilization of instruments has also been recommended (Ferenczy et al., 1989; Lou et al., 1991).

Sokal and Hermonat (1995) tested the inactivating effect of povidone–iodine against bovine papillomavirus in vitro. They found 90% inactivation with concentrations as low as 0.1%, 99.9% inactivation with 0.3% and 100% inactivation with 0.6% povidone–iodine. The authors suggested that topical formulations, especially for vaginal use, containing low concentrations of povidone–iodine might be useful in preventing HPV transmission. Iodine has serious disadvantages limiting its routine use, however. The brown colour can stain fabrics, iodine allergy is rather common, iodine may affect the thyroid gland and it may disturb normal microbial flora. The effective concentration in the study was ten times lower than that of commercially available formulations. Lower concentrations might solve at least some of these problems.

Heat disinfection is recommended for equipments contaminated with HPV or other viruses. Washing in at least 85 °C for 60 minutes or autoclaving will disinfect the articles from HPV. Viruses are also effectively inactivated by ionizing and nonionizing radiation by different mechanisms. Ionizing radiation causes a lethal break in a single-stranded RNA chain but in a double-stranded DNA chain, like the one in HPVs, only a small proportion of the single-strand breaks are lethal (White, 1994).

Ferenczy et al. (1989) tested objects used in the treatment of HPV infections for recovery of HPV DNA. HPV DNA was found in surgical gloves, biopsy forceps, and cryoprobe tips before and after disinfection. The rate of HPV DNA positivity was low after cleaning (Ferenczy et al., 1989). According to current recommendations, all instruments should be autoclaved and instruments which do not tolerate heat steam should be disinfected for three hours in detergents containing 2% glutaraldehyde and rinsed thoroughly with water afterwards.

Acknowledgments

Fig. 11.2 was provided courtesy of Dr Olli Ruuskanen.

REFERENCES

Abramson, A. L., Steinberg, B. M. & Winkler, B. (1987). Laryngeal papillomatosis: clinical, histopathologic and molecular studies. *Laryngoscope*, **97**, 678–85.

Alberico, S., Pinzano, R., Comar, M., Zocconi, E. & Guaschino, S. (1995). Juvenile laryngeal papillomatosis from an HPV-positive mother. A case report. *Clin. Exp. Obst. Gynecol.*, **22**, 243–6.

Alberico, S., Pinzano, R., Comar, M., Toffoletti, F., Maso, G., Ricci, G. & Guaschino, S. (1996). Maternal–fetal transmission of human papillomavirus. *Minerva Ginecol.*, **48**, 199–204.

Armbruster-Moraes, E., Ioshimoto, L. M., Leao, E. & Zugaib, M. (1994). Presence of human papillomavirus DNA in amniotic fluids of pregnant women with cervical lesions. *Gynecol. Oncol.*, **54**, 152–8.

Astori, G., Pipan, C., Muffato, G. & Botta, G. A. (1995). Detection of HPV-DNA in semen, urine and urethral samples by dot blot and PCR. *Microbiologica*, **18**, 143–9.

Backe, J., Roos, T., Mulfinger, L. & Martius, J. (1997). Prevalence of human papillomavirus DNA in cervical tissue. Retrospective analysis of 855 cervical biopsies. *Arch. Gynecol. Obstet.*, **259**, 69–77.

Barrasso, R., DeBrux, J., Croissant, O. & Orth, G. (1987). High prevalence of papillomavirus-associated penile intraepithelial neoplasia in sexual partners of women with cervical intraepithelial neoplasia. *N. Engl. J. Med.*, **317**, 916–23.

Barrett, T. J., Silbar, J. D. & McGinley, J. P. (1954). Genital warts – a venereal disease. *J.A.M.A.*, **154**, 333–4.

Bauer, H. M., Hildesheim, A., Schiffman, M. H., Glass, A. G., Rush, B. B., Scott, D. R., Cadell, D. M., Kurman, R. J. & Manos, M. M. (1993). Determinants of genital human papillomavirus infection in low-risk women in Portland, Oregon. *Sex. Transm. Dis.*, **20**, 274–8.

Bennett, R. S. & Powell, K. R. (1987). Human papillomaviruses: associations between laryngeal papillomas and genital warts. *Pediatr. Infect. Dis. J.*, **6**, 229–32.

Bergström, LaV. (1982). Laryngeal papillomatosis: recurrence after 33-year remission. *Laryngoscope*, **92**, 1160–3.

Beutner, K. R. (1987). Podophyllotoxin in the treatment of genital human papillomavirus infection: a review. *Semin. Dermatol.*, **6**, 10–18.

Bomholt, A. (1988). Juvenile laryngeal papillomatosis. *Acta Otol.*, **105**, 367–71.

Bosch, F. X., Manos, M. M., Munoz, N., Sherman, M., Jansen, A. M., Peto, J., Schiffman, M. H., Moreno, V., M., Kurman, R., Shah, K. V., Alihonou, E., Bayo, S., Mokhtar, H. C., Chichareon, S., Daudt, A., de Los Rios, E., Ghadirian, P., Kitniya, J. N. & Koulibaly, M. (1995). Prevalence of human papillomavirus in cervical cancer: a worldwide perspective. *J. Natl Cancer Inst.*, **87**, 796–802.

Burk, R. D., Kelly, P., Feldman, J., Bromberg, J., Vermund, S. H., Dehovitz, J. A. & Landesman, S. H. (1996). Declining prevalence of cervicovaginal human papillomavirus infection with age is independent of other risk factors. *Sex. Transm. Dis.*, **23**, 333–41.

Cason, J., Kaye, J. N., Jewers, R. J., Kambo, P. K., Bible, J. M., Kell, B., Shergill, B., Pakarian, F., Shanti-Raju, K. & Best, J. M. (1995). Perinatal infection and persistence of human papillomavirus types 16 and 18 in infants. *J. Med. Virol.*, **47**, 209–18.

Chan, P. J., Su, B. C., Kalugdan, T., Seraj, I. M., Tredway, D. R. & King, A. (1994). Human papillomavirus gene sequences in washed human sperm deoxyribonucleic acid. *Fertil. Steril.*, **61**, 982–5.

Chan, P. J., Kalugdan, T., Su, B. C., Su, B. C., Kalugdan, T., Seraj, I. M., Tredway, D. R. & King, A. (1995). Sperm as a noninvasive gene delivery system for perimplantation embryos [see comments]. *Fertil. Steril.*, **63**, 1121–4.

Chan, P. J., Seraj, I. M., Kalugdan, T. H. & King, A. (1996). Evidence for ease of transmission of human papillomavirus DNA from sperm to cells of the uterus and embryo. *J. Assist. Reprod. Genet.*, **13**, 516–19.

Chan, K. W., Wong, K. Y. & Srivastava, G. (1997). Prevalence of six types of human papillomavirus in inverted papilloma and papillary transitional cell carcinoma of the bladder: an evaluation by polymerase chain reaction. *J. Clin. Pathol.*, **50**, 1018–21.

Christensen, P-H., Jørgensen, K. & Grøntved, A. (1985). Larynxpapillomer hos børn. En 45 års opgørelse fra Fyns amt. *Ugeskr. Læger.*, **147**, 1110–13.

Cohen, S. R., Geller, K. A., Seltzer, S. & Thompson, J. W. (1980). Papilloma of the larynx and tracheobronchial tree in children. A retrospective study. *Ann. Otol.*, **89**, 497–503.

Cone, R., Beckmann, A., Aho, M., Wahlstrom, T., Ek, M., Corey, L. & Paavonen, J. (1991). Subclinical manifestations of vulvar human papillomavirus infection. *Int. J. Gynecol. Pathol.*, **10**, 26–35.

Contorni, M. & Leoncini, P. (1993). Typing of human papillomavirus DNAs by restriction endonuclease mapping of the PCR products. *J. Virol. Methods*, **41**, 29–36.

Cook, T. A., Cohn, A. M., Brunschwig, J. P., Goepfert, H., Butel, J. S. & Rawls, W. E. (1973). Laryngeal papilloma: etiologic and therapeutic considerations. *Ann. Otol. Rhinol. Laryngol.*, **82**, 649–55.

Costa, S., Syrjänen, S. M., Vendra, C., Chang, F., Gudia, G., Tervahauta, A., Hippelainen, M. & Syrjanen, K. (1992). Detection of human papillomavirus infections in the male sexual partners of women attending an STD clinic in Bologna. *Int. J. STD AIDS*, **3**, 338–46.

Cowsert, L. M. (1994). Treatment of papillomavirus infections: recent practice and future approaches. *Intervirology*, **37**, 226–30.

Cox, J. T., Lorincz, A. T., Schiffman, M. H., Sherman, M. E., Cullen, A. & Kurman, R. J. (1995). Human papillomavirus testing by hybrid capture appears to be useful in triaging women with a cytologic diagnosis of atypical squamous cells of undetermined significance. *Am. J. Obstet. Gynecol.*, **172**, 946–54.

Craigo, J., Hopkins, M. & DeLucia, A. (1995). Uterine cervix adenocarcinoma with both human papillomavirus type 18 and tumor suppressor gene p53 mutation from a woman having an intact hymen. *Gynecol. Oncol.*, **59**, 423–6.

Czegledy, J., Gergely, L. & Endrödi, I. (1989). Detection of human papillomavirus deoxyribonucleic acid by filter in situ hybridization during pregnancy. *J. Med.Virol.*, **28**, 250–4.

de Roda Husman, A. M., Walboomers, J. M. M., Hopman, E., Bleker, O. P., Helmerhorst, T. H. M. J., Rozendaal, L., Voorhorst, F. J. & Meyer, C. J. L. M. (1995a). HPV prevalence in cytomorphologically normal cervical scrapes of pregnant women as determined by PCR: the age-related pattern. *J. Med. Virol.*, **46**, 97–102.

de Roda Husman, A. M., Walboomers, J. M. M., Van den Brule, A. J. C., Meijer, C. J. L. M. & Snijders, P. J. F. (1995b). The use of general primers GP5 and GP6 elongated at their 3'ends with adjacent highly conserved sequences improves human papillomavirus detection by PCR. *J. Gen. Virol.*, **76**, 1057-62.

Derkay, C. S. (1995). Task force on recurrent respiratory papillomas. *Arch. Otolaryngol. Head Neck Surg.*, **121**, 1386–91.

Duggan-Keen, M. F., Brown, M. D., Stacey, S. N. & Stern, P. L. (1998). Papillomavirus vaccines. *Front. Biosci.*, **3**, 1192–208.

Evander, M., Edlund, K., Gustafsson, Å., Jonsson, M., Karlsson, R., Rydlander, E. & Wadell, G. (1995). Human papillomavirus infection is transient in young women: a population-based cohort study. *J. Infect. Dis.*, **171**, 1026–30.

Favre, M., Majewski, S., De Jesus, N., Malejczyk, M., Orth, G. & Jablonska, S. (1998). A possible vertical transmission of human papillomavirus genotypes associated with epidermodysplasia verruciformis. *J. Invest. Dermatol.*, **111**, 333–6.

Ferenczy, A. (1984). Treating genital condyloma during pregnancy with the carbon dioxide laser. *Am. J. Obstet. Gynecol.*, **148**, 9–12.

Ferenczy, A., Bergeron, C. & Richart, R. M. (1989). Human papillomavirus DNA in fomites on objects used for the management of patients with genital human papillomavirus infections. *Obstet. Gynecol.*, **74**, 950–4.

Ferenczy, A., Bergeron, C. & Richart, R. M. (1990). Human papillomavirus DNA in CO_2 laser-generated plume of smoke and its consequences to the surgeon. *Obstet. Gynecol.*, **75**, 114–18.

Fife, K. H. (1998). Human papillomavirus vaccine development. *Australas. J. Dermatol.*, **39**, 8–10.

Franco, E. L., Villa, L. L., Ruiz, A. & Costa, M. C. (1995). Transmission of cervical human papillomavirus infection by sexual activity: differences between low and high oncogenic risk types. *J. Infect. Dis.*, **172**, 756–63.

Fredericks, B. D., Balkin, A., Daniel, H. W., Schonrock, J., Ward, B. & Frazer, I. H. (1993). Transmission of human papillomaviruses from mother to child. *Aust. N.Z. J. Obstet. Gynaecol.*, **33**, 30–2.

Fuchs, P. G. & Pfister, H. (1994). Transcription of papillomavirus genomes. *Intervirology*, **37**, 159–67.

Galloway, D. A. (1992). Serological assays for the detection of HPV antibodies. *IARC. Sci. Publ.*, 147–61.

Galloway, D. A. & Jenison, S. A. (1990). Characterization of the humoral immune response to genital papillomaviruses. *Mol. Biol. Med.*, **7**, 59–72.

Garden, J. M., O'Banion, M. K., Shelnitz, L. S., Kinski, K. S., Bakus, A. D., Reichmann, M. E. & Sundberg, J. P. (1988). Papillomavirus in the vapor of carbon dioxide laser-treated verrucae. *J.A.M.A.*, **259**, 1199–202.

Gariglio, P., Benitez-Bribiesca, L., Berumen, J., Alcocer, J. M., Tamez, R. & Madrid, V. (1998). Therapeutic uterine–cervix cancer vaccines in humans. *Arch. Med. Res.*, **29**, 279–84.

Gibson, P. E., Gardner, S. D. & Best, S. J. (1990). Human papillomavirus types in anogenital warts of children. *J. Med. Virol.*, **30**, 142–5.

Gjooen, K., Olsen, A. O., Magnus, P., Grinde, B., Sauer, T. & Orstavik, I. (1996). Prevalence of human papillomavirus in cervical scrapes, as analyzed by PCR, in a population-based sample of women with and without cervical dysplasia. *APMIS*, **104**, 68–74.

Gloster, H. M. & Roenigk, R. K. (1995). Risk of acquiring human papillomavirus from the plume produced by the carbon dioxide laser in the treatment of warts. *J. Am. Acad. Dermatol.*, **32**, 436–41.

Gregoire, L., Arella, M., Campione Piccardo, J. & Lancaster, W. D. (1989). Amplification of human papillomavirus DNA sequences by using conserved primers. *J. Clin. Microbiol.*, **27**, 2660–5.

Griffiths, M., Penna, L. K. & Tovey, S. J. (1991). Aceto-white change of the glans penis associated with balanitis not human papillomavirus infection. *Int. J. STD AIDS*, **2**, 211–12.

Gross, G. (1987). Lesions of the male and female external genitalia associated with human papillomaviruses. In *Papillomaviruses and Human Disease*, ed. K. Syrjänen, L. Gissmann & L. G. Koss, pp. 197–235. Berlin, Heidelberg: Springer-Verlag.

Gutman, L. T., Herman-Giddens, M. E. & Phelps, W. C. (1993). Transmission of human genital papillomavirus disease: Comparsion of data from adults and children. *Pediatrics*, **91**, 31–8.

Haase, A. T., Retzel, E. F. & Staskus, K. A. (1990). Amplification and detection of lentiviral DNA inside cells. *Proc. Natl Acad. Sci. USA*, **87**, 4971–5.

Hajek, E. F. (1956). Clinical records: contribution to the etiology of laryngeal papilloma in children. *J. Laryngol. Otol.*, **70**, 166–168.

Hallden, C. & Majmudar, B. (1986). The relationship between juvenile laryngeal papillomatosis and maternal condylomata. *J. Reprod. Med.*, **31**, 804–87.

Handley, J. M., Maw, R. D., Bingham, E. A., Horner, T., Bharucha, H., Swann, A., Lawther, H. & Dinsmore, W. W. (1993). Anogenital warts in children. *Clin. Exp. Dermatol.*, **18**, 241–7.

Hartley, C., Hamilton, J., Birzgalis, A. R. & Farrington, W. T. (1994). Recurrent respiratory papillomatosis – the Manchester experience, 1974–1992. *J. Laryngol. Otol.*, **108**, 226–9.

Helmrich, G., Stubbs, T. M. & Stoerker, J. (1992). Fetal maternal laryngeal papillomatosis in pregnancy: a case report. *Am. J. Obstet. Gynecol.*, **166**, 524–5.

Hermonat, P. L., Han, L., Wendel, P. J., Quirk, J. G., Stern, S., Lowery, C. L. & Rechthin, T. M. (1997). Human papillomavirus is more prevalent in first trimester spontaneously aborted products of conception to elective specimens. *Virus Genes*, **14**, 13–17.

Hermonat, P. L., Kechelava, S., Lowery, C. L. & Korourian, S. (1998). Trophoblasts are the preferential target for human papilloma virus infection in spontaneously aborted products of conception. *Hum. Pathol.*, **29**, 170–4.

Hildesheim, A., Gravitt, P., Schiffman, M. H., Kurman, R. J., Barnes, W., Jones, S., Tchabo, J. G., Brinton, L. A., Copeland, C., Epp, J. & Manos, M. M. (1993). Determinants of genital human papillomavirus infection in low-income women in Washington, D.C. *Sex. Transm. Dis.*, **20**, 279–85.

Hildesheim, A., Schiffman, M. H., Gravitt, P. E., Glass, A. G., Greer, C. E., Zhang, T., Scott, D. R., Rush, B. B., Lawler, P., Sherman, M. E., Kurman, R. J. & Manos, M. M. (1994). Persistence of type-specific human papillomavirus infection among cytologically normal women. *J. Infect. Dis.*, **169**, 235–40.

Hippeläinen, M., Yliskoski, M., Syrjänen, S., Saastamoinen, J., Saarikoski, S. & Syrjänen, K.

(1994). Low concordance of genital human papillomavirus (HPV) lesions and viral types in HPV-infected women and their male sexual partners. *Sex. Transm. Dis.*, **21**, 76–82.

Hirschfield, L. S. & Steinberg, B. M. (1989). Clinical spectrum of HPV infection in the neonate and child. *Clin. Pract. Gynecol.*, **2**, 102–16.

Ho, L., Tay, S. K., Chan, S. Y. & Bernard, H. U. (1993). Sequence variants of human papillomavirus type 16 from couples suggest sexual transmission with low infectivity and polyclonality in genital neoplasia. *J. Infect. Dis.*, **168**, 803–9.

Hönig, J. F., Becker, H. J., Brinck, U. & Korabiowska, M. (1995). Detection of human papillomavirus DNA sequences in leukocytes: a new approach to identify hematological markers of HPV infection in patients with oral SCC. *Bull. Group. Int. Rech. Sci. Stomatol. Odontol.*, **38**, 25–31.

IARC (1995). *Monograph on the Evaluation of Carcinogenic Risks on Humans*. Vol. 64. *Papillomaviruses*. pp. 1–409. Lyon: IARC.

Inoue, M., Nakazawa, A., Fujita, M. & Tanizawa, O. (1992). Human papillomavirus (HPV) type 16 in semen of partners of women with HPV infection. *Lancet*, **339**, 1114–15.

Jalal, H., Sanders, C. M., Prime, S. S., Scully, C. & Maitland, N. J. (1992). Detection of human papilloma virus type 16 DNA in oral squames from normal young adults. *J. Oral Pathol. Med.*, **21**, 465–70.

Kashima, H. & Mounts, P. (1987). Tumors of the head and neck, larynx, lung and esophagus and their possible relation to HPV. In *Papillomaviruses and Human Disease*, ed. K. Syrjänen, L. Gissmann & L. G. Koss, pp. 138–57. Berlin, Heidelberg: Springer-Verlag.

Kashima, H. K., Kessis, T., Mounts, P. & Shah, K. (1991). Polymerase chain reaction identification of human papillomavirus DNA in CO_2 laser plume from recurrent respiratory papillomatosis. *Otolaryngol. Head Neck Surg.*, **104**, 191–5.

Kashima, H. K., Shah, F., Lyles, A., Glackin, R., Muhammad, N., Turner, L., van Zandt, S., Whitt, S. & Shah, K. (1992). A comparison of risk factors in juvenile-onset and adult-onset recurrent respiratory papillomatosis. *Laryngoscope*, **102**, 9–13.

Kataja, V., Syrjänen, S., Yliskoski, M., Hippeläinen, M., Väyrynen, M., Saarikoski, S., Mäntyjärvi, R., Jokela, V., Salonen, J. T. & Syrjänen, K. (1993). Risk factors associated with cervical human papillomavirus infections: a case-control study. *Am. J. Epidemiol.*, **138**, 735–45.

Kaye, J. N., Cason, J., Pakarian, F., Jewers, R. J., Kell, B., Bible, J., Raju, K. S. & Best, J. M. (1994). Viral load as a determinant for transmission of human papillomavirus type 16 from mother to child. *J. Med. Virol.*, **44**, 415–21.

Kaye, J. N., Starkey, W. G., Kell, B., Biswas, C., Raju, K. S., Best, J. M. & Cason, J., (1996). Human papillomavirus type 16 in infants: use of DNA sequence analyses to determine the source of infection. *J. Gen. Virol.*, **77**, 1139–43.

Kedzia, H., Gozdzicka Jozefiak, A., Wolna, M. & Tomczak, E. (1992). Distribution of human papillomavirus 16 in the blood of women with uterine cervix carcinoma. *Eur. J. Gynaecol. Oncol.*, **13**, 522–6.

Kirnbauer, R., Booy, F., Cheng, N., Lowy, D. R. & Schiller, J. T. (1992). Papillomavirus L1 major capsid protein self-assembles into virus-like particles that are highly immunogenic. *Proc. Natl Acad. Sci. USA*, **89**, 12180–4.

Kirnbauer, R., Taub, J., Greenstone, H., Rdoen, R., Durst, M., Gissmann, L., Lowry, D. R. & Schiller, J. T. (1993). Efficient self-assembly of human papillomavirus type 16 L1 and L1-L2 into virus-like particles. *J. Virol.*, **67**, 6929–36.

Koch, A., Hansen, S. V., Nielsen, N. M., Palefsky, J. & Melbye, M. (1997). HPV detection in children prior to sexual debut. *Int. J. Cancer*, **27**, 621–4.

Koss, L. G. (1987). Carcinogenesis in the uterine cervix and human papillomavirus infection. In *Papillomaviruses and Human Disease*, ed. K. Syrjänen, L. Gissmann & L. G. Koss, pp. 233–67. Berlin, Heidelberg: Springer-Verlag.

Kotloff, K. L., Wasserman, S. S., Russ, K., Shapiro, S., Daniel, R., Brown, W., Frost, A., Tabara, S. O. & Shah, K. (1998). Detection of genital human papillomavirus and associated cytological abnormalities among college women. *Sex. Transm. Dis.*, **25**, 243–50.

Koutsky, L. A., Galloway, D. A. & Holmes, K. K. (1988). Epidemiology of genital human papillomavirus infection. *Epidemiol. Rev.*, **10**, 122–63.

Koutsky, L. A. (1997). Epidemiology of genital human papillomavirus infection. *Am. J. Med.*, **102**, 3–8.

Krebs, H. B. (1991). Treatment of genital condylomata with topical 5-fluorouracil. *Dermatol. Clin.*, **9**, 333–41.

Kurvinen, K., Hietanen, S., Syrjänen, K. & Syrjänen, S. (1995). Rapid and effective detection of mutations in the p53 gene using nonradioactive single-strand conformation polymorphism (SSCP) technique applied on PhastSystem™. *J. Virol. Methods*, **51**, 43–54.

La Porta, R. F. & Taichman, L. B. (1982). Human papilloma viral DNA replicates as a stable episome in cultured epidermal keratinocytes. *Proc. Natl Acad. Sci. USA*, **79**, 3393–7.

Lai, Y. M., Yang, F. P. & Pao, C. C. (1996). Human papillomavirus deoxyribonucleic acid and ribonucleic acid in seminal plasma and sperm cells. *Fertil. Steril.*, **65**, 1026–30.

Lancaster, W. D. & Meinke, W. (1975). Persistence of viral DNA in human cell cultures infected with human papilloma virus. *Nature*, **256**, 434–6.

Ley, C., Bauer, H. M., Reingold, A., Schiffman, M. H., Chamebers, J. C., Tashiro, C. J. & Manos, M. M. (1991). Determinants of genital human papillomavirus infection in young women. *J. Natl. Cancer Inst.*, **83**, 997–1003.

Lindeberg, H. & Elbrønd, O. (1991). Malignant tumours in patients with a history of multiple laryngeal papillomas: the significance of irradiation. *Clin. Otolaryngol.*, **16**, 149–51.

Lindeberg, H., Syrjänen, S. M., Kärjä, J. & Syrjänen, K. (1989). Human papillomavirus type 11 DNA in squamous cell carcinomas and pre-existing multiple laryngeal papillomas. *Acta Otolaryngol.(Stockh.)*, **107**, 141–9.

Lou, Y-K., McKinnon, K. J., Ormsby, S. M., Nightingale, B. N. & Morris, B. J. (1991). Papillomavirus DNA and colposcopy instruments. *Lancet*, **338**, 1601–2.

Maitland, N. J., Cox, M. F., Lynas, C., Prime, S., Crane, I. & Scully, C. (1987). Nucleic acid probes in the study of latent viral disease. *J. Oral Pathol.*, **16**, 199–211.

Manos, M. M., Ting, Y., Wright, D. K., Lewis, A. S., Broker, T. R. & Wolinsky, S. M. (1989). Use of polymerase chain reaction amplification for the detection of genital human papillomaviruses. *Cancer Cells*, **7**, 209–14.

Massing, A. M. & Epstein, W. L. (1963). Natural history of warts. *Arch. Dermatol.*, **87**, 74.

Matsunaga, J., Bergman, A. & Bhatia, N. N. (1987). Genital condylomata acuminata in pregnancy: effectiveness, safety and pregnancy outcome following cryotherapy. *Br. J. Obstet. Gynaecol.*, **94**, 168–72.

Maxwell, G. L., Carlson, D. O., Zakarean, M., Veit, B. & Hoshaw, N. (1998). The absence of human papillomavirus in amniotic fluid. *J. Lower Genital Tract Dis.*, **2**, 151–4.

Maymon, R., Shulman, A., Maymon, B., Bekerman, A., Werchow, M., Faktor J. H. & Altaras, M. (1994). Penile condylomata: a gynecological epidemic disease: A review of the current approach and management aspects. *Obstet. Gynecol. Surv.*, **49**, 790–800.

McCance, D. J., Campion, M. J., Baram, A. & Singer, A. (1986). Risk of transmission of human papillomavirus by vaginal specula. *Lancet*, **ii**, 816–17.

McDonnell, P. J., McDonnell, J. M., Kessis, T., Green, W. R. & Shah, K. V. (1987). Detection of human papillomavirus type 6/11 DNA in conjunctival papillomas by in situ hybridization with radioactive probes. *Hum. Pathol.*, **18**, 1115–19.

Meisels, A. & Fortin, R. (1976). Condylomatous lesions of the cervix and vagina. Cytologic patterns. *Acta Cytol.*, **20**, 505–9.

Meisels, A., Morin, C., Casas Cordero, M. & Rabreau, M. (1983). Human papillomavirus (HPV) venereal infections and gynecologic cancer. *Pathol.Annu.*, **18**, 277–93.

Millikan, R. C. (1994). Epidemiologic evidence showing that human papillomavirus infection causes most cervical intraepithelial neoplasia [letter]. *J. Natl Cancer Inst.*, **86**, 392–3.

Monk, B. J., Cook, N., Ahn, C., Vasilev, S. A., Berman, M. L. & Wilczynski, S. P. (1994). Comparison of the polymerase chain reaction and southern blot analysis in detecting and typing human papillomavirus deoxyribonucleic acid in tumors of the lower female genital tract. *Diagn. Mol. Pathol.*, **3**, 283–91.

Moscicki, A. B., Palefsky, J., Smith, G., Siboshski, S. & Schoolnik, G. (1993). Variability of human papillomavirus DNA testing in a longitudinal cohort of young women. *Obstet. Gynecol.*, **82**, 578–85.

Mounts, P. & Shah, K. V. (1984). Respiratory papillomatosis: etiological relation to genital tract papillomaviruses. *Prog. Med. Virol.*, **29**, 90–114.

Nuovo, G. J., Gallery, F., MacConnell, P., Becker, J. & Bloch, W. (1991a). An improved technique for the in situ detection of DNA after polymerase chain reaction amplification. *Am. J. Pathol.*, **139**, 1239–44.

Nuovo, G. J., MacConnell, P., Forde, A. & Delvenne, P. (1991b). Detection of human papillomavirus DNA in formalin-fixed tissues by in situ hybridization after amplification by polymerase chain reaction. *Am. J. Pathol.*, **139**, 847–54.

Obalek, S., Jablonska, S., Favre, M., Walczak, L. & Orth, G. (1990). Condylomata acuminata in children: frequent association with human papillomaviruses responsible for cutaneous warts. *J. Am. Acad. Dermatol.*, **23**, 205–13.

Oriel, J. D. (1971). Natural history of genital warts. *Br. J. Vener. Dis.*, **47**, 1–13.

Ostrow, R. S., Zachow, K. R., Niimura, M., Okagaki, T., Muller, S., Bender, M. & Faras. A. J. (1986). Detection of papillomavirus DNA in human semen. *Science*, **231**, 731–33.

Pacheco, B. P., DiPaola, G., Ribas, J. M., Vighi, S. & Rueda, N. G. (1991). Vulvar infection caused by human papilloma virus in children and adolescents without sexual contact. *Adolesc. Pediatr. Gynecol.*, **4**, 136–42.

Padel, A. F., Venning, V. A., Evans, M. F., Quantrill, A. M. & Fleming, K. A. (1990). Human papillomaviruses in anogenital warts in children: typing by in situ hybridization. *Br. Med. J.*, **300**, 1491–4.

Pakarian, F., Kaye, J., Cason, J., Kell, B., Jewers, R., Derias, N. W., Faju, K. S. & Best, J. M. (1994). Cancer associated human papillomaviruses: perinatal transmission and persistence. *Br. J. Obstet. Gynaecol.*, **101**, 514–17.

Palefsky, J. M. (1995). Serologic detection of human papillomavirus-related anogenital disease: new opportunities and challenges. *J. Natl .Cancer Inst.*, **87**, 401–2.

Pao, C. C., Lin, S. S., Lin, C. Y., Maa, J. S., Lai, C. H. & Hsieh, T. T. (1991). Identification of human papillomavirus DNA sequences in peripheral blood mononuclear cells. *Am. J. Clin. Pathol.*, **95**, 540–6.

Pao, C. C., Tsai, P. L., Chang, Y. L., Hsieh, T. T. & Jin, J. Y. (1993). Possible non-sexual transmission of genital human papillomavirus infections in young women. *Eur. J. Clin. Microbiol. Infect. Dis.*, **12**, 221–2.

Pao, C. C., Hor, J. J., Wu, C. J., Shi, Y. F., Xie, X. & Lu, S. M. (1995). Human papillomavirus type 18 DNA in gestational trophoblastic tissues and choriocarcinomas . *Int. J. Cancer*, **15**, 505–9.

Phelps, W. C. & Alexander, K. A. (1995). Antiviral therapy for human papillomaviruses: rationale and prospects. *Ann. Intern. Med.*, **123**, 368–82.

Puranen, M., Syrjänen, K. & Syrjänen, S. (1996a) Transmission of human papillomavirus (HPV) infections is unlikely through the floor and seats of humid dwelling in countries of high-level hygiene. *Scand. J. Infect. Dis.*, **28**, 243–6.

Puranen, M., Yliskoski, M., Saarikoski, S., Syrjänen, K. & Syrjänen, S. (1996b). Vertical transmission of human papillomavirus from infected mothers to their newborn babies and persistence of the virus in the childhood. *Am. J. Obstet. Gynecol.*, **174**, 694–9.

Purola, E. & Savia, E. (1977). Cytology of gynecologic condyloma acuminatum. *Acta Cytol.*, **21**, 26–31.

Quick, C. A., Watts, S. L., Krzyzek, R. A. & Faras, A. J. (1980). Relationship between condylomata and laryngeal papillomata. Clinical and molecular virological evidence. *Ann. Otol. Rhinol. Laryngol.*, **89**, 467–71.

Rady, P. L., Chin, R., Arany, I., Hughes, T. K. & Tyring, S. K. (1993). Direct sequencing of consensus primer generated PCR fragments of human papillomaviruses. *J. Virol. Methods*, **43**, 335–50.

Rando, R. F., Lindheim, S., Hasty, L., Sedlacek, T. V., Woodland, M. & Eder, C. (1989). Increased frequency of detection of human papillomavirus deoxyribonucleic acid in exfoliated cervical cells during pregnancy. *Am. J. Obstet. Gynecol.*, **161**, 50–5.

Rock, B., Naghashfar, Z., Barnett, N., Buscema, J., Woodruff, J. D. & Shah, K. (1986). Genital tract papillomavirus infection in children. *Arch. Dermatol.*, **122**, 1129–32.

Rogo, K. O. & Nyansera, P. N. (1989). Congenital condylomata acuminata with meconium staining of amniotic fluid and fetal hydrocephalus: case report. *East Afr. Med. J.*, **66**, 411–13.

Roman, A. & Fife, K. H. (1989). Human papillomaviruses: are we ready to type? *Clin. Microbiol. Rev.*, **2**, 166–90.

Schiffman, M. H. (1992). Recent progress in defining the epidemiology of human papillomavirus infection and cervical neoplasia. *J. Natl. Cancer Inst.*, **84**, 394–8.

Schiffman, M. H., Bauer, H. M., Hoover, R. N., Glass, A. E., Cadell, D. M., Rush, B. B., Scott, D.

R., Sherman, M. E., Kurman, R. J. Weholder, S., Stanton, C. K. & Manos, M. M. (1993). Epidemiologic evidence showing that human papillomavirus infection causes most cervical intraepithelial neoplasia. *J. Natl. Cancer Inst.*, **85**, 958–64.

Schiffman, M. H. (1994). Epidemiology of cervical human papillomavirus infections. *Curr. Top. Microbiol. Immunol.*, **186**, 55–81.

Schneider, A., Hotz, M. & Gissmann, L. (1987). Increased prevalence of human papillomaviruses in the lower genital tract of pregnant women. *Int. J. Cancer*, **40**, 198–201.

Schneider, A., Kirchmayr, R., de Villiers, E-M. & Gissmann, L. (1988). Subclinical human papillomavirus infections in male sexual partners of female carriers. *J. Urol.*, **140**, 1431–34.

Schneider, A., Kirchhoff, T., Meinhardt, G. & Gissmann, L. (1992). Repeated evaluation of human papillomavirus 16 status in cervical swabs of young women with a history of normal Papanicolaou smears. *Obstet.Gynecol.*, **79**, 683–8.

Schneider, V., Kay, S. & Lee, H. M. (1983). Immunosuppression as a high risk factor in the development of condyloma accuminatum and squamous neoplasia of the cervix. *Acta Cytol.*, **27**, 220–4.

Schwartz, D. B., Greenberg, M. D., Daoud, Y. & Reid, R. (1988). Genital condylomas in pregnancy: use of trichloroacetic acid and laser therapy. *Am. J. Obstet. Gynecol.*, **158**, 1407–16.

Sedlacek, T. V., Lindheim, S., Eder, C., Hasty, L., Woodland, M., Ludomirsky, A. & Rando, R. F. (1989). Mechanism for human papillomavirus transmission at birth. *Am. J. Obstet. Gynecol.*, **161**, 55–9.

Shah, K., Kashima, H., Polk, B. F., Shah, F., Abbey, H. & Abramson, A. (1986). Rarity of cesarean delivery in cases of juvenile-onset respiratory papillomatosis. *Obstet. Gynecol.*, **68**, 795–9.

Shah, K. V., Stern, W. F., Shah, F. K., Bishai, D. & Kashima, H. (1998). Risk factors for juvenile onset recurrent respiratory papillomatosis. *Pediatr. Inf. Dis. J.*, **17**, 372–6.

Simma, B., Burger, R., Uehlinger, J., Ghelfi, D., Hof, E., Dangel, P., Briner, J. & Fanconi, S. (1993). Squamous-cell carcinoma arising in a non-irradiated child with recurrent respiratory papillomatosis. *Eur. J. Pediatr.*, **152**, 776–8.

Smith, E. M., Johnson, S. R., Cripe, T. P., Perlman, S., McGuinness, G., Jiang, D., Cripe, L. & Turek, L. P. (1995). Perinatal transmission and maternal risks of human papillomavirus infection. *Cancer Detect. Prevent.*, **19**, 196–205.

Snijders, P. J., van den Brüle, A. J., Schrijnemakers, H. F., Snow, G., Meijer, C. J. & Walboomers, J. M. (1990). The use of general primers in the polymerase chain reaction permits the detection of a broad spectrum of human papillomavirus genotypes. *J. Gen. Virol.*, **71**, 173–81.

Snoeck, R., Wellens, W., Desloovere, C., van Randst, M., Ryder, R. W., Heyward, W. L. & Reeves, W. C. (1998). Treatment of severe laryngeal papillomatosis with intralesional injections of cidofovir [(S)-1-(3-hydroxy-2-phosphonylmethoxypropyl) cytosine]. *J. Med. Virol.*, **54**, 219–25.

Soares, V. R., Nieminen, P., Aho, M., Vesterinen, E., Vaheri, A. & Paavonen, J. (1990). Human papillomavirus DNA in unselected pregnant and non-pregnant women. *Int. J. STD AIDS*, **1**, 276–8.

Sokal, D. C. & Hermonat, P. L. (1995). Inactivation of papillomavirus by low concentrations of povidone-iodine. *Sex. Transm. Dis.*, **22**, 22–4.

St Louis, M. E., Icenogle, J. P., Manzila, T., Kamenga, M., Ryder, R. W., Heyward, W. L. &

Reeves, W. C. (1993). Genital types of papillomavirus in children of women with HIV-1 infection in Kinshasa, Zaire. *Int. J. Cancer*, **54**, 181–4.

Stanley, M. A., Chambers, M. A. & Coleman, N. (1995). Immunology of human papillomavirus infection. In *Genital Warts. Human Papillomavirus Infection*, ed. A. Mindel, pp. 253–70. London: Edward Arnold.

Strong, M., Vaughan, C. W., Healy, B., Cooperband, S. & Clemente, M. (1976). Recurrent respiratory papillomatosis. *Ann. Otol. Rhinol. Laryngol.*, **85**, 508–16.

Stumpf, P. G. (1980). Increasing occurrence of condylomata acuminata in premenarchal children. *Obstet. Gynecol.*, **56**, 262–4.

Syrjänen, K J. (1989a). Epidemiology of human papillomavirus (HPV) infections and their associations with genital squamous cell cancer. *APMIS*, **97**, 957–70.

Syrjänen, K J. (1989b). Histopathology, cytology, immunohistochemistry and HPV typing techniques. In *Genital Papilloma Virus Infection: A Survey for the Clinician*, ed. G. von Grogh & E. Rylander, pp. 33–67. Karlstad, Sweden: Conpharm AB.

Syrjänen, K. J. (1990). Natural history of genital HPV infections. *Papillomavirus Rep.*, **1**, 1–5.

Syrjänen, K. J. (1992). Genital human papillomavirus (HPV) infections and their associations with squamous cell cancer: reappraisal of the morphologic, epidemiologic and DNA data. In *Progress in Surgical Pathology*, ed. C. M. Fenoglio-Preiser, M. Wolff & F. Rilke, pp. 217–40. New York: Field & Wood.

Syrjänen, K. J. (1995). Association of human papillomavirus with penile cancer. In *Genital Warts. Human Papillomavirus Infection*, ed. A. Mindel, pp. 163–97. London: Edward Arnold.

Syrjänen, K. J. & Syrjänen, S. M. (1990). Epidemiology of human papilloma virus infections and genital neoplasia. *Scand. J. Infect. Dis.*, **69**, 7–17.

Syrjänen K. J. & Syrjänen, S. (2000) *Papillomavirus Infections in Human Pathology*. Wiley, London, Paris. pp. 1–620.

Syrjänen, K. J., Väyrynen, M., Castren, O., Yliskoski, M., Mäntyjarvi, R., Pyrhönen, S., & Saarikoski, S. (1984). Sexual behaviour of women with human papillomavirus (HPV) lesions of the uterine cervix. *Br. J. Vener. Dis.*, **60**, 243–8.

Syrjänen, K. J., Väyrynen, M., Saarikoski, S. Mäntyjarvi, R., Parkkinen, S., Hippeläinen, M. & Castren, O. (1985). Natural history of cervical Human papillomavirus (HPV) infections based on prospective follow-up. *Br. J. Obstet. Gynaecol.*, **92**, 1086.

Syrjänen, K. J., Gissmann, L. & Koss, L. G. (1987). *Papillomaviruses and Human Disease.*, pp. 1–518. Berlin; New York: Springer-Verlag.

Syrjänen, K. J., Hakama, M., Saarikoski, S., Väyrynen, M., Yliskoski, M., Syrjänen, S., Kataja, V. & Castren, O. (1990). Prevalence, incidence, and estimated life-time risk of cervical human papillomavirus infections in a nonselected Finnish female population. *Sex. Transm. Dis.*, **17**, 15–19.

Syrjänen, K. J., Kataja, V., Yliskoski, M., Chang, F., Syrjänen, S. & Saarikoski, S. (1992). Natural history of cervical HPV lesions with special emphasis on the biologic relevance of the Bethesda System. *Obstet. Gynecol.*, **79**, 675.

Syrjänen, S. M. (1987). Human papillomavirus infections in the oral cavity. In *Papillomaviruses and Human Disease*, ed. K. J. Syrjänen, L. Gissmann & L. G. Koss, pp. 104–37. Heidelberg: Springer-Verlag.

Syrjänen, S. M. (1990). Basic concepts and practical applications of recombinant DNA techniques in detection of human papillomavirus (HPV) infection. Review article. *APMIS*, **98**, 95–110.

Tang, C-K., Shermeta, D. W. & Wood, C. (1978). Congenital condylomata acuminata. *Am. J. Obstet. Gynecol.*, **131**, 912–13.

Tseng, C-J., Lin, C-Y., Wang, R-L., Chen, L. J., Chang, Y. L., Hsieh, T. T. & Pao, C. C. (1992). Possible transplacental transmission of human papillomaviruses. *Am. J. Obstet. Gynecol.*, **166**, 35–40.

Tseng, C. J., Liang, C. C., Soong, Y. K. & Pao, C. C. (1998). Perinatal transmission of human papillomavirus in infants: relationship between infection rate and mode of delivery. *Obstet. Gynecol.*, **91**, 92–6.

Valente, P. T., Hurt, M. A. & Jelen, I. (1991). Human papillomavirus – associated vulvar verrucous carcinoma in a 20-year-old with an intact hymen. A case report. *J. Reprod. Med.*, **36**, 213–16.

Watts, D. H., Koutsky, L. A., Holmes, K. K., Goldman, D., Kuypers, J., Kiviat, N. B. & Galloway, D. A. (1998). Low risk of perinatal transmission of human papillomavirus: results from a prospective cohort study. *Am. J. Obstet. Gynecol.*, **178**, 365–73.

Wheeler, C. M., Parmenter, C. A., Hunt, W. C., Becker, T. M., Greer, C. E., Hildesheim, A. & Manos, M. M. (1993). Determinants of genital human papillomavirus infection among cytologically normal women attending the University of New Mexico student health center. *Sex. Transm. Dis.*, **20**, 286–9.

Wheeler, C. M., Greer, C. E., Becker, T. M., Hunt, W. C., Anderson, S. M. & Manos, M. M. (1996). Short-term fluctuations in the detection of cervical human papillomavirus DNA. *Obstet. Gynecol.*, **88**, 261–8.

White, D. O. (1994). *Medical Virology*, 4th edn. pp. 13–15. San Diego: Academic Press.

Wu, T. C. (1995). Immunology of the papilloma virus in relation to cancer. *Curr. Opin. Immunol.*, **6**, 746–54.

Yell, J. A., Sinclair, R., Mann, S., Fleming, K. & Ryan, T. J. (1993). Human papillomavirus type 6-induced condylomata: an unusual complication of intertrigo. *Br. J. Dermatol.*, **128**, 575–7.

Yliskoski, M., Saarikoski, S., Syrjänen, K., Syrjänen, S. M. & Castren, O. (1989). Cryotherapy and CO_2-laser vaporization in the treatment of cervical and vaginal human papillomavirus (HPV) infections. *Acta Obstet. Gynecol. Scand.*, **68**, 619–25.

Yliskoski, M., Saarikoski, S. & Syrjänen, K. (1991). Conization for CIN associated with human papillomavirus infection. *Arch. Gynecol. Obstet.*, **249**, 59–65.

Yoder, M. G. & Batsakis, J. G. (1980). Squamous cell carcinoma in solitary laryngeal papilloma. *Otolaryngol. Head Neck Surg.*, **88**, 745–8.

Zehbe, I., Sällström, J. F., Evander, M., Edlund, K., Rylander, E., Wadell, E. & Wilander, E. (1996). Non-radioisotopic detection and typing of human papillomaviruses (HPVs) by use of polymerase chain reaction and single-strand conformation polymorphism (PCR–SSCP). *Diagn. Mol. Pathol.*, **5**, 206–13.

zur Hausen, H. (1994). Molecular pathogenesis of cancer of the cervix and its causation by specific human papillomavirus types. *Curr. Top. Microbiol. Immunol.*, **186**, 131–56.

12

HIV-1 infection

Glenda Gray, James McIntyre and Marie-Louise Newell

Introduction

More than 33 million people were living with HIV by the end of 1998. According to UNAIDS estimates, 22.5 million of these were in Africa (67%), and 6.7 million in South and Southeast Asia (20%). Close to six million new infections are occurring each year, with 10% of these in children, the majority as a result of mother-to-child transmission (MTCT) (UNAIDS, 1998). An estimated one and a half to two million HIV-infected women will become pregnant each year, with 1600 children each day infected by mother-to-child transmission.

In Europe, the increase in heterosexually acquired HIV infection in women of childbearing age has been paralleled by increasing numbers of infected children. Antenatal HIV prevalence in Europe is generally below 5 per 1000 deliveries, although variable: higher in selected groups and inner cities. In a number of countries in Africa south-of-the-Sahara, 10–25% of pregnant women are infected, with rates of over 40% reported in parts of Southern Africa (US Bureau of the Census, 1999; Stanecki & Way, 1999). Southeast Asia has seen a rapid rise in infection rates in some areas.

HIV infected children most commonly present early in life with non-specific clinical manifestations. About one-quarter of infected children will develop AIDS in the first year of life, but the progression of disease in the remainder is much slower. In developed countries about 75% of infected children are alive by age 5 years, and in developing countries about 40% (French Pediatric HIV Infection Study Group and European Collaborative Study, 1997). HIV/AIDS has increased infant and child mortality dramatically in the most affected African countries, and is expected to lead to a doubling of under-5 mortality by 2010 in southern African countries. In contrast, successful prevention interventions in parts of the USA, Europe and other developed countries have reduced mother-to-child transmission rates to below 5% and almost complete elimination of vertical infection is being viewed as a possibility in the future (Mofenson, 1999).

Human immunodeficiency virus

The human immunodeficiency virus (HIV) is a retrovirus, which has as its main target cell the helper/inducer T-lymphocytes. The destruction of these lymphocytes results in immunosuppression and increased susceptibility to common infections and AIDS. There are at least two types of HIV of which HIV-1 is the most prevalent and pathogenic. HIV-2 is uncommon in Western countries, less transmissible and in this section we refer to HIV-1 (Adjorlolo Johnson et al., 1994). HIV infection is transmitted in three ways: sexually, through contaminated blood and vertically from mother to child.

Mother-to-child transmission

Mother-to-child transmission (MTCT) is the dominant mode of acquisition of infection for children. However, in countries where safe blood supply is not available, and where medically used needles and syringes are in short supply and reuse is routine, acquisition of infection through blood transfusion or contaminated needles and syringes remains a strong possibility.

Estimates of the rates of vertical transmission vary between studies and between population groups. Historically, the rate of vertical transmission in Europe was 15–20%, in the USA 15–30% and in Africa and Asia 25–45% (Working Group on Mother-to-Child Transmission of HIV, 1995). The introduction of antiretroviral treatment in pregnancy and other interventions has further reduced rates in developed countries. Differences between populations in the rate of mother-to-child transmission are related to differences in the distribution of risk factors associated with increased transmission.

Early in utero HIV infection is rare, and the importance of intrapartum acquisition of infection is generally acknowledged (European Mode of Delivery Collaboration, 1999). The exchange of blood between mother and child during labour and at the time of delivery, and the detection of virus in cervical secretions, make acquisition of infection at this stage plausible. Postnatal transmission of infection through breastfeeding can occur in infants born to women with established infection, as well as in infants born to mothers who become infected postnatally (Dunn et al., 1992).

Risk factors for vertical transmission

Mother-to-child transmission is associated with maternal factors or factors surrounding the delivery as well as with breastfeeding. These are summarized in Table 12.1. Maternal factors linked with increased likelihood of transmission include genetic factors, which may be associated with immune response (such as the HLA

Table 12.1. Factors associated with mother-to-child transmission of HIV

Vital	Viral load
	Viral genotype and phenotype
	Viral resistance
Maternal	Immunological status
	Nutritional status
	Clinical status
	Behavioural factors
	Antiretroviral treatment
Obstetrical	Mode of delivery
	Prolonged rupture of membranes
	Intrapartum haemorrhage
	Obstetrical procedures
	Invasive fetal monitoring
Fetal	Prematurity
	Genetic
	Multiple pregnancy
Infant	Breastfeeding
	Gastrointestinal tract factors
	Immature immune system

Adapted from World Health Organization (1999).

system). The presence of other sexually transmitted diseases and chorioamnionitis may increase the HIV load in the cervical tract and cause increased exposure to infection for the fetus (Goldenberg et al., 1998). A mother who has recently become infected, with a primary infection, might be more likely to transmit the infection, as her viral load is likely to be higher than in established infection. Similarly, the viral load is increased in advanced disease and the risk of transmission higher than in the clinically latent stage of infection. Recently, it has become possible to measure directly the effect of viral load. Several small studies have reported an increase in transmission rate with increasing viral load, although there is no threshold below which transmission does not occur (Borkowsky, et al., 1994; Fang et al., 1995; Dickover et al., 1996). A strong association between viral load and the risk of transmission was seen in Thailand, for both in utero and intrapartum transmission. In this study, transmitting mothers had 4.3-fold higher median plasma HIV RNA level at delivery than did non-transmitters ($P < 0.001$) (Shaffer et al., 1999a,b; Mock et al., 1999). It has been suggested that some clades or viral subtypes may be more likely to be transmitted than others, but quantitative evidence is lacking. Clade C in particular may have a higher rate of transmission (Renjifo et al., 1999).

Placental factors have been implicated in mother-to-child transmission of HIV (Temmerman et al., 1995; St Louis et al., 1993; Goldenberg et al., 1998). Infection of the placenta with HIV-1 has been reported, and CD4+ is expressed on Hofbauer cells and possibly trophoblasts which are thus susceptible to infection (Douglas & King, 1992). An association between increased transmission and the presence of chorioamnionitis was described early in the epidemic and other placental infections and non-infectious conditions such as abruptio placentae have also been implicated, (Boyer et al., 1994). Smoking and drug use, both associated with increased transmission, may influence transmission through placental disruption: even in the absence of these risk factors, breaks in the placental surface can occur at any stage of pregnancy and may be related to transmission, although the significance of these may, in turn, depend upon the maternal viral load (Burton et al., 1996). In areas of high malaria prevalence, placental involvement is common. Malarial infestation of the placenta with *P. falciparum* has been associated with poorer survival in infants born to HIV-1 positive mothers in Malawi, which may represent increased transmission rates (Bloland et al., 1995) and with higher rates of transmission from mother to child in Kenya (Nahlen et al., 1998). Prematurity has been linked to increased likelihood of transmission (European Collaborative Study 1999). The time between rupture of membranes and delivery, as well as the duration of the second stage of labour influence the exposure of the infant to HIV-infected maternal fluids, and may, therefore, affect the transmission risk (Burns et al., 1994; Landesman et al., 1996).

Information is accumulating on HIV viral load in the genital tract (Mostad & Kreiss, 1996; Kreiss et al., 1994) and possible associations with viraemia, and advanced disease. Henin et al. (1993) in a cross-sectional study estimated the prevalence of viral excretion in cervico-vaginal secretions of 55 women. Excretion of HIV was significantly higher in pregnant than in non-pregnant women, nearly 40% of whom had evidence of virus replication. More recently, studies have concentrated on the detection of actively replicating virus, HIV–RNA, and with increased sensitivity of the tests, cervical HIV–RNA can be detected in the majority of samples (Goulston et al., 1996). In the study by Goulston et al. (1996), cervical shedding of HIV RNA was associated with increased levels of plasma RNA, but this finding needs to be confirmed in larger studies. In a study in Nairobi the presence of DNA in the genital tract was associated with severe immunosuppression and severe vitamin A deficiency (John et al., 1997). The presence of sexually transmitted infections or other causes of inflammation and the local immune response may affect viral shedding (Landers, 1996).

As labour and delivery have been suggested as times of high risk for vertical transmission of HIV from mother to child, much attention has focused on the method of delivery as being an important time for intervention. Elective caesarean delivery has been shown to reduce the rate of transmission probably because of a reduced exposure to contaminated blood or cervical secretions (European Mode of Delivery Collaboration, 1999; International Perinatal HIV Group, 1999). Other modifications to obstetric practice, such as avoiding unnecessary episiotomy and avoiding the use of penetrating scalp electrodes have also been suggested (World Health Organization, 1999).

Breastfeeding

HIV can be transmitted from mother to child through breast milk (Van de Perre et al., 1991). Although HIV has been detected in breastmilk (Nduati et al., 1995; Ruff et al., 1994; Lewis et al., 1998), the exact mechanism by which transmission occurs is not fully understood. The risk of breastmilk transmission of HIV may be dependent on the size of the viral inoculum, the amount of cell-free and cell-associated HIV present in colostrum or breastmilk, the presence of antiviral substances and polyanionic milk proteins in breastmilk, the infant's individual susceptibility and local specific immune responses to HIV. Little is understood about the correlation between HIV RNA levels in plasma and breastmilk and its relation to transmission. Nduati et al. demonstrated an association between maternal immunosuppression and the prevalence and concentration of breastmilk HIV-1 DNA in a group of HIV infected women in Nairobi (Nduati et al., 1995).

HIV elicits a local humoral immune response in breastmilk. Both colostrum and mature breast milk of HIV infected women contain secretory IGA and secretory IgM to HIV antigens, including antibodies to the env-encoded surface glycoproteins. Van der Perre et al. (1993) found in a study looking at breastmilk samples of HIV infected women in Rwanda that lack of persistence of HIV specific IgM in breastmilk collected at 18 months was associated with a higher risk of transmission. The local immune response is likely to affect transmission of HIV through breastmilk.

It is presently unclear whether infection takes place through cell-free HIV in breastmilk or through cell-associated HIV. Cell-free and cell-associated HIV have both been detected in both colostrum and breastmilk. Cell-free virus could penetrate the mucosal lining of the gastrointestinal tract of infants by infecting cells, or directly into the blood stream via mucosal breaches.

Studies using animal models to explore potential mechanisms of transmission have demonstrated that it is possible to infect neonatal rhesus monkeys with simian immunodeficiency virus and kittens with feline immunodeficiency virus by applying cell-free virus on the mucosa. This may suggest that cell-free HIV in breastmilk could infect cells of the intestinal mucosa. In addition, Bomsel (1997) demonstrated in an in vitro study that HIV infected cells stimulated enterocytes to engulf HIV particles presented by HIV infected cells in the intestinal lumen, which may suggest that both cell-free and cell-associated HIV play a role in breastmilk transmission.

Presently it is unknown whether colostrum is more infectious than breastmilk. It is also unclear whether damage to the intestinal tract of the infant, caused by the early introduction of other foods, could increase its permeability and thus result in increased rates of acquisition of infection for the infant (Tess et al., 1997). The immature gastrointestinal tract of the newborn may facilitate transmission, however, this is not a requirement as transmission has been reported in infants who begin breastfeeding outside the neonatal period (Datta et al., 1994).

Transmission of HIV through breastmilk can occur in situations where the mother acquired the infection shortly after delivery, but also in established maternal infection. Based on a meta-analysis of limited evidence, it has been estimated that the additional risk of acquisition of infection through breastfeeding is between 7% and 22%, and in observational studies from South Africa, Brazil and Europe breastfeeding doubled the overall vertical transmission rate (European Collaborative Study, 1994; Mayaux et al., 1995; Gray et al., 1996; Newell et al., 1997; Tess et al., 1997). Transmission may be less related to the amount of exposure and more related to time of exposure, infectivity of milk or specific susceptibility of the infant. It has been suggested that the risk of vertical transmission may be particularly high for infants who receive other foods as well as breastmilk (Coutsoudis et al., 1999a), and there is little evidence to suggest that the risk of transmission is associated with duration of breastfeeding (de Martino et al., 1992; Tess et al., 1997). None of the studies to date on HIV transmission and breastfeeding has explored differences in transmission associated with variations in breastfeeding practices. In a posthoc subgroup analysis by Coutsoudis et al., no increase in risk of HIV transmission was observed in the first three months of age amongst infants who were exclusively breastfed compared to infants who where exclusively formula fed, with the highest rates observed among mixed feeders (Coutsoudis et al., 1999a). The mechanism by which exclusive breastfeeding may reduce the risk of postnatal transmission is unknown. Several mechanisms may be postulated to explain the protective effects of exclusive breastfeeding in HIV-1 transmission. These may be related to reduced exposure to dietary antigens and enteric pathogens that may cause inflammatory processes that facilitate HIV transmission across the gut mucosa, specific components of breastmilk, maternal hormonal or immunological factors or alterations in the integrity of epithelial tight junctions in the mammary gland.

Hypothesis of timing of transmission

A working definition of the timing of vertical transmission in non-breastfeeding populations has been proposed by Bryson and colleagues in which an infant is defined as infected intrauterine if there is a positive result of a culture or DNA–polymerase chain reaction (PCR) test on a sample drawn in the first 48 hours after birth (Bryson et al., 1992). Intrapartum acquisition of infection is assumed if there is a negative culture or PCR test in the first week of life, followed by a positive sample before 3 months of age. However, this definition is not based on experimental data, and the underlying assumption may not hold true if negative early specimens could be due to sequestration of the virus in an inaccessible location (such as lymph nodes or CNS). Furthermore, in breastfeeding populations infants are additionally exposed to HIV through breastmilk, and it is not possible to distinguish intrapartum from early postnatal acquisition of infection on the basis of virological tests.

There have been several attempts to quantify the relative contribution of each of these routes, using different methodological approaches (Dunn et al., 1995; Rouzioux et al., 1995; Busch & Satten, 1997; Kuhn et al., 1996; Kalish et al., 1997; Chouquet et al., 1997). The results of these exercises are consistent, and indicate that, in non-breastfeeding populations, about 70% of vertical infection is acquired in the peripartum period (Table 12.2). This is probably a lower estimate as the observed proportion positive at birth will underestimate the true proportion with intrauterine infection, as a transmission event shortly before delivery may not have sufficient time for infection to be established and to produce a positive culture at birth, or because of sequestration of the virus (De Rossi et al., 1992, 1997; Kalish et al., 1997). In breastfeeding populations results from similar exercises again suggest that the risk of transmission is likely to be higher during labour and delivery than during gestation (Simonon et al., 1994; Bertolli et al., 1996).

Acquisition of infection after 3–6 months of age through breastfeeding may contribute substantially to the overall rate of infection in breastfeeding populations. The results from Rwanda and Zaire already suggested that about 5% of children born to HIV infected mothers only became infected after 3 months of age, and the relative contribution of this to the overall rate of vertical transmission was 12–20% (Simonon et al., 1994; Bertolli et al., 1996). Late postnatal acquisition of infection was further confirmed in a study in Ivory Coast by Ekpini et al. (1997) who defined late postnatal transmission to have taken place when a child had a negative PCR at 3 or 6 months or age, followed by either or both a positive PCR at 9 months or older, or by persistently positive serology beyond 15 months of age. Among the 45 children born to HIV-1 positive mothers whose PCR results were

Table 12.2. Time to first positive PCR or culture

Non-breastfeeding populations					
	n	birth	2 wks	3 wks	1 mth
Dunn et al. (1995)	271	38%	93%	94%	96%
Kuhn et al. (1996)	120	22%	73%	90%	>95%
Chouquet et al. (1997)	135	25%	80%	93%	>95%
Kalish et al. (1997)	140	27%	88%	89%	89%
Breastfeeding populations					
	in utero	intrapartum +early postpartum	>3 mths	total VTR	
Simonon et al. (1994)	7.7%	12.7%	4.9%	25.3%	
Bertolli et al. (1996)	6%	18%	4%	26%	

negative at or before 6 months of age, four (9%) became HIV infected. The estimated rate of late postnatal transmission with account taken of loss to follow-up and weaning patterns was 12% (95% 3–23%) or 9.2 per 100 child–years of breastfeeding (Ekpini et al., 1997).

To provide a more reliable estimate of late postnatal transmission of HIV through breastfeeding, a meta-analysis of data from four cohorts from industrialized and four cohort from developing countries was undertaken by the Ghent International Working Group on mother-to-child transmission of HIV-1 (Leroy et al., 1998). Results from this analysis indicate an overall risk of acquisition of infection after 3 months of age of about 3 per 100 child–years of breastfeeding, with the similarity between individual studies on HIV-1. Miotti et al. (1999) reported, from a study in Malawi, a cumulative infection rate while breastfeeding from month one to the end of months 5, 11, 17 and 23 of 3.5%, 7%, 8.9% and 10.3% respectively. Incidence per month was 0.7% during months 1–5, 0.6% during months 6–11 and 0.3% during age 12–17 months. In this setting an uninfected infant breastfed by an HIV infected mother had a 10.3% risk of becoming infected (Miotti et al., 1999).

However, in many settings in the developing world, the disadvantages of artificial feeding in terms of morbidity and mortality may outweigh the reduction in the risk of HIV infection (Nicoll et al., 1995). To further quantify the additional risk of transmission and to better understand the timing of transmission through breastfeeding, a randomized controlled trial of breast vs. formula feeding was undertaken in Nairobi, Kenya. Preliminary results suggest nearly a doubling in the rate of vertical transmission (Nduati et al., 1999).

There are limited data on age-specific risks of morbidity and mortality in infants who are not breastfed, or optimally breastfed, or given mixed feeding irrespective of the mother's HIV status. In the randomized trial in Nairobi, mortality at 2 years of age was similar in the formula (20%) and breastfed (24%) group, indicating a relatively high risk in the non-breastfed group (Nduati et al., 1999). In a modelling exercise, assuming different infant feeding practices, infant mortality rates, varying antenatal HIV seroprevalence and HIV incidence postnatally, and HIV transmission rates through breastfeeding, Kuhn and Stein (1997) contributed to the debate about feeding alternatives for infants born to HIV-infected women in less developed countries. Complete avoidance of breastfeeding by the whole population always produced the worst outcome. The lowest frequency of adverse outcomes (HIV infection or infants deaths) occurred if no HIV-infected women breastfed and all HIV-negative women breastfed optimally, when infant mortality rates are less than 100 per 1000 and assuming a relative risk of dying in non-breastfed infants of 2.5 compared to breastfed infants. If the absolute rate of late postnatal transmission of HIV infection through breastfeeding was 7% or more, early cessation of breastfeeding (3 months after the delivery) by HIV-infected mothers may be beneficial, even at high infant mortality rates (Kuhn & Stein 1997). However, they clearly showed that where HIV infected women were not identified antenatally sustained promotion of breastfeeding is desirable.

In a cost-effectiveness analysis, Soderlund et al. (1999) found that the appropriateness of exclusive formula feeding was highly cost effective only in settings with high HIV seroprevalence and reasonable levels of child survival, and dangerous where infant mortality was higher than 70–140/1000. In addition their model showed that allowed breastfeeding early on, to be replaced by formula feeding at 4 or 7 months seemed likely to save fewer lives and offered poorer value for money.

Mode of delivery

Elective caesarean section has been associated with a reduced risk of transmission in a number of studies. Initially evidence from the European Collaborative Study (1994) suggested a halving in the risk of vertical transmission in children delivered by elective caesarean section. A subsequent 1994 meta-analysis of data from 11 prospective perinatal transmission studies, including 3202 mother–child pairs showed a 20% reduction in the risk of vertical transmission after caesarean section delivery (Dunn et al., 1994). No allowance was made for emergency vs. elective caesarean section or for any other variables known to be associated with vertical transmission.

A more recent meta-analysis included five European and ten North American prospective studies totalling over 8500 mother–infant pairs, and included information regarding elective and emergency procedures and other variables. Elective caesarean section reduced the risk of mother-to-child transmission by more than 50%, after adjusting for antiretroviral therapy, birth weight and maternal infection stage (International Perinatal HIV Group, 1999).

A French study showed a transmission rate of 0.8% in women who had received long-course antiretroviral treatment and had an elective caesarean section, compared with 6.6% with vaginal delivery (Mandelbrot et al., 1998), while a similar study in Switzerland reported no transmission in 45 women who received long-course zidovudine and had an elective caesarean section (Kind et al., 1998).

A randomized controlled trial of mode of delivery in Europe randomized more than 400 women to either elective caesarean section delivery or planned vaginal delivery. Three out of 170 infants (1.8%) born to women in the caesarean section group were HIV infected compared with 21 out of 200 (10.5%) born to women in the vaginal delivery group, representing a treatment effect odds ratio of 0.2 (95% confidence intervals 0.1–0.6) (European Mode of Delivery Collaboration, 1999). Two-thirds of the women taking part in this trial received zidovudine during pregnancy, and in this subgroup 0.8% of babies born to the women allocated to caesarean section were HIV infected compared with 4.3% of those born to women allocated vaginal delivery. This gives an odds ratio of 0.2 (95% confidence intervals 0–1.7). For women who did not receive zidovudine during pregnancy the odds ratio for transmission was also 0.2 suggesting that the protective effect of caesarean section persists independent of the antiretroviral treatment.

In this trial, there were no serious adverse complications in either group. Postpartum fever was reported more commonly in women delivered by caesarean section although the overall incidence was low. Some earlier reports have shown higher rates of complications in HIV-positive women who have had elective caesarean sections (Semprini et al., 1995; Bulterys et al., 1996). This possibility of increased morbidity must be taken into account when considering caesarean section, along with the availability of safe operating facilities and the effect on other maternity services. Based on the randomized trial and meta-analysis evidence, there is now sufficient justification to recommend elective caesarean section deliveries for HIV infected women, in those settings where this can be done safely.

To avoid acquisition of infection during birth, cleansing of the birth canal with an antiseptic and/or viricidal agent has been proposed (Consensus Workshop Siena, 1995). The agent should inactivate HIV, have little or no local or systemic toxicity, and be simple to apply. The agent used should, in addition, be safe for the infant. It is not entirely clear what the most effective and safe agent is, neither is it clear whether there would be a benefit of the agent over and above the action of lavage.

Little information is available regarding HIV viral load in the vagina and cervix, and possible associations with viraemia, and advanced disease. Evidence from a small number of women studied suggests that viral load in vagina/cervix is increased during pregnancy, although less than half of pregnant women are thought to harbour virus in the vagina/cervix. The expected effect of vaginal lavage on reduction of vertical transmission is therefore limited. However, as an intervention it is relatively cheap and easy to apply, and may thus be attractive in many settings. In a clinical trial in Malawi on the use of cleansing of the birth canal with chlorhexidine (Biggar et al., 1996), there were no adverse reactions to the intervention procedure. However, the birth canal cleansing had no significant impact on HIV transmission rates, except when membranes were ruptured more than four hours before delivery. These results would indicate that either birth canal exposure is not important in the acquisition of infection for the baby, or that the cleansing was not done to maximum effect. Similar findings have been reported recently from a trial in Mombasa, Kenya (M. Temmerman, personal communication, 1999). An important finding from the Malawi trial was the sharp reduction in infant morbidity and mortality due to a decrease in neonatal sepsis, which in itself may be sufficient reason to advocate its introduction generally (Taha et al., 1997; Hofmeyr & McIntyre, 1997).

Antiretroviral therapy

Antiretroviral drugs decrease maternal viral load and/or inhibit viral replication in the infant, thereby decreasing the risk of transmission. This hypothesis was confirmed in 1994 by the results from an American–French trial (PACTG 076) (Connor et al., 1994). In this randomized placebo-controlled trial, in a non-breastfeeding population, treatment with ZDV (100 mg 5 times daily) or placebo was started between 14 and 34 weeks of pregnancy (median 26 weeks). Women also received intravenous ZDV or placebo during labour and the infants received oral ZDV (2 mg/kg 4 times daily) or placebo for 6 weeks. All women had CD4+ counts > 200 per cubic mm, were symptom free and had not previously received ZDV. The first interim analysis on 356 mother–infant pairs demonstrated a rate of mother-to-child transmission of 25.5% in the placebo group, and 8.3% in the ZDV group. Treatment with ZDV achieved a 67.5% reduction in transmission risk. The drug was well tolerated in the short term in the pregnant women and the neonates. These trial results have subsequently been confirmed in observational studies, suggesting the generalizibility to the larger population of infected women. However, the optimum timing and method of therapeutic interventions is not yet known, neither is there much information regarding the long-term effect of zidovudine treatment on children or on the effect of temporary zidovudine treatment for the management of subsequent pregnancies in these women. Evidence that in utero exposure to zidovudine does not appear to produce any unexpected long-term effects has been provided from a follow-up study among the uninfected children born to women participating in ACTG076 (Culnane et al., 1999). This study reported follow-up information from 122 uninfected children in the zidovudine group and 112 uninfected children in the placebo group. Median age of the children at time of last follow-up was 4.2 years with a range of 3.2–5.6 years. No differences could be detected in any parameters of growth, cognitive and developmental function assessed by the Bailey Scales of Infant Development, immunological function, cardiac function or ophthalmologic function and there were no late deaths or malignancies detected in this group. In France, eight uninfected children born to HIV infected mothers were diagnosed with mitochondrial abnormalities and serious clinical disease. Two of these died. All eight had been exposed in utero, intrapartum and neonatally to prophylactic antiretroviral therapy with zidovudine with or without lamivudine (Blanche et al., 1999). Although a causal association is biologically plausible, further assessment of the toxic effect of these drugs is required to obtain definitive proof of such a link.

Long-course or combination antiretroviral treatment is unaffordable for developing country settings and several trials have investigated the use of shorter, more affordable interventions. The Bangkok Perinatal AZT Study, was a randomized placebo-controlled trial to evaluate the safety and efficacy of a short-regimen of oral zidovudine [ZDV] administered during late pregnancy and labour to reduce the risk for perinatal HIV transmission. The regimen was 300 mg ZDV orally twice daily from 36 weeks' gestation until the onset of labour and 300 mg every 3 hours from the onset of labour until delivery. All women were advised not to breastfeed and were provided with infant formula, and it is important to bear in mind that these results are directly applicable only to formula-fed infants. Transmission in the treatment group was 9.4% (95% confidence interval, 5.2–13.5%) and 18.9% (95% confidence interval, 13.2–24.2%) in the placebo group, representing a 50% reduction in transmission risk (95% confidence interval, 15.4–70.6%) (Shaffer et al., 1999a, b).

Two West African trials support the efficacy of short course zidovudine treatment. A trial in Côte d'Ivoire randomized women to receive the same treatment regimens as the Bangkok study. In this trial, however, over 95% of infants were breastfed (Wiktor et al., 1999). The relative risk of transmission in the placebo group was 0.63 (95% confidence intervals 0.38–1.06), representing a 37% reduction. A further trial of short regimen in more than 350 women conducted in Burkina Faso and Côte d'Ivoire compared oral zidovudine, given as a single loading dose of 600 mg at the onset of labour followed by oral zidovudine started between 36 and 38 weeks' gestation at 300 mg twice daily, followed by a single loading dose of 600 mg at the onset of labour followed by oral zidovudine 300 mg twice a day to the mother continued until 7 days after delivery compared to placebo (Dabis et al., 1999). More than 85% of infants in this study were breastfed for longer than 3 months. Transmission rate at 6 months was reduced by 38% (95% confidence intervals 5–60%), with no evidence of 'catch up transmission' in the treated group during the period of breastfeeding, and preliminary evidence suggests that this effect holds until at least 15 months (Leroy et al., 1999).

The UNAIDS PETRA trial investigated a combination of zidovudine and 3TC (lamivudine), and was undertaken in predominantly breastfeeding populations in five sites in South Africa, the United Republic of Tanzania and Uganda. This trial compared the effectiveness of three different drug regimens with placebo. Arm A received zidovudine and 3TC from 36 weeks' gestation, during labour and for 1 week postpartum to mother and child. Arm B received zidovudine and 3TC from the onset of labour and for one week postpartum to mother and child. Arm C received zidovudine and 3TC during labour only. Over 1790 women were recruited in all. Interim early efficacy results at 6 weeks of age of the infant have been reported, in which the risk of transmission by 6 weeks of age in Arm A was 8.6%, in Arm B 10.8%, in Arm C 17.7% and in the placebo group 17.2% (Saba et al., 1999). Long-term follow-up results have not yet been released.

Another possible approach to reducing transmission through drug treatment is the use of non-nucleoside reverse transcriptase inhibitors (NNRTI). Nevirapine is a NNRTI with potent antiretroviral activity and a favourable safety profile but in which there is rapid development of drug resistance limiting the duration of its effect. Of particular interest is that the drug achieves high circulating levels that are long-lasting, raising the possibility of dosing regimens. The HIVNET 012 trial in Uganda gave one dose of 200 mg nevirapine orally to women at the onset of labour and one dose of 2 mg/kg to the baby within 72 hours, compared to intrapartum zidovudine and one week zidovudine treatment to the child. Almost all babies were breastfed. In the nevirapine treatment group, the transmission rate at 14–16 weeks was 13.1% compared with 25.1% in the comparison group. The efficacy of nevirapine was 47% (95% CI 20–64). Side effects were similar in the two regimens, which were both well tolerated (Guay et al., 1999). A trial is ongoing in the USA, Europe and Brazil to evaluate the additional effect of nevirapine on the rate of vertical transmisison in women who already receive other antiretroviral therapy or who are delivered by elective caesarean section (PACTG 316). Results are expected by late 2000. In South Africa, a trial is ongoing to compare nevirapine with the PETRA arm B.

The HIVNET 012 results provide the most feasible option yet for the prevention of mother-to-child transmission in developing countries, at an estimated cost of around $4.00 for the drug. Infrastructure development, including the provision of counselling, testing and better maternity services will be required to enable HIV-positive women in these countries to benefit.

Supplementation with vitamin A

Based on the findings from studies in Malawi (Semba et al., 1995) and the USA (Greenberg et al., 1997) that HIV infected women who were severely deficient for Vitamin A were at increased risk to transmit the infection to their infant and from a Kenyan study demonstrating an association between severe maternal vitamin A deficiency and a substantial increase in HIV–DNA in breast milk in immunocompromised women (Nduati et al., and others 1995), several randomized trials have started (in Malawi, Zimbabwe, South Africa and Tanzania) to evaluate the effect of micronutrient supplementation with vitamin A in reducing the risk of vertical transmission (Greenberg et al., 1997). Vitamin A is essential for maintaining the integrity of the mucosal surfaces, for modulating healthy antibody responses and for the function and growth of T and B cells. Supplementation with vitamin A during pregnancy and lactation may prove to be an inexpensive, simple and effective way of diminishing transmission to infants. However, preliminary results from these trials demonstrated no decrease in vertical transmission of HIV in women receiving multivitamins with or without vitamin A (Fawzi, 1999). In a randomized clinical trial of vitamin A in Durban, South Africa, Coutsoudis et al. (1999b) demonstrated no difference in the risk of HIV transmission by 3 months of age between vitamin A(20.3%;95%CI, 15.7–24.9) and placebo (22.3%; 95%CI, 17.5–27.1).

Immunotherapy

Maternal immune response, humoral and/or cellular, to HIV infection may play a role in preventing perinatal transmission, although results from various studies are conflicting (Consensus Workshop Sienna, 1995). Passive immunization has been investigated in a small trial, but currently no effectiveness trials are ongoing. Concern has been expressed regarding the use of blood products from HIV infected donors, and the cost of production. Furthermore, there is unease about the possible adverse effects on the infant, and the effect of passive immunisation on viral load and the immune system will need to be carefully assessed.

Active immunization is the most attractive approach because it can potentially induce a long-lasting immunity in the mother, and it may also induce fetal immunity. Several phase I trials have been carried out in the USA (Consensus Workshop Sienna, 1995), but there have not been any large efficacy trials.

Screening tests

Current serological tests for HIV-specific IgG antibody are of high specificity and sensitivity. Antibody tests include enzyme-linked immunoabsorbent assay tests (ELISA) and simple /rapid tests. The simple and rapid tests can be performed outside a laboratory setting and will give results within a short period of time. The newer tests available are as reliable as ELISA tests. Sera found to be reactive for anti-HIV on screening should be confirmed with a different ELISA or rapid test or Western blot, depending on the local testing algorithm. For diagnostic purposes it is prudent to obtain a repeat sample from the woman to confirm infection.

The majority of infected women seroconvert within 6–8 weeks after infection, although in some cases antibody may not appear until 6–9 months later. Thus a negative antibody test is reliable only if the woman has not been exposed to the virus in the previous 6 months. However, a false-negative test result may occur if the woman is tested in the window period between infection and seroconversion.

Diagnosis of HIV infection in the infant

The diagnosis of HIV infection in infants is complicated by the presence of passively acquired maternal antibody, which may persist for up to 18 months. An earlier diagnosis can made by virus culture, polymerase chain reaction (PCR), the detection of p24 antigen or IgA. Culture of HIV is the definitive method of diagnosis but it is slow, expensive and limited to specialized laboratories. An ELISA for detection of p24 antigen is the most commonly used antigen test; more recently this test has been improved through acid or heat dissociation of antibody–antigen complexes. The polymerase chain reaction (PCR) is a method of amplification of DNA sequences in a cell-free system. The technique is sensitive and of particular value in infants born to HIV seropositive mothers where serological diagnosis is not helpful in determining infection status. PCR sensitivity in the first few days of life is about 40% and increases rapidly to about 100% by 1 month of age (Dunn et al., 1995).

Natural history of vertically acquired HIV infection

The natural history of HIV infection in children is variable and tends to be more rapidly progressive when compared with adults. Before the widespread use of antiretroviral therapy, 30% of infected infants presented before 6 months of age and 17–25% died within the first 18 months of life. In the developed world, without antiretroviral therapy, 75% of children were alive at 6 years of age, with 50% still alive at 9 years of age, despite having low CD4 counts (Rogers et al., 1994; French Pediatric HIV Infection Study Group and European Collaborative Study, 1997).

Table 12.3. Risk for rapid progressive HIV disease in infants

Advanced maternal HIV disease

High maternal viral load

Maternal p24 antigenimia

Timing of infection

Viral strain

Gestational age

Prematurity

Symtomatic in early infancy

Positive HIV culture or PCR at birth

High viral load in early infancy

Early opportunistic infection

Early-onset encephalopathy

Failure to thrive

Early onset diarrhoea

Early onset of CMV infection

Progression of HIV infection in children may depend upon the timing of transmission, the inoculum of virus, the phenotype of the virus and immune functioning (Table 12.3). The timing of viral detection in the newborn period may serve as a prognostic indicator of subsequent clinical course. Several prospective cohorts have observed significant associations between early viral detection (in utero infection) and rapid disease progression in infancy. Kuhn et al. (1999) evaluated 432 infants born to mothers infected with HIV. HIV was detected by PCR or culture within the first 2 days of life in 19/67 (28%) infants with a calculated relative risk for progression to AIDS or death of 2.6 (CI, 1.5–4.6). In children with virus detectable 48 hours after birth, 29% had died or developed AIDS by 1 year of age.

Mayaux reported a three-fold risk increase for early disease progression among infants with early viral detection. Infants who were determined to be infected in the intrapartum period also appear to have rapid increases in HIV RNA with peak levels occurring between 4 and 6 weeks of age with some of these infants developing a rapid progression of HIV disease (Mayaux et al., 1996)

There is at this stage no demonstrable RNA threshold that can differentiate rapid from slow progressors in the first few months of life. Risk of disease progression has been shown to be related to high viral loads (100 000 copies/ml) especially if CD4 counts are low (Mofenson et al., 1997).

Two related properties of the virus are syncitium induction and macrophage tropism. In adults and children, macrophage tropism has been associated with a non-progressive clinical state. In contrast the syncitium inducing and CD4 lymphocyte tropic phenotypes have been observed with the development of symptomatic progressive disease (De Rossi et al., 1997). There is an association between the human leukocyte antigen (HLA) system and genetic susceptibility to HIV. The discovery of the co-receptors CXCR4, CCR5, CCR2 and CCR3 and the effects of their mutants has led to clear evidence of genetic variability in host susceptibility. Homozygosity to the CCR5 gene confers protection against non-syncitium inducing or macrophage-tropic HIV strains, and that heterozygosity is associated with a slower disease progression in children and adults (Mummidi et al., 1998; Vallat et al., 1998; Misrahi et al., 1998).

In 1996, in the USA the median age of children with AIDS was 8 years. Survival of children with AIDS appears to be bimodal with approximately 10–20% of infected children being 'rapid progressors' usually dying of AIDS before 4 years of age, while the remaining 80–90% of children have survival patterns more typical of adults with AIDS, with a mean survival of approximately 9–10 years (Rogers et al., 1994). Survival of children infected with HIV in Africa appears to be much shorter than that seen in Europe and the United States. In Uganda the infant mortality rate for children with laboratory diagnosis of HIV infection was 336/1000. Median survival of children in the Ugandan cohort was 21 months with 66.2% of children dying by 36 months of age (Marum et al., 1996).

In Zimbabwe, HIV infected women had a perinatal mortality rate 2.1 times greater, a still birth rate 1.6 times greater and a neonatal mortality rate 2.7 times greater than HIV uninfected women (Zijenah et al., 1998). Neonates born to HIV infected women had an increased mortality rate (133/1000) compared with neonates born to HIV uninfected women (40/1000) in Abidjan (Lucas et al., 1996) and decreased 12-month survival (61 vs. 97%) in Brazzaville (Lallemant et al., 1989).

In Haiti, Halsey et al. (1990) found that infants born to HIV infected women had a significantly lower mean birth weight (2944 g vs. 3111g; P=0.001), were more likely to weigh less than 2500 g at birth and were more likely to be less than 37 weeks' gestation than were infants born to HIV uninfected women. In Asia, follow-up of children infected with HIV in the Bangkok perinatal HIV-transmission study measured mortality rates of 18% at 12 months and 30% at 24 months. In this cohort, most of the paediatric deaths were caused by pneumonia (Chotpityayasunondh et al., 1996).

Conclusion

In developed countries, with the introduction of antiretroviral therapy, modification of obstetric practice, and avoidance of breastfeeding, the rate of vertical transmission will decrease significantly to levels below 5%, making antenatal HIV screening a top priority. The situation for developing countries is more difficult: high HIV seroprevalence rates, inadequate health facilities and lack of resources continue to make HIV one of the major causes of infant mortality. The use of ultra-short course antiretrovirals, as demonstrated in the Uganda nevirapine trial, provides a relatively inexpensive way to reduce the transmission risk. The challenge for developing country health services is to strengthen the maternity service to include HIV testing, counselling, improve obstetric care and find ways to promote safe infant feeding options. The main target of any public health effort remains, however, the prevention of acquistion of infection in women of child-bearing age.

REFERENCES

Adjorlolo-Johnson, G., De Cock, K. M., Ekpini, E., Vetter, K. M., Sibailly, T., Brattegaard, K., Yavo, D., Doorly, R., Whitaker, J. P., Kestens, L. et al.(1994). Prospective comparison of mother-to-child transmission of HIV-1 and HIV-2 in Abidjan, Ivory Coast. *J.A.M.A.*, **272**, 462–6.

Bertolli, J., St. Louis, M. E., Simonds, R. J., Nieburg, P. I., Kamenga, M., Brown, C., Tarande, M., Quinn, T. & Ou, C. Y. (1996). Estimating the timing of mother-to-child transmission of human immunodeficiency virus in a breastfeeding population in Kinshasa, Zaire. *J. Infect. Dis.*, **174**, 722–6.

Biggar, R. J., Miotti, P. G., Taha, T. E., Mtimavalye, L., Broadhead, R., Justesen, A., Yellin, F., Liomba, G., Miley, W., Waters, D., Chiphangwi, J. D. & Goedert, J. J. (1996). Perinatal intervention trial in Africa: effect of birth canal cleansing intervention to prevent HIV transmission. *Lancet*, **347**, 1647–50.

Blanche, S., Tardieu, M., Rustin, P., Slama, A., Barret, B., Firtion, G., Ciraru-Vigneron, N., Lacroix, C., Rouzioux, C., Mandelbrot, L., Desguerre, I., Rotig, A., Mayaux, M. & Delfraissy, J. F. (1999). Persistent mitochondrial dysfunction and perinatal exposure to antiretroviral nucleoside analogues. *Lancet*, **354**, 1084–9.

Bloland, P. B., Wirima, J. J., Steketee, R. W., Chilima, B., Hightower, A. & Breman, J. G. (1995). Maternal HIV infection and infant mortality in Malawi: evidence for increased mortality due to placental malaria infection. *AIDS*, **9**, 721–6.

Bomsel, M. (1997). Transcytosis of infectious human immunodeficiency virus across a thigh human epithelial cell line barrier. *Nature Med.*, **3**, 42–7.

Borkowsky, W., Krasinski, K., Cao, Y., Ho, D., Pollack, H., Moore, T., Chen, S. H., Allen, M. & Tao, P-T. (1994). Correlation of perinatal transmission of human immunodeficiency virus type 1 with maternal viremia and lymphocyte phenotypes. *J. Pediatr.*, **125**, 345–51.

Boyer, P. J., Dillon, M., Navaie, M., Deveikis, A., Keller, M., O'Rourke, S. & Bryson, Y. J. (1994). Factors predictive of maternal–fetal transmission of HIV-1. *J.A.M.A.*, **217**, 1925–30.

Bryson, Y. J., Luzuriaga, K., Sullivan, J. L. & Wara, D. W. (1992). Proposed definitions for in utero versus intrapartum transmission of HIV-1. *N. Engl. J. Med.*, **327**, 1246–7.

Bulterys, M., Chao, A., Dushimimana, A. & Saah, A. (1996). Fatal complications after caesarean section in HIV infected women. *AIDS*, **10**, 923–4.

Burns, D., Landesman, S., Muenz, L. R., Nugent, R. P., Goedert, J. J., Minkoff, H., Walsh, J. H., Mendez, H., Rubinstein, A. & Willoughby, A. (1994). Cigarette smoking, premature rupture of membranes, and vertical transmission of HIV-1 among women with low CD4+ levels. *J. Acquir. Immune Defic. Syndr.*, **7**, 718–26.

Burton, G. J., O'Shea, S., Rostron, T., Mullen, J. E., Aiyer, S., Skepper, J. N., Smith, R. & Banatvala, J. (1996). Physical breaks in the placental trophoblastic surface: significance in vertical transmission of HIV. *AIDS*, **10**, 1294–5.

Busch, M. P. & Satten, G. A. (1997). Time course of viremia and antibody seroconversion following human immunodeficiency virus exposure. *Am. J. Med.*, **102**(5B), 117–24.

Centers for Disease Control and Prevention. (1998). Public health service task force recommendations for the use of antiretroviral drugs in pregnant women infected with HIV-1 for maternal health and for reducing perinatal HIV-1 transmission in the United States. *MMWR*, **47** (RR-2), 1–27.

Chotpitayayasunondh, T., Chearskul, S., Suteewarn, W. Wanprapa, N., Sangtaweesin, V., Batter, V., Kalish, M., Nieburg, P., Mastro, T. D. & Shaffer, N. (1996) Natural history and mortality of perinatal HIV-1 infection, Bangkok, Thailand [abstract] XI International Conference on AIDS, Vancouver, **2**,133–4.

Chouquet, C., Burgard, M., Richardson, S., Rouzioux, C. & Costagliola, D. (1997). Timing of mother-to-child HIV-1 transmission and diagnosis of infection based on polymerase chain reaction in the neonatal period by a non-parametric method. *AIDS*, **11**, 1183–99.

Connor, E. M., Sperling, R. S., Gelber, R., Kiselev, P., Scott, G., O'Sullivan, M. J., Van Dyke, R., Bey, M., Shearer, W. & Jacobson, R. L. (1994). Reduction of maternal–infant transmission of human immunodeficiency virus type 1 with zidovudine treatment. *N. Engl. J. Med.*, **331**, 1173–80.

Consensus Workshop Sienna. (1995). Strategies for prevention of perinatal transmission of HIV infection. *J. Acquir. Immune Defic. Syndr. Hum. Retrovirol.*, **8**, 161–78.

Coutsoudis, A., Pillay, K., Spooner, E., Kuhn, L. & Coovadia, H. M. (1999a). Influence of infant-feeding patterns on early mother-to-child transmission of HIV-1 in Durban, South Africa: a prospective cohort study. *Lancet*, **354**, 471–6.

Coutsoudis, A., Pillay, K., Spooner, E., Kuhn, L. & Coovadia, H. M. (1999b). Randomised trial testing the effect of Vitamin A supplementation on pregnancy outcomes and early mother-to-child transmission in Durban, South Africa. South African Vitamin A Study Group. *AIDS*, **12**, 1517–24.

Culnane, M., Fowler, M., Lee, S. S., McSherry, G., Brady, M., O'Donnell, K., Mofenson, L., Gortmaker, S. L., Shapiro, D. E., Scott, G., Jimenez, E., Moore, E. C., Diaz, C., Flynn, P. M., Cunningham, B. & Oleske, J. (1999). Lack of long-term effects of in-utero exposure to zidovudine in children born to HIV-infected women. *J.A.M.A.*, **281**, 151–7.

Dabis, F., Msellati, P., Meda, N., Welffens-Ekra, C., You, B., Manigart, O., Leroy, V., Simonon, A., Cartoux, M., Combe, P., Ouangre, A., Ramon, R., Ky-Zerbo, O., Montcho, C., Salamon, R., Rouzioux, C., Van de Perre, P. & Mandelbrot, L. (1999). 6-month efficacy, tolerance, and acceptability of a short regimen of oral zidovudine to reduce vertical transmission of HIV in breastfed children in Cote d'Ivoire and Burkina Faso: a double-blind placebo-controlled multicentre trial. *Lancet*, **353**, 786–92.

Datta, P., Embree, J. E., Kreiss, J. K., Ndinya-Achola, J. O., Braddick, M., Temmerman, M., Nagelkerke, N. J. D., Maitha, G., Holmes, K. K., Piot, P. et al. (1994). Mother-to-child transmission of human immunodeficiency virus type 1: report from the Nairobi study. *J. Infect. Dis.*, **170**, 1134–40.

de Martino, M., Tovo, P.-A., Tozzi, A. E., Pezzotti, P., Galli, L., Livadiotti, S., Caselli, D., Massironi, E., Ruga, E., Fioredda, F. et al. (1992). HIV-1 transmission through breastmilk: appraisal of risk according to duration of feeding. *AIDS*, **6**, 991–7.

De Rossi, A., Ometto, L., Mammano, F., Zanotto, C., Giaquinto, C. & Chieco-Bianchi, L. (1992). Vertical transmission of HIV-1: lack of detectable virus in peripheral blood cells of infected children at birth. *AIDS*, **6**, 1117–20.

De Rossi, A., Ometto, L., Masiero, S., Zanchetta, M. & Chieco-Bianchi, L. (1997). Viral phenotype in mother-to-child HIV transmission and disease progression of vertically acquired HIV-1 infection. *Acta Paediatr. Suppl.*, **421**, 22–8.

Dickover, R. E., Garratty, E. M., Herman, S. A., Sim, M-S., Plaeger, S., Boyer, P. J., Keller, M., Deveikis, A., Stiehm, R. & Bryson, Y. J. (1996). Identification of levels of maternal HIV-1 RNA associated with risk of perinatal transmission. *J.A.M.A.*, **275**, 599–605.

Douglas, G. C. & King, B. F. (1992). Maternal–fetal transmission of human immunodeficiency virus: a review of possible routes and cellular mechanisms of infection. *Clin. Infect. Dis.*, **15**, 678–91.

Dunn, D., Brandt, C. D., Krivine, A., Cassol, S. A., Roques, P., Borkowsky, W., de Rossi, A., Denamur, E., Ehrnst, A., Loveday, C. et al. (1995). The sensitivity of HIV-1 DNA polymerase chain reaction in the neonatal period and the relative contributions of intra-uterine and intra-partum transmission. *AIDS*, **9**, F7–F11.

Dunn, D., Newell, M. L., Ades, A. & Peckham, C. S. (1992). Risk of human immunodefiency virus type 1 transmission through breastfeeding. *Lancet*, **340**, 585–8.

Dunn, D., Newell, M. L., Mayaux, M. J., Kind, C., Hutto, C., Goedert, J. & Andiman, W., Perinatal AIDS Collaborative Transmission Studies. (1994). Mode of delivery and vertical transmission of HIV-1: a review of prospective studies. *J. Acquir. Immune Defic. Syndr.*, **7**, 1064–6.

Ekpini, E., Wiktor, S. Z., Satten, G. A., Adjorlolo, G., Sibailly, T., Ou, C. Y., Karon, J. M., Brattegaard, K., Whitaker, J. P., Gnaore, E. et al. (1997). Late postnatal mother-to-child transmission of HIV-1 in Abidjan, Cote d'Ivoire. *Lancet*, **349**, 1054–9.

European Collaborative Study. (1994). Caesarean section and risk of vertical transmission of HIV-1 infection. *Lancet*, **343**, 1464–7.

European Collaborative Study (1996). Vertical transmission of HIV-1: maternal immune status and obstetric factors. *AIDS*, **10**, 1675–81.

European Collaborative Study. (1999). Maternal viral load and vertical transmission of HIV-1: an important factor but not the only one. *AIDS*, **13**, 1377-85.

European Mode of Delivery Collaboration. (1999). Elective caesarean-section versus vaginal delivery in prevention of vertical HIV-1 transmission: a randomised clinical trial. *Lancet*, **353**, 1035-9.

Fang, G., Burger, H., Grimson, R., Tropper, P., Nachman, S., Mayers, D., Weislow, O., Moore, R., Reyelt, C., Hutcheon, N. et al. (1995). Maternal plasma human immunodefiency virus type 1 RNA level: a determinant and projected threshold for mother-to-child transmission. *Proc. Natl Acad. Sci. USA*, **92**, 12100–4.

Fawzi, W. (1999). Micronutrients and HIV transmission. The second conference on global strategies for the prevention of HIV transmission from mothers to infants, Montreal, September 5–6 1999. Abstract 019.

French Pediatric HIV Infection Study Group and European Collaborative Study (1997). Morbidity and Mortality in European children vertically infected by HIV-1. *J. Acquir. Immune Defic. Syndr. Hum. Retrovirol.*, **14**, 442–50.

Goldenberg, R. L., Vermund, S. H., Goepfert, A. R. & Andrews, W. W. (1998). Choriodecidual inflammation: a potentially preventable cause of perinatal HIV-1 transmission? *Lancet*, **352**, 1927–30.

Goulston, C., Stevens, E., Gallo, D., Mullins, J. I., Hanson, C. V. & Katzenstein, D. (1996). Human immunodeficiency virus in plasma and genital secretions during the menstrual cycle. *J. Infect. Dis.*, **174**, 858–61.

Gray, G. E., McIntyre, J. A. & Lyons, S. F. (1996). The effect of breastfeeding on vertical transmission of HIV-1 in Soweto, South Africa [Abstract]. XI International Conference on AIDS, Vancouver Th.C.415,237.

Greenberg, B. L., Semba, R. D., Vink, P. E., Farley, J. J., Sivapalsingam, M., Steketee, R. W., Thea, D. M. & Schoenbaum, E. E. (1997). Vitamin A deficiency and maternal–infant transmission of HIV in two metropolitan areas in the United States. *AIDS*, **11**, 325–32.

Guay, L. A., Musoke, P., Fleming, T., Bagenda, D., Allen, M., Nakabitito, C., Sherman, J., Bakaki, P., Ducar, C., Deseyve, M., Emel, L., Mirochnick, M., Fowler, M. G., Mofenson, L., Miotti, P., Dransfield, K., Bray, D., Mmiro, F. & Brooks Jackson J. (1999). Intrapartum and neonatal single-does nevirapine compared with zidovudine for prevention of mother-to-child transmission of HIV-1 in Kampala, Uganda: HIVNET 012 randomised trial. *Lancet*, **354**, 795–802.

Halsey, N. A., Boulos, R., Holt, E. & Ruff, A. (1990). Transmission of HIV-1 infections from mothers to infants in Haiti. Impact on childhood mortality and malnutrition. *J.A.M.A.*, **264**, 2088–92.

Henin, Y., Mandelbrot, L., Henrion, R., Pradineaud, R. & Montagnier, L. (1993). HIV in the cervicovaginal secretions of pregnant and non-pregnant women. *J. Acquir. Immune Defic. Syndr.*, **6**, 72–5.

Hofmeyr, G. J. & McIntyre, J. A. (1997). Preventing perinatal infections. Need for a simple, inexpensive, safe intervention that can be used routinely in all women. *Br. Med. J.*, **315**, 199–200.

International Perinatal HIV Group. (1999). The mode of delivery and the risk of vertical transmission of human immunodeficiency virus type 1–a meta-analysis of 15 prospective cohort studies. The International Perinatal HIV Group. *N. Engl. J. Med.*, **340**, 977–87.

John, G. C., Nduati, R. W., Mbori-Ngacha, D., Overbaugh, J., Welch, M., Richardson, B. A., Ndinya-Achola, J., Bwayo, J. J., Krieger, J., Onyango, F. et al. (1997). Genital shedding of human immunodeficiency virus type 1 DNA during pregnancy: association with immunosuppression, abnormal cervical or vaginal discharge, and severe vitamin A deficiency. *J. Infect. Dis.*, **175**, 57-62.

Kalish, L. A., Pitt, J., Lew, J., Landesman, S., Diaz, C., Hershow, R., Blaine Hollinger, F., Pagano, M., Smeriglio, V., Moye, J. et al. (1997). Defining the time of fetal or perinatal acquisition of human immunodeficiencey virus type I infection on the basis of age at first positive culture. *J. Infect. Dis.*, **175**, 712–15.

Kind, C., Rudin, C., Siegrist, C. A., Wyler, C. A., Biedermann, K., Lauper, U., Irion, O., Schupbach, J. & Nadal, D. (1998). Prevention of vertical HIV transmission: additive protective effect of elective caesarean section and zidovudine prophylaxis. Swiss Neonatal HIV Study Group. *AIDS*, **12**, 205–10.

Kreiss, J., Willerford, D. M., Hensel, M., Emonyi, W., Plummer, F., Ndinya-Achola, J., Roberts, P. L., Hoskyn, J., Hillier, S. & Kiviat, N. (1994). Association between cervical inflammation and cervical shedding of human immunodeficiency virus DNA. *J. Infect. Dis.*, **170**, 1597-601.

Kuhn, L. & Stein, Z. (1997) Infant survival, HIV infection and feeding alternatives in less-developed countries. *Am. J. Public Health*, **87**, 926–31.

Kuhn, L., Abrams, E. J., Chincilla, M., Tsai, W. Y., Thea, D. M. & New York City Perinatal HIV Transmission Collaborative Study Group. (1996). Sensitivity of HIV-1 DNA polymerase chain reaction in the neonatal period. *AIDS*, **10**, 1181–2.

Kuhn, L., Steketee, R. W., Weedon, J., Abrams, E. J., Lambert, G., Bamji, M., Schoenbaum, E., Farley, J., Nesheim, S. R., Palumbo, P., Simonds, R. J. & Thea, D. M. (1999). Distinct risk factors for intrauterine and intrapartum human immunodeficiency virus transmission and consequences for disease progression in infected children. Perinatal AIDS collaborative Transmission Study. *J. Infect. Dis.*, **179**, 52–8.

Lallemant, M., Lallemant-Le-Coeur, S., Cheynier, D., Nzingoula, S., Jourdain, G., Sinet, M., Dazza, M. C., Blanche, S., Griscelli, C. & Larouze, B. (1989). Mother-child transmission of HIV-1 in infants and infant survival in Brazzaville, Congo. *AIDS*, **3**, 643–6.

Landers, D. V. (1996). Nutrition and immune function II: maternal factors influencing transmission. *J. Nutr.*, **126**, S2637–40.

Landesman, S. H., Kalish, L. A., Burns, D., Minkoff, H., Fox, H. E., Zorrilla, C., Garcia, P., Fowler, M. G., Mofenson, L., Tuomala, R. et al. (1996). Obstetrical factors and the transmission of human immunodeficiency virus type 1 from mother-to-child. *N. Engl. J. Med.*, **334**, 1617–23.

Leroy, V., Newell, M. L., Dabis, F., Peckham, C., Van de Perre, P., Bulterys, M., Kind, C., Simonds, R. J., Wiktor, S. & Msellati, P. for the Ghent International Working Group on Mother-to-child transmission of HIV (1998). International multicentre pooled analysis of late postnatal mother-to-child transmission of HIV-1 infection. *Lancet*, **352**, 597–600.

Leroy, V., Meda, N., Roman, R., Welffens-Ekra, C., Mandelbrot, L., Combe, P., Van de Perre, P. & Dabis, F. for the DITRAME Study Group (1999). Postnatal HIV transmission risk in a trial assessing the efficacy of a short regimen of oral zidovudine in West Africa. Abstract 15ET3–3, p. 118. *XIth International Conference on AIDS and STDs in Africa*: Lusaka,

Lewis, P., Nduati, R., Kreiss, J. K., John, G. C., Richardson, B. A., Mbori-Ngacha, D., Ndinya-Achola, J. & Overbaugh, J. (1998). Cell free human immunodeficiency virus type 1 in breastmilk. *J. Infect. Dis.*, **177**, 34–9.

Lucas, S. B., Peacock, C. S., Hounnou, A., Brattegaard, K., Koffi, K., Honde, M., Andoh, J., Bell, J. & De Cock, K. M. (1996). Disease in children infected with HIV in Abidjan, Cote d'Ivoire *Br. Med. J.*, **312**, 335–8.

Mandelbrot, L., Le Chenadec, J., Berrebi, A., Bongain, A., Benifla, J. L., Delfraissy, J. F., Blanche, S. & Mayaux, M. J. (1998). Perinatal HIV-1 transmission: interaction between zidovudine prophylaxis and mode of delivery I the French Perinatal Cohort. *J.A.M.A.*, **280**, 55–60.

Marum, L., Bagenda, D., Guay, L. et al. (1996). Three-year mortality in a cohort of HIV-1 infected and uninfected Ugandan children. *XIth International Conference on AIDS &STDs* Vancouver, July 1996 Abstract WeB312.

Mayaux, M. J., Blanche, S., Rouzioux, C., Le Chenadec, J., Chambrin, V., Firtion, G., Allemon, M. C., Vilmer, E., Vigneron, N. C., Tricoire, J. et al. (1995). Maternal factors associated with perinatal HIV-1 transmission: the French Cohort Study: 7 years of follow-up observation. *J. Acquir. Immune Defic. Syndr. Hum. Retrovirol.*, **8**, 188–94.

Mayaux, M. J., Burgard, M., Teglas, J. P., Cottalorda, J., Krivine, A., Simon, F., Puel, J., Tamalet, C., Dormont, D., Masquelier, B., Doussin, A., Rouzioux, C. & Blanche, S. (1996) Neonatal characteristics in rapidly progressive perinatally acquired HIV-1 disease. *J.A.M.A.*, **275**, 606–10.

Miotti, P. G., Taha, T. E. T., Kumwenda, N. I., Broadhead, R., Mtimavalye, L. A. R., Van der Hoeven, L., Chiphangwi, J. D., Liomba, G. & Biggar, R. J. (1999). HIV transmission through breastfeeding. *J.A.M.A.*, **282**, 744–9.

Misrahi, M., Teglas, J. P., N'Go, N., Burgard, M., Mayaux, M. J., Rouzioux, C., Delfraissy, J. F. & Blanche, S. (1998). CCR5 chemokine receptor variant in HIV-1 mother-to-child transmission and disease progression in children. French Pediatric HIV Infection Study Group. *J.A.M.A.*, **279**, 277–80.

Mock, P. A., Shaffer, N., Bhadrakom, C., Siriwasin, W., Chotpitayasunondh, T., Chearskul, S., Young, N. L., Roongpisuthipong, A., Chinayon, P., Kalish, M. L., Parekh, B. & Mastro, T. D. (1999). Maternal viral load and timing of mother-to-child HIV transmission, Bangkok, Thailand. Bangkok Collaborative Perinatal HIV Transmission Study Group. *AIDS*, **13**, 407–14.

Mofenson, L. M. (1999). Short-course zidovudine for prevention of perinatal infection. *Lancet*, **353**, 766–7.

Mofenson, L. M., Korelitz, J. , Meyer, W. A. 3rd, Bethel, J., Rich, K., Pahwa, S., Moye, J. Jr, Nugent, R. & Read, J. (1997). The relationship between serum human immunodeficiency virus type 1(HIV)RNA levels, CD4 lymphocyte percent, and long-term mortality risk in HIV-1 infected children. *J. Infect. Dis.*, **175**, 1029–38.

Mostad, S. B. & Kreiss, J. K. (1996). Shedding of HIV-1 in the genital tract. *AIDS*, **10**, 1305–15.

Mummidi, S., Ahuja, S. S., Gonzalez, E., Anderson, S. A., Santiago, E. N., Stephan, K. T., Craig, F. E., O'Connell, P., Tryon, V., Clark, R. A., Dolan, M. J. & Ahuja, S. K. (1998). Genealogy of the CCR5 locus and chemokine system gene variants associated with altered rates of HIV-1 disease progression. *Nature Med.*, **4**, 786–93.

Nduati, R. W., John, G. C., Richardson, B. A., Overbaugh, J., Welch, M., Ndinya-Achola, J., Moses, S., Holmes, K., Onyango, F. & Kreiss, J. K. (1995). Human immunodeficiency virus type-1 infected cells in breastmilk: association with immunosuppression and vitamin A deficiency. *J. Infect. Dis.*, **172**, 1461–8.

Nduati, R., John, G., Ngacha, D. A., Richardson, S., Overbaugh, J., Mwatha, A., Achola, J., Fleming, T., Onyango, F. & Kreiss, J. (1999). Breastfeeding transmission of HIV-1: a randomised clinical trial. Abstract 13ET5-2, page 16. *XIth International Conference on AIDS and STDs in Africa*, Lusaka, September.

Newell, M. L., Gray, G. & Bryson, Y. J. (1997). Prevention of mother-to-child transmission of HIV-1 infection. *AIDS*, **11**(Suppl A), S165–72.

Nicoll, A., Newell, M. L., Van Praag, E., Van de Perre, P. & Peckham, C. (1995). Infant feeding policy and practice in the presence of HIV-1 infection. *AIDS*, **9**,107–19.

Renjifo, B., Essex, M., Mwakagile, D., Hunter, D., Msamanga, G., Spiegelman, D., Garland, M., Hertarmark, E. & Fawzi, W. (1999). Differences in vertical transmission between HIV phenotypes. The second conference on global strategies for the prevention of HIV transmission from mothers to infants, Montreal, September 5–6 1999. Abstract 099.

Rogers, M. F., Caldwell, M. B., Gwinn, M. L. & Simonds, R. J. (1994). Epidemiology of pediatric human immunodeficiency virus in the United States. *Acta Paediatr. Suppl.*, **400**, 5–7.

Rouzioux, C., Costagliola, D., Burgard, M., Blanche, S., Mayaux, M. J., Griscelli, C. & Valleron, A. J. HIV Infection in Newborns French Collaborative Study Group. (1995). Estimated timing of mother-to-child human immunodeficiency virus type 1 (HIV-1) transmission by use of a Markov model. *Am. J. Epidemiol.*, **142**, 1330–7.

Ruff, A. J., Coberly, J., Halsey, N. A., Boulos, R., Desormeaux, J., Burnley, A., Joseph, D. J., McBrien, M., Quinn, T., Losikoff, P., et al (1994). Prevalence of HIV-1 DNA and p24 antigen in breastmilk and correlation with maternal factors. *J. Acquir. Immune Defic. Syndr.*, **7**, 68–73.

Saba, J. on behalf of the PETRA Trial Study Team. (1999). Interim analysis of early efficacy of three short ZDV/3TC regimens to prevent mother-to-child transmission of HIV-1: the PETRA trial. *6th Conference on Retroviruses and Opportunistic Infections*, Chicago IL, Jan 31–Feb 4, 1999 (abstract 57).

Semba, R. D., Miotti, P. G., Chiphangwi, J. D., Liomba, G., Yang, L. P., Saah, A. J., Dallabetta, G. A. & Hoover, D.R. (1995). Infant mortality and maternal vitamin A deficiency during human immunodeficiency virus infection. *Clin. Infect. Dis.*, **21**, 966–72.

Semprini, A. E., Castagna, C., Ravizza, M., Fiore, S., Savasi, V., Muggiasca, M. L., Grossi, E., Guerra, B., Tibaldi, C., Scaravelli, G. et al. (1995). The incidence of complications after caesarean section in 156 HIV positive women. *AIDS*, **9**, 913–17.

Shaffer, N., Chuachoowong, R., Mock, P. A., Bhadrakom, C., Siriwasin, W., Young, N. L., Chotpitayasunondh, T., Chearskul, S., Roongpisuthipong, A., Chinayon, P., Karon, J., Mastro, T. D. & Simonds, R. J. (1999a). Short-course zidovudine for perinatal HIV-1 transmission in Bangkok, Thailand: a randomised controlled trial. Bangkok Collaborative Perinatal HIV Transmission Study Group. *Lancet*, **353**, 773–80.

Shaffer, N., Roongpisuthipong, A., Siriwasin, W., Chotpitayasunondh, T., Chearskul, S., Young, N. L., Parekh, B., Mock, P. A., Bhadrakom, C., Chinayon, P., Kalish, M. L., Phillips, S. K., Granade, T. C., Subbarao, S., Weniger, B. G. & Mastro, T. D. (1999b). Maternal virus load and perinatal human immunodeficiency virus type 1 subtype E transmission, Thailand. Bangkok Collaborative Perinatal HIV Transmission Study Group. *J. Infect. Dis.*, **179**, 590–9.

Simonon, A., Lepage, P., Karita, E., Hitimana, D. G., Dabis, F., Msellati, P., Van Goethem, C., Nsengumuremyi, F., Bazubagira, A. & Van de Perre, P. (1994). An assessment of the timing of mother-to-child transmission of human immunodeficiency virus type 1 by means of polymerase chain reaction. *J. Acquir. Immune Defic. Syndr.*, **7**, 952–7.

Soderlund, N., Zwi, K., Kinghorn, A. & Gray, G. (1999). Prevention of vertical transmission of HIV: analysis of cost effectiveness of options available in South Africa *Br. Med. J.*, **318**, 1650–6.

St Louis, M. E., Kamenga, M., Brown, C., Nelson, A. M., Manzila, T., Batter, V., Behets, F., Kabagabo, U., Ryder, R. W., Oxtoby, M., et al (1993) Risk for perinatal HIV-1 transmission according to maternal immunologic, virologic and placental factors. *J.A.M.A.*, **169**, 2853–9.

Stanecki, K. A. & Way, P. O. (1999). Focus on HIV/AIDS in the developing world. In *US Bureau of the census, Report WP/98, World Population Profile*, 1998, Washington DC: US Government Printing Office.

Steketee, R., Nahlen, B. Avisi, J., van Eijk, A., Otienc, J., Misore, A., Rayfield, M. & Udhayakumar, K. Association between placental malarial infection and increased risk of mother to infant transmission of HIV-1 in western Kenya. 12th World AIDS Conference, Geneva, 28 June–3 July 1998, Abstract 23268.

Taha, T. E., Biggar, R. J., Broadhead, R. L., Mtimavalye, L. A., Justesen, A. B., Liomba, G. N., Chiphangwi, J. D. & Miotti, P. G. (1997). The effect of cleansing the birth canal with antiseptic solution on maternal and neonatal morbidity and mortality in Malawi: clinical trial. *Br. Med. J.*, **315**, 65–9.

Temmerman, M., Nyong'o, A. O., Bwayo, J., Fransen, K., Coppens, M. & Piot, P. (1995). Risk factors for mother-to-child transmission of human immunodeficiency virus-1 infection. *Am. J. Obstet. Gynecol.*, **172**, 700–5.

Tess, B. T., Rodrigues, L. C., Newell, M. L., Dunn, D. T., Lago, T. D. G. for the Sao Paolo Collaborative Study of Vertical Transmission of HIV-1. (1997). Infant feeding and risk of mother-to-child transmission of HIV-1 in Sao Paolo State, Brazil. *J. Acquir. Immune Defic. Syndr. Hum. Retrovirol.* **19**, 189–94.

UNAIDS. (1998). *AIDS Epidemic Update: December 1998.* Geneve: Joint United Nations Programme on HIV/AIDS.

US Bureau of the Census (1999). *Recent HIV Seroprevalence Levels by Country:* February 1999. Research Note No.26, Washington DC: US Government Printing Office.

Vallat, A.V., De Girolami, U., He, J., Mhashilkar, A., Marasco, W., Shi, B., Gray, F., Bell, J., Keohane, C., Smith, T. W. & Gabuzda, D. (1998). Localization of HIV-1 co-receptors CCR5 and CXCR4 in the brain of children with AIDS. *Am. J. Pathol.*, **152**, 167–78.

Van de Perre, P., Simonon, A., Msellati, P., Hitimana, D. G., Vaira, D., Bazubagira, A., Van Goethem, C., Stevens, A. M., Karita, E., Sondag-Thull, D., et al. (1991). Postnatal transmission of human immunodeficiency virus type 1 from mother to infant. A prospective cohort study in Kigali, Rwanda. *N. Engl. J. Med.*, **325**, 593–8.

Van de Perre, P. Simonon, A., Hitimana, D. G., Dabis, F., Msellati, P., Mukamabano, B., Butera, J. B., Van Goethem, C., Karita, E. & Lepage, P. (1993). Infective and anti-infective properties of breastmilk from HIV-1 infected women. *Lancet*, **341**, 914–18.

Wiktor, S. Z., Ekpini, E., Karon, J. M., Nkengasong, J., Maurice, C., Severin, S. T., Roels, T. H., Kouassi, M. K., Lackritz, E. M., Coulibaly, I. M. & Greenberg, A. E. (1999). Short-course oral zidovudine for prevention of mother-to-child transmission of HIV-1 in Abidjan, Côte d'Ivoire: a randomised trial. *Lancet*, **353**, 781–85.

Working Group on Mother-to-Child Transmission of HIV. (1995). Rates of mother-to-child transmission of HIV-1 in Africa, America, and Europe: results from 13 perinatal studies. *J. Acquir. Immune Defic. Syndr. Hum. Retrovirol.*, **8**, 506–10.

World Health Organization. (1998). Recommendations on the safe and effective use of short-course ZDV for the prevention of mother-to-child transmission of HIV *Wkly. Epidemiol. Rec.*, **73**, 313–20.

World Health Organization. (1999). *HIV in Pregnancy: A Review.* Occasional Paper Number 2. WHO/CHS/RHR/99.15; UNAIDS 99.35E. Geneva: World Health Organization.

Zijenah, L., Mbizvo, M. T., Kasule, J., Nathoo, K., Munjoma, M., Mahomed, K., Maldonado, Y., Madzime, S. & Katzenstein, D. (1998). Mortality in the first 2 years among infants born to human immunodeficiency virus infected women in Harare, Zimbabwe. *J. Infect. Dis.*, **178**, 109–13.

13

Syphilis: prevention, diagnosis and management during pregnancy and infancy

Suzanne D. Delport and Robert C. Pattinson

Introduction

Congenital syphilis is a serious and preventable disease, which remains an important cause of infant morbidity and mortality (Sciarra, 1997; Finelli et al., 1998). *Treponema pallidum* can be transmitted from an infected woman to her fetus, particularly when the mother presents with syphilis in the primary, secondary or early latent stage (Fiumara, 1952). In adults the primary lesion appears at the initial site of the infection about 3 weeks after exposure, followed by a more generalized illness involving skin rashes and condylomatalata after 6–12 weeks (secondary syphilis). If untreated, this stage is self-limited and the patient usually progresses to a latent stage of infection during which the only evidence of syphilis is positive serology. During the early latent phase (within 2 years of onset) organisms can be seeded intermittently into the blood stream.

Transmission from mother to infant can occur after at any stage of pregnancy, so that early antenatal serological screening with treatment of infected women prevents most cases of congenital syphilis (Sanchez et al., 1996). Detection in late pregnancy is less effective, but may prevent some of the sequelae. Untreated syphilis in pregnancy may result in significant perinatal mortality and morbidity, the risk depending on the stage of infection in the mother and levels of spirochetes in the blood stream (Wendel, 1988; Larkin et al., 1998). During the first 2 years of untreated latent maternal infection an estimated 20% of infants will die in utero or in the neonatal period, 20% will be premature but otherwise normal, 40% will be infected and damaged and 20% will be uninfected (McDermott et al., 1993). If a woman has a primary or secondary infection in pregnancy, it is unlikely that she will deliver a normal term infant. After the second year of maternal infection, the probability of fetal infection diminishes, and transmission is rare after the fourth year.

Congenital syphilis still occurs in both developed and developing countries despite the availability of cheap tests to diagnose maternal syphilis and an effective, cheap drug to treat the disease. Morbidity and mortality due to congenital syphilis is preventable if screening for maternal syphilis is performed during pregnancy and women found to be infected are treated without delay.

Prevalence

The magnitude of the problem of syphilis worldwide is not fully recognized since estimates depend to a large extent on the prevalence in women attending antenatal clinics, which may not be representative of the general population. The estimated prevalence in the antenatal population varies between 0.2% in developed countries to 13% in developing countries. Although tests for syphilis have been routinely performed for decades in many developed countries, there is little information on the number of women identified and treated during pregnancy, or on the incidence of congenital syphilis. The only surveillance data in the UK come from aggregate returns from genitourinary medicine clinics. As cases are not validated, stillbirths and intrauterine deaths are not included and since some infected children may be seen only by paediatricians, and not by genitourinary physicians, these figures do not reflect the true incidence.

Over the 1982–1992 period, changes in the incidence of acquired and congenital syphilis have been reported from both developed and developing countries which highlight the importance of monitoring trends. In the USA the rate of congenital syphilis among infants increased from 4.3 per 100 000 in 1982 to 94.7 per 100 000 in 1992. This closely reflected the increase in primary and secondary syphilis in women of childbearing age (Rolfs & Nakshima, 1990), which was related to social deprivation, drug use, exchange of sex for drugs and failure to receive antenatal care. Primary and secondary syphilis rates started to drop in 1991 and congenital syphilis rates declined from 1992. There was a 78.2% decrease in rates of congenital syphilis from 1992 to 1998, although rates remain disproportionately high in the southeastern USA and in minority populations (Centers for Disease Control and Prevention 1999; St Louis & Wasserheit, 1998).

High rates of syphilis have been reported from many African areas and from Eastern Europe, although a decline was shown in rates in Nairobi in the 1990s (Temmerman et al., 1999). Table 13.1 shows reported rates of syphilis seroprevalence in antenatal women.

Pathophysiology – maternal syphilis

Syphilis is caused by *Treponema pallidum*, a spirochaete below the resolution of the light microscope. Humans are the natural host and sexual contact provides the

Table 13.1. Reported syphilis seroprevalence in pregnant women

Reference	Country	Year	Prevalence
Newell et al., 1999	UK (London)	1996	0.206%
	UK (elsewhere)		0.024%
Valadez et al., 1999	Kenya (rural)	1989–1992	1.89%–12.82%
Temmerman et al., 1999	Kenya (Nairobi)	1993	6.5%
		1994	7.2%
		1995	7.3%
		1996	4.5%
		1997	3.8%
Kambarami et al., 1998	Zimbabwe (rural)	1993	9.8%
Kilmarx et al., 1998	Thailand	1996	0.5%
Meda et al., 1997	Burkina Faso	1994	3.6%
Sangare et al., 1997	Burkina Faso (national)	1994/1995	2.5%
Diallo et al., 1997	Cote d'Ivoire	1997	1.1%
Scott-Wright et al., 1997	Belize	1997	2.8%
Wilkinson et al., 1997	South Africa (rural)	1997	6.5%
Mwakagile et al., 1996	Tanzania (urban)	1996	4.0%
Folgosa et al., 1996	Mozambique	1996	7%

usual means of transmission between adults. The clinical manifestations of primary, secondary and latent syphilis are not altered by pregnancy. A primary infection is manifested by a chancre, which occurs approximately 3 weeks after contact. Chancres are commonly not recognised in women because they are asymptomatic and occur in the vagina or cervix. They are clearly demarcated ulcers 0.5–2 cm in diameter and are associated with regional enlarged lymph nodes. If untreated, chancres heal spontaneously within 3–8 weeks. Secondary syphilis appears 4–10 weeks after the initial appearance of the chancre. Treponemes from a chancre disseminate and a skin rash develops. The latter may be macular, papular, follicular, papulosquamous or pustular. The lesions are symmetrical, non-pruritic and involve the trunk and the palms and soles. Superficial mucosal erosions may involve the oral cavity, vulva, vagina or cervix. Papules may become exuberant and wart-like if situated in warm, moist areas and are then called condylomata lata, which are highly infectious. The spirochaetaemia from secondary syphilis causes constitutional symptoms such as fever, anorexia, headache, fatigue and arthralgia, associated with a non-tender lymphadenopathy. Other complications such as hepatitis, glomerulonephritis, nephrotic syndrome, osteitis, iritis or meningitis may occur during secondary syphilis.

Latent syphilis is characterized by an absence of clinical signs and positive serological tests for syphilis. Ongoing organ destruction may occur. Early latent syphilis refers to a period of 2 years after onset when the patient is at risk for relapsing secondary syphilis and is still infectious. Latent syphilis refers to a period of 2 years thereafter. Untreated, one-third of patients will remain in the latent phase and one-third will have clinical manifestations of the disease; of those in the last group, one-third each has neurosyphilis, cardiovascular syphilis and late benign syphilis.

Serological diagnosis of syphilis during pregnancy

Screening and confirmatory tests for syphilis are both varied and complex (Tables 13.2 and 13.3). Serological screening is performed on blood samples collected at the first antenatal visit, by standard tests such as the Venereal Disease Research Laboratory (VDRL) or the rapid plasma reagin (RPR) test (Larsen et al., 1990; Young, 1992, 1998). Since these are non-specific tests and detect non-treponemal antibodies, all positive or dubious results require confirmation by a specific treponemal test such as the *Treponema pallidum* immobilization test (TPI) and the fluorescent treponemal antibody absorption (FTA-ABS) test. Other treponemal infections such as yaws, bejel and pinta are serologically indistinguishable.

Serological tests should be assessed in combination with historical, epidemiological and clinical knowledge of the patient. Total reliance on a serological test for the diagnosis of syphilis may result in an incorrect diagnosis. Identification of antibodies produced after infection by *T. pallidum* is possible with either a cardiolipin–lecithin–cholesterol antigen or a treponema-derived antigen, forming the basis for non-treponemal and treponemal tests, respectively.

Non-treponemal tests

The non-treponemal tests are flocculation tests. The basic antigen used in most tests contains cardiolipin, cholesterol and lecithin. Modifications of the antigen have been made by stabilizing the suspension and by adding visualizing agents. All the non-treponemal tests measure IgG and IgM antibodies, can be used as qualitative tests for screening and as quantitative tests to follow treatment of the patient, are similar in sensitivity and specificity and are performed in a similar manner.

Five non-treponemal tests are currently considered standard tests for syphilis. The microscopic tests are the Venereal Disease Research Laboratory (VDRL) slide test and the unheated serum reagin (USR) test. The macroscopic tests are the rapid plasma–reagin (RPR) circle card test, the reagin screen test (RST) and the toludine red unheated serum test (TRUST). The VDRL antigen is the only one that has not

Table 13.2. Serological tests used in the diagnosis and treatment of syphilis

Test	Type of test	Clinical application
Rapid plasma reagin (RPR) test	Non-treponemal (non-specific) On-site card test Macroscopic test thus can be used in clinics Cheap	Diagnosis of activity, used in screening but also in diagnosis of active disease Quantitative Success of treatment/ re-infection
Venereal Disease Research Laboratory (VDRL)	Non-treponemal (non-specific) Not on-site More sensitive test because a microscope is used to assess the presence of flocculation. Thus is used on CSF. Must be done in a laboratory.	Diagnosis of activity, used in screening but also in diagnosis of active disease Quantitative Success of treatment/ re-infection
Treponemal pallidum Microhaemagglutination (MHA-TP)	Treponemal Specific Not on-site Expensive	Exclusion of false-positive non-treponemal tests Serofast (positive lifelong) Qualitative test
Fluorescent treponemal pallidum antibody absorption test (FTA–ABS)	Treponemal Specific Not on-site Expensive	Exclusion of false positive non-treponemal tests Serofast (positive lifelong) Qualitative IgM may be positive in the very early stages of syphilis

been stabilized by the addition of the disodium salt of ethylene–diaminetetraacetic acid (EDTA) to eliminate daily antigen preparation. The RPR and TRUST antigens contain sized particles (charcoal and red paint pigment respectively) to aid in the visualization of the antigen–antibody reaction. The RST test uses a lipid-soluble dye that stains the antigen. The RPR card test is the most widely used non-treponemal test.

A reactive non-treponemal test may indicate past or present infection. A reactive test may also be false positive. A non-reactive test may be interpreted as no current infection or as an effectively treated infection. A non-reactive test does not rule out incubating syphilis. A fourfold increase in titre (for example 1:16 to 1:64) indicates infection, re-infection or treatment failure. A fourfold decrease in titre indicates adequate therapy. A twofold increase (example 1:16 to 1:32) or decrease

Table 13.3. Changes in serology in mother over time in relation to stages of syphilis

Stage	Non-treponemal tests (RPR, VDRL)	Treponemal tests (MHA-TP, FTA–ABS)
Incubation period (6 weeks)	Negative	Negative
Primary syphilis	Negative	FTA–ABS IgM positive early, then disappears FTA–ABS IgG positive MHA-TP positive
Secondary syphilis	Positive	Positive
Early latent syphilis (first 2 years)	Positive	Positive
Late latent syphilis (after 2 years)	Positive (titre lower than early latent syphilis)	Positive
Tertiary	Negative (low titre)	Positive
Treated syphilis	Negative after 6 months	Positive (serofast)
Re-infection	Positive after previous negativity or fourfold increase in titre	Positive
Failed treatment	Failure of titre to decrease fourfold over 3–6 months	Positive

(example 1:16 to 1:8) in titre is interpreted as a stable titre to accommodate interobserver variation. Non-treponemal test misinterpretation can occur if more than one type of non-treponemal test (for example RPR and VDRL) is used to follow treatment. Up to a fourfold difference in end-point titres can occur with different non-treponemal tests.

The overall sensitivity of the non-treponemal tests is approximately 90%. Up to 28% of patients with primary syphilis, however, will have a non-reactive result on their initial visit. In approximately 30% of cases with late untreated syphilis, the non-treponemal test will be non-reactive. Specificity for the non-treponemal tests is around 98%.

Women with suspected primary stage lesions whose non-treponemal tests are non-reactive, should be retested after one week and one month. The non-treponemal tests are always reactive with secondary syphilis. Titres will be 1:16 or greater regardless of the test method used. Non-treponemal test titres in early latent syphilis are similar to those in secondary syphilis. As the length of the latent stage increases the titre decreases. Adequate treatment of primary and secondary syphilis will lead to a fourfold decline in titres after 3 months and will continue to decline until little or no reaction is detected after 1 and 2 years, respectively.

Women treated in the latent stage will show a more gradual decline in titre. In approximately 50% of women with late latent syphilis, low titres will persist even after two years or may change little.

False-negative results of non-treponemal tests are because of the prozone phenomenon. The latter occurs when agglutination is inhibited due to an excess of antibody in the serum, and should be suspected if serological results do not substantiate a clinical diagnosis. It may occur in 1–2% of women with secondary syphilis. Reactivity will occur after dilution of serum.

All non-treponemal tests will occasionally exhibit false-positive reactions at a rate of 1–2% in the pregnant and general population. Acute false-positive reactions lasting less than 6 months occur after febrile illnesses and immunisations. Chronic false-positive reactions are associated with autoimmune diseases and chronic infections such as leprosy. Ten per cent of intravenous drug users will have false-positive results. Ninety per cent of the false-positive results will have titres less than 1:8. Low titres are, however, also seen in late latent syphilis. In low-risk populations, over 50% of the reactive non-treponemal tests may be false-positive.

Treponemal tests

The treponemal tests are used for confirmatory testing of non-treponemal tests. Four treponemal tests are standard tests for syphilis: the fluorescent treponemal antibody absorption (FTA-ABS) test, the FTA-ABS double staining (DS) test, the microhaemagglutination assay for antibodies to *T. pallidum* (MHA-TP) and the haemagglutination treponemal test for syphilis (HATTS). All treponemal tests detect treponemal cellular components. The treponemal tests are qualitative tests and cannot be used to monitor the efficacy of treatment. The sensitivity of the FTA–ABS test is 98% compared with 95% for the other treponemal tests, the major difference being in the primary stage. The specificity is 98% for the FTA–ABS test and 99% for the other three treponemal tests.

A reactive treponemal test indicates past or present infection, since reactivity remains for life. A non-reactive test indicates no infection – past or present. The greatest value of the treponemal tests is the differentiation between true-positive and false-positive non-treponemal tests.

Screening for maternal syphilis

Screening aims to prevent congenital syphilis by the treatment of pregnant seropositive women with penicillin, which is highly effective (Bergstrom et al., 1994). Infants with suspected congenital syphilis should be examined clinically during their first months of life, and they should be treated if maternal treatment was suboptimal or if there is a suspicion of active infection in the child. Congenital syphilis has become a relatively rare condition in developed countries and most doctors in the UK will never have seen a case (Ewing et al., 1985).

All women should be screened for syphilis at the time that their pregnancy is diagnosed and treated immediately if indicated. In order to implement this principle in practice, women in developing countries must be screened on site during their first visit to an antenatal clinic and treated before they leave the clinic (Delport & van den Berg, 1998; Wilkinson, 1998; Wilkinson & Sach, 1998). In developed countries with an effective recall system, the tests can be done in a laboratory.

Screening should be repeated in the third trimester and at delivery in populations with a high incidence of syphilis. If the first visit occurred after the first trimester, re-screening during the third trimester is unnecessary, but screening at delivery should still take place. The RPR card test, developed originally for field conditions, is a suitable test for on-site screening for syphilis. It is inexpensive, simple, rapid and convenient. It is reliable with a sensitivity and specificity during on-site testing reported as 80% and 99%, respectively. With a syphilis prevalence of 6.6%, the positive and negative predictive values will be 78.8% and 98.5%, respectively. Thus only positive on-site tests need to be verified at a central laboratory to identify false positive on-site tests. The results of on-site negative tests do not need verification, because the negative predictive value is high.

On-site testing will, in addition, detect with a sensitivity of 100% all women with RPR titres of 1:16 and more whose fetuses are at greatest risk of dying from congenital syphilis (Delport & van Denberg, 1998). If the on-site RPR test is positive, the woman should be counselled and treated. Blood should be sent to a laboratory for verification of the result. She should return after 1 week for confirmation of her result and documentation on her handheld medical notes (motherhood card), further counselling and treatment if indicated. A referral letter to a clinic for sexually transmitted diseases must be given to the woman to hand to her partner. If the result of the on-site test is doubtful, the woman should be counselled and blood sent to a laboratory. She should return in a week for treatment if indicated.

The sensitivity of the on-site RPR test is highest in the high RPR titre ranges of 1:8 and higher. On-site testing will therefore miss women with very low RPR titres such as 1:2 and 1:4. These low titres may be due to serofast low titres, declining titres as a result of successful treatment of syphilis or biological false positive tests and are thought not to place the fetus at risk of congenital syphilis since active maternal syphilis is not present. Some clinicians would not treat these women. Serological screening for syphilis is cost-effective even if the prevalence of maternal syphilis is as low as 0.005%.

The rate of seroconversion in pregnancy appears to be low. However, women at risk of syphilis who are screened in the first trimester and found to be negative should be re-screened at the beginning of the third trimester to exclude seroconversion. This practice will identify women who have undiagnosed syphilis due to inadequate screening during pregnancy, women who seroconverted and women with a re-infection. Untreated women with RPR titres of 1:8 or more have active syphilis and are in need of treatment.

Treatment of maternal syphilis

Treatment before 20 weeks of gestation virtually eliminates the possibility of congenital syphilis, barring re-infection. Patients should be screened and treatment started – if indicated – at the time pregnancy is detected. For primary, secondary and latent syphilis less than one year's duration benzathine penicillin G, 2.4 million units should be administered intramuscularly. For latent syphilis of unknown duration, benzathine penicillin-G 2.4 million units are administered intramuscularly weekly for 3 successive weeks. Women with proven penicillin allergy are desensitized on an inpatient basis by using an oral phenoxymethyl penicillin suspension regimen followed by the appropriate benzathine penicillin schedule for the stage of syphilis (Hollier & Cox, 1998; Birnbaum et al., 1999; Chisholm et al., 1997) see (Table 13.4).

The expected serologic response is a fourfold drop in titre after 3 months for primary and after 6 months for secondary syphilis. In patients with persistent high non-treponemal titres, treatment failure or re-infection should be considered.

Congenital syphilis

Syphilis and pregnancy outcome

T. pallidum crosses the placenta and may result in fetal infection, preterm delivery or stillbirth. Congenital syphilis has been traditionally divided into two stages. When clinical features of the disease are apparent in the first 2 years of life, and a direct result of active infection and inflammation, the disease is designated as early congenital syphilis. After 2 years it is termed late congenital syphilis, and presents with malformations and stigmata that represent the scars induced by initial lesions of early syphilis or reactions to persisting or ongoing inflammation. The most common neonatal presentation includes hepatomegaly, jaundice and osteochondritis; lymphadenopathy, pneumonia and myocarditis are less common clinical manifestations. Clinical features may not become apparent until 2–12 weeks of age. The most common clinical manifestation of late congenital syphilis is interstitial keratitis, occurring in about 40% of affected children, usually between 6 and 14 years. Bone and joint lesions, and disease leading to deafness and neurological involvement may result in a minority of children.

Table 13.4. Penicillin allergy: oral desensitization protocol

Dosage (U\ml)[a]	Amount[b] ml	Amount[b] U	Cumulative dose (U)
1000	0.1	100	100
1000	0.2	200	300
1000	0.4	400	700
1000	0.8	800	1500
1000	1.6	1600	3100
1000	3.2	3200	6300
1000	6.4	6400	12 700
10 000	1.2	12 000	24 700
10 000	2.4	24 000	48 700
10 000	4.8	48 000	96 700
80 000	1.0	80 000	176 700
80 000	2.0	160 000	336 700
80 000	4.0	320 000	656 700
80 000	8.0	640 000	1 296 700

[a] Interval between doses, 15 minutes; elapsed time 3 hours and 35 minutes; cumulative dose 1.3 million unit.

[b] The specific amount of penicillin V suspension was diluted in approximately 30 ml of water and then given orally.

Diagnosis of congenital syphilis is difficult, even when infection is suspected, because many infected infants are asymptomatic at birth and the presence of maternal antibody makes infants' serology difficult to interpret. Definitive proof with the identification of *T. pallidum* is rare since the organism cannot be cultured and few infants have skin lesion to produce a specimen for dark field microscopy (Ewing et al., 1985). As a result, good reporting criteria for congenital syphilis are difficult to formulate. The CDC definition of congenital syphilis includes infants with clinical evidence of active infection, asymptomatic infants and stillbirths (Centers For Disease Control, 1992). All infants at risk require a full clinical evaluation at birth and follow-up until non-treponemal and treponemal tests are negative and maternal antibody has disappeared.

T. pallidum readily crosses the placenta at any stage during pregnancy. The fetal risks for congenital infection depend on the degree of maternal spirochaetaemia and duration of infection prior to delivery. When primary or secondary syphilis is untreated, 50% of the infants will be either stillborn, premature or die during the neonatal period. In the event of early latent syphilis, up to 60% of neonates will be normal with 40% having congenital syphilis. In untreated late latent syphilis, only

Table 13.5. Risk of vertical transmission

Stage of syphilis	Perinatal infection (%)
Primary	50
Secondary	50
Latent	
Early latent	40
Late latent	10
Tertiary	0

10% of infants will have congenital syphilis. Table 13.5 summarizes the risk of transmission.

Kassowitz's law, which states that with each succeeding pregnancy the effect on the fetus will be less severe until eventually an unaffected infant will be born, relates to the maternal immune response which will eventually protect the fetus from infection.

The placenta is involved secondarily after the initial spirochaetaemia in the fetus. Macroscopically, the placenta is enlarged disproportionately. Congenital syphilis in utero may present with abnormalities on cardiotocography such as type II decelerations and loss of baseline variability. Non-immune hydrops fetalis due to intrauterine hemolysis should raise the suspicion of congenital syphilis.

The Jarisch–Herxheimer reaction following treatment of maternal syphilis during pregnancy may have further adverse effects on the fetus. The occurrence of the reaction reflects the maternal stage of syphilis, occurring most commonly in the primary and secondary stages of the disease. Patients may experience increased uterine activity associated with fever, hypotension, tachycardia, myalgia and headache which occur at an average of 5 hours after treatment. A transient change in fetal well-being is evidenced by transient late decelerations associated with reaction-induced contractions. If the fetus is severely affected, preterm labour, delivery or fetal death may ensue. Tocolysis may have to be undertaken in this setting because these fetuses might benefit more if delivered and treated with parenteral penicillin (Rodriguez et al., 1996).

Early congenital syphilis

This diagnosis should be considered in any infant whose mother had suboptimal antenatal care regarding syphilis surveillance and treatment during pregnancy. Prematurity associated with intrauterine growth retardation is a common finding associated with congenital syphilis. The effect of syphilis on the growth of the fetus seems, however, to be related to the timing and severity of the fetal infection.

Infants may have a normal birthweight with clinical signs or have no clinical signs at birth, only to develop them one to three months after birth.

Clinical manifestations

Significant differences occur in the clinical manifestations among neonates and postneonates. The mortality rate can be fivefold higher among neonates.

Hepatosplenomegaly

Nearly all infants have hepatosplenomegaly with equal frequency amongst neonates and older infants. Hepatomegaly may occur in the absence of splenomegaly but the reverse rarely occurs. Jaundice can be present in up to one-third of patients but is a more common manifestation during the neonatal period, and is commonly a conjugated hyperbilirubinaemia caused by a syphilitic hepatitis.

Mucocutaneous manifestations

A skin rash is more common in infants after the neonatal period. The most common cutaneous lesion is an erythematous maculopapular rash that becomes coppery-brown and involves the palms and soles. In neonates desquamation of the palms and soles is the most common cutaneous manifestation of congenital syphilis. Bilateral symmetrical hypopigmented skin lesions, which involve the buttocks, upper and lower extremities and the diaper area, may also occur.

Rhinitis (snuffles) occurs in the minority (10%) of neonates and is more common after the neonatal period. A mucous discharge develops which teems with spirochaetes. The discharge may become blood-tinged.

Joint swellings and pseudoparesis

These occur with great rarity in neonates. Pseudoparesis occurs associated with painful osteochondritis in older infants. Although the latter is symmetric radiologically, only one extremity may be painful. More commonly the infant appears extremely irritable and keeps his extremities relatively still. On passive movement during examination, pain is elicited.

Generalized lymphadenopathy

Generalized enlargement of lymph nodes occurs in at least 50% of patients. Non-tender generalized lymphadenopathy in early infancy should arouse a suspicion of congenital syphilis.

Ocular manifestations

Chorioretinitis, salt and pepper fundus, glaucoma, uveitis and chancres of the eyelids have been described. The frequency of syphilitic involvement of the eye in early congenital syphilis is unknown.

Gastrointestinal manifestations

Neonates may present with an intestinal malfunction resulting from a mechanical obstruction. An atresia or stenosis may be present or a meconium ileus or plug resulting from an intestinal motility disturbance due to syphilitic enterocolitis. The latter is aggravated in the presence of inspissated meconium secondary to a pancreatic exocrine deficiency due to syphilitic pancreatitis.

Renal manifestations

The clinical picture may be that of a nephrotic syndrome or an acute glomerulonephritis.

Central nervous system

Acute syphilitic leptomeningitis forms part of the clinical syndrome of congenital syphilis and is characterized by cerebrospinal fluid abnormalities. The latter includes an increase in protein, a normal glucose level, an increase in mononuclear cells and a positive VDRL test.

Chronic meningovascular syphilis may have a protracted course resulting in progressive hydrocephalus, cranial nerve palsies or vascular lesions of the brain. The hydrocephalus is low grade, progressive and communicating because of obstruction of the basal cisterns. It usually develops towards the end of the first year.

Haematological abnormalities

A Coombs-negative haemolytic anaemia is a common manifestation of the disease during the early neonatal period. A lymphocytosis during the early neonatal period when polymorphonucluear leukocytes should predominate commonly occurs and may be associated with an absolute neutropaenia. Polychromasia and erythroblastaemia with up to 500 nucleated red blood cells per 100 leukocytes may in the presence of anaemia lead to confusion with erythroblastosis fetalis. A leukemoid reaction is possible and may be so severe as to mimic a diagnosis of congenital leukaemia. Thrombocytopaenia occurs and is related to decreased platelet survival rather than to insufficient production.

Radiological changes

Bony involvement is the most common and frequent manifestation of congenital syphilis. The lesions are not due to inflammatory changes, but are dystrophic in nature because of a disturbance in enchondral and periosteal bone formation. The metaphysis, diaphysis and periosteum are involved with sparing of epiphyses. The earliest and most characteristic changes occur in the metaphysis in the form of radiopaque bands, porotic zones, combinations of the two, saw tooth appearance or a lateral bone deficiency. Metaphyseal dystrophy is the most common radiological finding in neonates. Lesions in long bones are located on the lateral aspects of the metaphyses. The tibia may show metaphyseal defects on the medial side. If the defect occurs bilaterally it is called Wimberger's sign.

A 'celery stick' appearance of alternating longitudinal bands of translucency and relative density results from irregularity of the endosteal and periosteal aspects of the cortex. This finding is also seen in congenital rubella and cytomegalovirus infection. Periosteal dystrophy seen as a single or multiple periosteal layering is the most common radiological finding. It occurs, however, very rarely at birth. Involvement of the metacarpals and proximal phalanges of the hand is rarely seen. Dactylitis occurs after the neonatal period. Single bone involvement is extremely rare. Bony lesions heal without residual deformity and seem to be uninfluenced by whether treatment was received.

Serologic tests

Non-treponemal (e.g. RPR) and treponemal (e.g. MHA-TP) tests are used for the serologic diagnosis in the infant as well. Since these tests measure IgG, they will reflect passively transferred antibodies from the mother. A rising RPR titre performed in an untreated infant will indicate a congenital infection, while a declining titre (without treatment) reflects declining passively acquired IgG and no congenital infection. A minority of infants with congenital syphilis have higher RPR titres than the mother.

The FTA–ABS IgM test measures IgM that does not cross the placenta. However it is falsely negative in 20–39% of cases and falsely positive in up to 10% of cases and cannot be used in the diagnosis of congenital syphilis. Table 13.6 summarizes serological tests in neonates. New tests under investigation are the FTA–ABS 19S, IgM ELISA, Western blot and a PCR test. None has a sensitivity greater than 88% and their cost and sophistication preclude routine use.

Disease identification and treatment

Symptomatic infants

The diagnosis of congenital syphilis is straightforward in a symptomatic infant born to a woman with untreated or inadequately treated syphilis. Radiological abnormalities and a reactive non-treponemal test are invariably present. These infants should receive a 10–14-day uninterrupted course of crystalline penicillin G 150 000 units/kg intravenously daily in two divided doses or procaine penicillin G 50 000 units/kg intramuscularly once daily for 10 days.

Asymptomatic infants

Infants who are born to inadequately treated women and are clinically asymptomatic form the majority of potentially infected infants. Radiographs in these

Table 13.6. Serology in the neonate

Clinical picture	Non-treponemal tests (RPR, VDRL)	Treponemal tests (MHA-TP, FTA-ABS)	Diagnosis
Clinical signs present in neonate e.g. hepatosplenomegaly Inadequate maternal treatment	RPR positive (titre lower, equalling or exceeding maternal titre)	MHA-TP positive, FTA–ABS IgG positive FTA–ABS IgM positive or negative	Congenital syphilis
Neonate clinically normal, term and appropriately grown Inadequate maternal treatment	RPR positive (titre equalling or lower than maternal titre performed concurrently)	MHA-TP positive FTA–ABS IgG positve FTA–ABS IgM positive or negative	Asymptomatic congenital syphilis (risk 4.1%) or no infection Treat with benzathine penicillin G. Untreated, the RPR titre of infected infants will be higher after 1–3 months. If the titre declines over 1–3 months, infection is ruled out. (See treatment section)
Neonate clinically normal, term and appropriately grown (>2.5kg) Adequate maternal treatment	RPR positive (equalling or lower than maternal titre – performed concurrently)	TPHA positive FTA–ABS IgG positve FTA–ABS IgM positive or negative	Non-infection

infants are invariably normal and serological tests for syphilis are non-contributory because of passively acquired maternal IgG. The guidelines of the Centers of Disease Control relating to the management of these asymptomatic infants are cumbersome and difficult to apply in settings which are inadequately resourced with regard to manpower and finances and where follow-up of infants is unreliable. Longitudinal follow-up of untreated asymptomatic infants showed that the treatment history of the mother and clinical evaluation of the infant could be used to predict the risk of asymptomatic congenital syphilis (Delport, 1994). Term, appropriately grown, asymptomatic infants born to women who received any number of benzathine penicillin G injections more than 1 month before delivery have no risk of having asymptomatic (occult) congenital syphilis. No special investigations in the form of serology or radiographs need to be performed on the infants and no follow-up is necessary. However, term, appropriately grown, asymptomatic infants born to women whose treatment was initiated during the last month of pregnancy or who received no treatment during pregnancy have a risk of around 4% of having asymptomatic (occult) congenital syphilis. These infants should receive one dose of benzathine penicillin G 50 000 units/kg intramuscularly. Low birthweight asymptomatic infants born to women who received inadequate treatment still pose a diagnostic and therapeutic dilemma. Treatment as for symptomatic infants may be the safest option.

REFERENCES

Bergstrom, S., Hojer, B., Liljestrand, J. & Tunell, R. (1994). *Perinatal Health Care with Limited Resources*, pp. 10–12. London: Macmillan.

Birnbaum, N. R., Goldschmidt, R. H. & Buffett, W. O. (1999). Resolving the common clinical dilemmas of syphilis. *Am. Fam. Physician*, **59**, 2233–40, 2245–6.

Centers for Disease Control. (1992). *Congenital Syphilis Case Investigation and Reporting Form Instructions.* Atlanta: Centers for Disease Control.

Centers for Disease Control and Prevention (1999). Congenital syphilis – United States, 1998. *Morb. Mortal. Wkly. Rep.*, **48**, 757–61.

Chisholm, C. A., Katz, V. L., McDonald, T. L. & Bowes, W. A. Jr. (1997). Penicillin desensitization in the treatment of syphilis during pregnancy. *Am. J. Perinatol.*, **14**, 553–4.

Delport, S. D. (1994). Missed opportunities for the prevention of congenital syphilis and a proposed solution. PhD Thesis, Univ. of Pretoria, Pretoria.

Delport, S. D. & van den Berg, J. H. (1998). On-site screening for syphilis at an antenatal clinic. *S. Afr. Med. J.,* **88**, 43–4.

Diallo, M. O., Ettiegne-Traore, V., Maran, M., Kouadio, J., Brattegaard, K., Makke, A., Van Dyck, E., Laga, M. & De Cock, K. M. (1997). Sexually transmitted diseases and human immunodeficiency virus infections in women attending an antenatal clinic in Abidjan, Côte d'Ivoire. *Int. J. STD AIDS*, **8**, 636–8.

Ewing, C. I., Roberts, C., Davidson, D. C. & Arya, O. P. (1985). Early congenital syphilis still occurs. *Arch, Dis. Child*, **60**, 1128–33.

Finelli, L., Berman, S. M., Koumans, E. H. & Levine, W. C. (1998). Congenital syphilis. *Bull. World Health Organ.* **76**, 126–8.

Fiumara, N. (1952). The incidence of prenatal syphilis at the Boston City Hospital. *N. Engl. J. Med.*, **247**, 48–52.

Folgosa, E., Bique-Osman, N., Gonzalez, C., Hagerstrand, I. Bergstrom, S. & Ljungh, A. A. (1996). Syphilis seroprevalence among pregnant women and its role as a risk factor for still birth in Maputo, Mozambique, *Genitourin. Med.*, **72**, 339–42.

Hollier, L. M. & Cox, S. M. (1998). Syphilis. *Semin. Perinatol.*, **22**, 323–31.

Kambarami, R. A., Manyame, B. & Macq, J. (1998). Syphilis in Murewa District, Zimbabwe: an old problem that rages on. *Cent. Afr. J. Med.*, **44**, 229–32.

Kilmarx, P. H., Black, C. M., Limpakarnjanarat, K., Shaffer, N., Yanpaisarn, S., Chaisilwattana, P., Siriwasin, W., Young, N. L., Farshy, C. E., Mastro, T. D. & St Louis, M. E. (1998). Rapid assessment of sexually transmitted diseases in a sentinel population in Thailand: prevalence of chlamydial infection, gonorrhoea, and syphilis among pregnant women – 1996. *Sex. Transm. Infect.*, **74**, 189–93.

Larkin, J. A., Lit, L., Toney, J. & Haley, J. A. (1998). Recognizing and treating syphilis in pregnancy. *Medscape Wom. Health,* **3**, 5.

Larsen, S. A., Hunter, E. F. & Kraus, S. J. (1990). *A Manual of Tests for Syphilis.* Washington DC: American Public Health Association.

McDermott, J., Steketee, R., Larsen, S. & Wirima, J. (1993). Syphilis-associated perinatal and infant mortality in rural Malawi. *Bull. World Health Organ.*, **71**, 773–80.

Meda, N., Sangare, L., Lankoande, S., Sanou, P. T., Compaore, P. I., Catraye, J., Cartoux, M. & Soudre, R. B. (1997). Pattern of sexually transmitted diseases among pregnant women in Burkina Faso, west Africa: potential for a clinical management based on simple approaches. *Genitourin. Med.*, **73**, 188–93.

Mwakagile, D., Swai, A. B., Sandstrom, E., Urassa, E., Biberfeld, G. & Mhalu, F. S. (1996). High frequency of sexually transmitted diseases among pregnant women in Dar es Salaam, Tanzania: need for intervention. *East Afr. Med. J.*, **73**, 675–8.

Newell, M. L., Thorne, C., Pembrey, L., Nicoll, A., Goldberg, D. & Peckham, C. (1999). Antenatal screening for hepatitis B infection and syphilis in the UK. *Br. J. Obstet. Gynaecol.*, **106**, 66–71.

Rodriguez, A. C., Meyer, W. J. & Watrobka, T. (1996). The Jarisch–Herxheimer reaction in pregnancy: a nursing perspective. *J. Obstet. Gynecol. Neonatal. Nurs.*, **25**, 383–6.

Rolfs, R. T. & Nakshima, A. K. (1990). Epidemiology of primary and secondary syphilis in the United States, 1981 through 1989. *J.A.M.A.*, **264**, 1432–7.

Sanchez, P. J., Wendel, G. D. & Norgard, M. V. (1996). IgM antibody to *Treponema pallidum* in cerebrospinal fluid of infants with congenital syphilis. *Am. J. Dis. Child.*, **146**, 1171–5.

Sangare, L., Meda, N., Lankoande, S., Van Dyck, E., Cartoux, M., Compaore, I. P., Catraye, J., Sanou, P. T. & Soudre, R. (1997). HIV infection among pregnant women in Burkina Faso: a nationwide serosurvey. *Int. J. STD AIDS*, **8**, 646–51.

Sciarra, J. J. (1997). Sexually transmitted diseases: global importance. *Int. J. Gynaecol. Obstet.*, **58**, 107–19.

Scott-Wright, A., Hakre, S., Bryan, J. P., Jaramillo, R., Reyes, L. G., Cruess, D., Macarthy, P. O. & Gaydos, J. C. (1997). Hepatitis B virus, human immunodeficiency virus type-1, and syphilis among women attending prenatal clinics in Belize, Central America. *Am. J. Trop. Med. Hyg.*, **56**, 285–90.

St Louis, M. E. & Wasserheit, J. N. (1998). Elimination of syphilis in the United States. *Science*, **281**, 353–4.

Temmerman, M., Fonck, K., Bashir, F., Inion, I., Ndinya-Achola, J. O., Bwayo, J., Kirui, P., Claeys, P. & Fansen, L. (1999). Declining syphilis prevalence in pregnant women in Nairobi since 1995: another success story in the STD field? *Int. J. STD AIDS*, **10**, 405–8.

Valadez, J. J., Loolpapit, P. M., Nyangao, A. & Dikir, F. (1999). HIV and syphilis serostatus of antenatals in traditional Maasai pasturalist communities in Kajiado District, Kenya: 1989–1992. *Trop. Doct.*, **29**, 94–8.

Villar, J. & Bergsjo, P. (1997). Scientific basis for the content of routine antenatal care I. Philosophy, recent studies, and power to eliminate or alleviate adverse maternal outcomes. *Acta Obstet. Gynecol. Scand.*, **76**, 1–14.

Wendel, G. D. (1988). Gestational and congenital syphilis. *Clin. Perinatol.*, **15**, 287–303.

Wilkinson, D. (1998). Screening for syphilis in pregnant women. *Trop. Doct.*, **28**, 120.

Wilkinson, D. & Sach, M. (1998) Improved treatment of syphilis among pregnant women through on-site testing: an intervention study in rural South Africa. *Trans. R. Soc. Trop. Med. Hyg.*, **92**, 348.

Wilkinson, D., Sach, M. & Connolly, C. (1997). Epidemiology of syphilis in pregnancy in rural South Africa: opportunities for control. *Trop. Med. Int. Health*, **2**, 57–62.

Yetman, R. J., Risser, W. L., Barth, B. A., Risser, J. M., Hwang, L. Y. (1998). Problems in physician's classification and reporting of congenital syphilis. *Int. J. STD AIDS*, **9**, 765–8.

Young, H. (1992). Syphilis: new diagnostic directions. *Int. J. Sex. Transm. Dis. AIDS*, **3**, 391–413.

Young, H. (1998). Syphilis. Serology. *Dermatol. Clin.*, **16**, 691–8.

14

The other sexually transmitted diseases

Paolo Miotti and Gina Dallabetta

Introduction

This chapter discusses aspects of five reproductive tract infections (RTIs) on maternal and infant health. The five RTIs considered are gonorrhoea, chlamydial infection, genital mycoplasma infection, trichomoniasis and bacterial vaginosis. These infections are very common in resource-constrained settings and are the cause of significant morbidity for women and their children. Syphilis and HIV are discussed in other chapters.

Neisseria gonorrhoeae infection in pregnancy

Epidemiology

Globally, the prevalence of gonococcal cervical infections in pregnant women varies widely geographically (Table 14.1). In Western Europe and Canada, the prevalence of gonorrhoea in pregnant women is very low. In the USA prevalence in pregnant women varies widely. In sub-Saharan Africa, Asia, Latin America and the Caribbean, gonococcal infection prevalence rates in pregnant women and family planning clinic attenders vary widely, but are also much higher than in industrialized areas. Overall, the burden of gonococcal infection in developing countries is increasing due to its rising prevalence and to the increasing cost of treatment, after the widespread emergence of resistance to inexpensive antibiotic therapy (Ison et al., 1998).

Risk factors for gonococcal infection appear to be the same in pregnant as in non-pregnant women. Studies in North America have shown that individuals with the highest rate of detected gonorrhoea live in urban areas, are young, non-white, unmarried, of low socio-economic status and with a prior history of gonorrhoea (Barnes & Holmes, 1984). Studies from developing countries have shown that cervical gonococcal and/or chlamdyial infection correlates with young age, un-married status, number of recent sexual partners, and behavioural and occupa-tional characteristics of the male partners (Ryan et al., 1998a; Costello Daly et al.,

Table 14.1. Prevalence of reproductive tract infections in antenatal clinic (ANC) and family planning (FP) clinic attendees

Region	Country	Population	N. gonorrhoeae	C. trachomatis	T. vaginalis	Bacterial vaginosis
Africa						
	Gabon, 1994–95 [1]	ANC	1.9	9.9	10.7	22.9
	Zaire, 1990 [2]	ANC	1.1	1.6	18.4	
	Tanzania, 1992–93 [3]	ANC	2.1	6.6	27.4	
	Kenya, 1987 [4]	ANC	10	8		
	Kenya, 1994 [5]	ANC	2.4	8.8	19.9	20.6
	Kenya, 1997 [6]	FP	2.1	3.8	10	
	Tanzania, 1991–92 [7]	ANC	4.2		14.3	
	Tanzania, 1994 [8]	ANC	2.3	5.9	16	24
	Tanzania, 1995 [9]	FP	1.6	6.7	21.6	
	Burkina Faso, 1994 [10]	ANC	1.6	3.1	14.0	12.9
	Botswana, 1990 [11]	ANC	14		48	
	Nigeria [12]	ANC	4	3	16	11
	Rwanda, 1992–93 [13]	ANC	4.7	4.5	15.5	
	South Africa, 1987 [14]	ANC	5.7	11.4	49.2	
	South Africa, 1994 [15]	FP	3	12	18	29
	Malawi, 1989–90 [16]	ANC	5	3	32	
	Morocco, 1995–96 [17]	FP	3.2	2.6	6.6	18.5
Latin America/Caribbean						
	Haiti, 1993 [18]	ANC	4.0	12.1	34.7	30.8
	Jamaica, 1995 [19]	FP	2.7	12.2	11.5	
	Peru, 1997 [20]	FP	0.3	22.4	14.9	61.4
	Brazil, 1991–92 [21]	FP	0	6.7	1.7	25.8
Asia						
	Bangladesh, 1996 [22]	PHC	0.2	1.2	0.9	17
	Fiji, 1997 [23]	FP	0.4	19.5	11	
	Thailand, 1996 [24]	ANC	0.2	5.7		
	Papua New Guinea, 1995 [25]	Community	1.5	26.4	46.5	9.1
	Cambodia, 1996 [26]	RHC	3	3.1	1.0	12.7
	Indonesia, 1992–93 [27]	ANC	0.5	8	5	
North America						
	Colorado 1991–92 [28]	ANC	0.6	8.5	9.8	30.9
	Wisconsin, 1990 [29]	FP	0.4	6.9		

[1]Bourgeois et al. (1998); [2]Vuylsteke et al. (1993); [3] Mayaud et al. (1995); [4]Braddick et al. (1990); [5] Thomas et al. (1996); [6]Temmerman et al. (1998a); [7]Gertig et al. (1997); [8]Mayaud et al. (1998); [9]Kapiga et al. (1998); [10]Meda et al. (1997); [11]Sheller et al. (1990); [12]Erwin (1993); [13]Leroy et al. (1995); [14]O'Farrell et al. (1989); [15]Schneider et al. (1998); [16]Dallabetta et al. (1993); [17]Ryan et al. (1998); [18]Behets et al. (1995); [19]Behets et al. (1998); [20]Sánchez et al. (1998); Teles et al. (1997); [22]Hawkes et al. (1997); [23]Mathai et al. (1998); [24]Kilmarx et al. (1998); [25]Passey et al. (1998); [26]Ryan & Gorbach (1997); [27] Linnan (1995); [28]McGregor et al. (1995); [29]Addiss et al. (1993).

Table 14.2. Maternal reproductive tract infections (RTI): consequences of untreated infections and control strategies

RTI	Consequences of untreated Infections at delivery	Control strategies

Neisseria gonorrhoeae	Adverse pregnancy outcome:
	  Abortion 2–35%
	  Perinatal death 2–11%
	  Prematurity 13–67%
	  Premature rupture of membranes 21–75%
	  Prenatal distress 5–10%
	Maternal postpartum infection 14–50%
	(gonococcal and/or chlamydial infection)
	Neonatal infection
	  Conjunctivitis/ophthalmia 30–47%
	  Disseminated disease – rare (0–1%)
		Prevention of gonococcal infection in the mother (all complications)
		Screening and treatment of maternal gonorrhoea (all complications)
		– universal screening and treatment
		– selective screening and treatment
		– universal presumptive therapy (mass therapy)
		– selective presumptive therapy
		Ocular prophylaxis immediately after birth (for conjunctivitis/ophthalmia)
		Diagnosis and treatment of gonococcal ophthalmia neonatorum (reasonable in very low prevalence setting with good health services)

Chlamydia trachomatis	Adverse pregnancy outcome:
	  inconclusive data
	Maternal postpartum infection 14–50%
	(gonococcal and/or chlamydial infection)
	Neonatal infection
	  Conjuctivitis/ophthalmia 15–44%
	  Pneumonia 1–22%
		Prevention of chlamydial infection in the mother (all complications)
		Screening and treatment of maternal chlamydial infection (all complications)
		– universal screening and treatment
		– selective screening and treatment
		– universal presumptive therapy (mass therapy)
		– selective presumptive therapy
		Ocular prophylaxis immediately after birth (for conjunctivitis/ophthalmia)
		Diagnosis and treatment of chlamydial complications (conjunctivitis/ophthalmia and pneumonia)

Mycoplasmas	Adverse pregnancy outcome (inconclusively proven to date)
	  Spontaneous abortion
	  Infertility
	  Premature rupture of membranes
	  Chorioamnionitis
	  Prematurity
	Neonatal infections
	  Respiratory tract infections
	  Meningitis
		No control strategy recommended due to inability to establish causal role of mycoplasmas in the presence of other pathogens

Table 14.2. (*cont.*)

RTI	Consequences of untreated infections at delivery	Control strategies
Trichomonas vaginalis	Adverse pregnancy outcome (% increase over BV negative women):	Prevention of trichomonal Infection in the mother (all complications)
	Prematurity 4–10%	Screening and treatment of maternal
	Premature rupture of membranes 15%	trichomoniasis (all complications)
	Maternal postpartum infection 2%	Presumptive treatment of symptomatic
	Neonatal infection/colonization	women
	Vaginal colonization of female infants 5%	
	Vaginitis/Urinary tract infection rare	
Bacterial vaginosis	Adverse pregnancy outcome (% increase over BV negative women):	Screening and treatment of women with high risk pregnancies
	Chorioamnion/amnion infection 5–13%	Screening and treatment of all pregnant
	Prematurity 2–12%	women (benefit unknown)
	Premature rupture of membranes 3–12%	Presumptive treatment of symptomatic
	Maternal postpartum infection 12–23%	women
	Neonatal infection	
	No data	

1998). These epidemiological characteristics may be useful in designing more cost-effective screening programmes (Mertz et al., 1997).

Consequences of infection on maternal and child health

Several reports have shown an association between maternal gonococcal infection and prematurity, premature rupture of membranes, and fetal and perinatal death (Table 14.2) (Sarrel & Pruett, 1968; Amstey & Steadman, 1976; Temmerman et al., 1992; Charles et al., 1970; Handsfield et al., 1973; Israel et al., 1975; Edwards et al., 1978; Elliot et al., 1990). Recent studies from Africa suggest that gonococcal infection may be responsible for a substantial proportion of premature deliveries in areas where gonococcal infection prevalence is high (Temmerman et al., 1992; Elliot et al., 1990).

Endometritis is the most common postpartum maternal infection. Cervical gonococcal or chlamydial infection accounts for a significant proportion, 14 to 50%, of postpartum infections in developing countries (Perine et al., 1980; Temmerman et al., 1988; Plummer et al., 1987). The magnitude of the contribution of postpartum infections to secondary infertility in these settings, however, has not been adequately documented. Infections in neonates present either with infections at mucosal sites (e.g. conjunctivitis/ophthalmia, urethritis, vaginitis, proctitis, pharyngitis or rhinitis, contaminated orogastric contents, scalp abscesses due to fetal monitors) or as disseminated disease (polyarthritis or sepsis) (Kleiman & Lamb, 1973; Holmes et al., 1971; Barton & Shuja, 1981; Kirkland & Storer, 1931; Hunter, 1939; D'Auria, 1978; Fransen et al., 1986). The most common complication of gonococcal infection in the neonate is gonococcal ophthalmia neonatorum. From a public health viewpoint, it is the most important neonatal infection because, if untreated, the infection can lead rapidly to blindness (Laga et al., 1989). Two prospective studies in Africa estimated the transmission rate of gonococcal infection from mother to child in the absence of ocular prophylaxis as 47% in Nairobi, Kenya and 30% in Yaounde, Cameroon (Laga et al., 1986a,b; Galega et al., 1984). The resulting incidence of gonococcal ophthalmia neonatorum was 3.6 and 4 per 100 live births, respectively. By comparison, the incidence rates of gonococcal ophthalmia neonatorum in industrialized countries averaged about 0.06 % (Laga et al., 1986a,b).

Diagnosis
Infection in the mother

Routine screening of pregnant women is warranted in high prevalence areas. Routine screening is recommended in the USA, while many countries in Europe no longer perform it because of the very low prevalence of disease. Screening, however, is not practised in developing countries because of lack of diagnostic facilities and cost. The most commonly reported symptoms for urogenital gonococcal infection in women include abnormal vaginal discharge, dysuria, menorrhagia and/or intermenstrual uterine bleeding ranging from minimal to severe (McCormick et al., 1977; Curran et al., 1975). The associated clinical signs of purulent or mucopurulent discharge, erythema and oedema of the zone of ectopy and easily induced cervical bleeding are quite specific, but insensitive (Bourgeois et al., 1998; Curran et al., 1975; Ryan et al., 1998b). Syndrome management has been recommended as a means to identify and treat symptomatic women with cervical gonococcal or chlamydial infection in resource-constrained settings (World Health Organization, 1994). This approach, however, is limited by the large percentage of infected women without symptoms and the non-specific nature of the symptoms (Dallabetta et al., 1998). Under optimal conditions, Gram stains of cervical discharge to detect gonococci have a reported sensitivity of 40–65% and a specificity of up to 97% (Spiegel, 1991). Isolation of *Neisseria gonorrhoeae* with culture is the standard technique for the definitive diagnosis of gonococcal disease, has a diagnostic sensitivity of 80 to 95% under optimal conditions and allows for antimicrobial testing (Schmale et al., 1969). Nucleic acid-based tests, either nucleic acid hybridization or nucleic acid amplification, eliminate problems posed by transport of cultures and have sensitivities that are equal or better than culture techniques (Ching et al., 1995; Panke et al., 1991; Hale et al., 1993). Nucleic acid amplification techniques also perform well when used with first-void urine specimens and allow for screening of women in settings where genital examinations are not possible (Smith et al., 1995).

Infection in neonates

Conjunctival infection in the newborn usually begins 1–13 days after birth, although later cases have been reported (Fivush et al., 1980). It is important to consider gonococcal conjunctivitis in all cases of infant conjunctivitis, regardless of severity or age of onset, since prolonged incubation after perinatal exposure is difficult to distinguish from postnatal acquisition. Typically, gonococcal conjunctivitis presents with bilateral purulent discharge and hyperaemic and oedematous conjunctivae and eyelids. Infiltrations begin near the border of the cornea and the sclera and can rapidly enlarge and ulcerate leading to perforation of the globe and vision loss (Laga et al., 1989). The presence of Gram-negative intracellular diplococci in a conjunctival Gram stain is highly sensitive and specific for gonococcal infection (Winceslaus et al., 1987). This simple test allows for the institution of therapy quickly and can be performed even in places where laboratory facilities are minimal. Where feasible, Gram-stain should be supplemented with standard culture techniques for the isolation of *N. gonorrhoeae*. In children, rapid, non-culture systems such as enzyme immunoassay tests and nucleic acid detection tests have not been fully evaluated.

Gonococcaemia in the neonatal period most commonly manifests itself as polyarticular septic arthritis (Kohen, 1974). Typically, it presents with the infant's refusal to move a limb. Infections of the hip are particularly problematic to diagnosis and must be ruled out with particular care. Diagnosis is made using the usual methods for sepsis evaluation including blood cultures and arthrocentesis with culture.

Treatment and management

Infection in the mother

Uncomplicated gonococcal cervical infection is ideally treated with a single dose of an antibiotic approved for use in pregnancy. Single-dose regimens that are currently recommended are ceftriaxone 125 mg intramuscularly, cefixime 400 mg orally or spectinomycin 2 g intramuscularly (Centers for Disease Control, 1997; World Health Organization, 1991). Co-therapy for possible chlamydial infection with erythromycin (erythromycin base 250 mg tablet four times daily for 14 days or erythromycin ethylsuccinate 800 mg four times daily for 7 days), or azythromycin 1 g single dose should also be given as presumptive co-therapy for chlamydial infection if no chlamydial testing was performed. Due to the risk of re-infection, intensive partner referral and treatment efforts are warranted. Women with an identified gonococcal infection in pregnancy should be followed closely and re-screened if possible.

Infections in the neonate

Infants with gonococcal ophthalmia should be hospitalized and treatment instituted promptly. Recommended therapies include ceftriaxone 25–50 mg/kg intramuscularly as a single dose not to exceed 125 mg, kanamycin 25 mg/kg intramuscularly as a single dose or spectinomycin 25 mg/kg as a single dose (Centers for Disease Control, 1997; World Health Organization, 1986; Laga et al., 1986). Removal of purulent material from eyelids and the application of 1% tetracyline ointment every 4 hours for 7–14 days is also recommended if ceftriaxone is not used (World Health Organization, 1986). Since co-infection with chlamydial infection is possible, systemic therapy with erythromycin should be considered if chlamydial testing cannot be done (World Health Organization, 1986). Infants with systemic disease (e.g. arthritis, septicaemia) should be hospitalized and treated with intravenous antibiotics, for example ceftriaxone 25–50 mg/kg/day in a single dose for 7 days.

Prevention and control

Four control strategies are possible for the prevention and control of gonococcal ophthalmia neonatorum (Laga et al., 1989):

 (i) prevention of gonococcal infection in the mother
 (ii) diagnosis and treatment of maternal gonococcal infection
 (iii) ocular prophylaxis of infant at birth
 (iv) diagnosis and treatment of gonococcal ophthalmia neonatorum

Prevention of gonococcal infection in the mother may be pursued by behaviour modification in the mother or the couple, including reduction of high-risk sexual encounters and use of barrier methods. Although primary prevention strategies to reduce STDs have not been generally successful in the past, HIV/AIDS prevention efforts with the same prevention messages appear to have reduced STD prevalence in Thai men (and presumably their partners) (Hannenberg et al., 1994). However, even in the best circumstances, STD prevalence is only reduced and other elements are required for the effective prevention and control of gonococcal ophthalmia neonatorum.

Screening and treatment of maternal gonococcal infection is an approach that offers the benefits of reducing all maternal and infant complications related to gonococcal infection. Screening can be done in all women attending antenatal clinics or done selectively based on epidemiological risk assessment, symptoms or physical exam findings. Selective screening increases the cost-effectiveness of screening programs. Alternatively, another potential strategy would be presumptive treatment (mass treatment) of all antenatal women or presumptive treatment of higher risk women based on screening criteria. This approach has been promoted as a means to provide STD care to pregnant women in high prevalence settings, where detection of infection is impossible (Temmerman et al., 1995; Wawer et al., 1999).

Ocular prophylaxis of infant at birth interrupts the transmission of *N. gonorrhoeae* from the maternal cervix to the newborn's eyes. Three different regimens have been recommended for prophylaxis: (i) silver nitrate 1% eye drops, (ii) tetracycline 1% eye ointment, or (iii) erythromycin 0.5% eye ointment (World Health Organization, 1986; Laga et al., 1988; Chen, 1992). Povidone–iodine 2.5% eye drops have also been shown to be effective (Isenberg et al., 1995).

The diagnosis and treatment of gonococcal ophthalmia neonatorum as the sole control strategy for the disease is appropriate in settings with excellent health services and very low incidence of the disease. However, early diagnosis and appropriate treatment is important everywhere because cases of ophthalmia do occur even in the presence of a comprehensive ocular prophylaxis programme. Ocular prophylaxis is the most widely applicable and cost-effective of the four strategies for preventing gonococcal ophthalmia in newborns. The cost-effectiveness and operational feasibility of the strategies has not been evaluated when the entire spectrum of maternal gonococcal infection complications is considered.

Chlamydia trachomatis infection in pregnancy

Epidemiology

With a recent (1995) estimate of 89 million incident infections worldwide, *C. trachomatis* infection is the second most common sexually transmitted disease, after trichomoniasis (Gerbase et al., 1998). Globally, the prevalence of *C. trachomatis* in antenatal and family planning settings varies widely but is almost universally more prevalent than gonorrhoea (Table 14.1). Due to the difficulty in diagnosis and the frequency of asymptomatic infections, this number of incident infections is undoubtedly an underestimate of the true *C. trachomatis* incidence. In higher-risk groups in the USA, for example in urban women, women of low socio-economic status and ethnic minority background and adolescents, cervical infection has been documented in a high percentage of screened women, with a median of approximately 15% (Cates & Wasserheit, 1991).

Consequences of infection on maternal and child health

Screening of at-risk populations is important because *C. trachomatis* can have severe consequences in women, with outcomes such as pelvic inflammatory disease, ectopic pregnancy, infertility and in children, with outcomes such as infant conjunctivitis and pneumonia. Since most women infected with *C. trachomatis* are asymptomatic, screening remains the optimal way to identify those at risk. Infection is transmitted from mother to infant during vaginal delivery, although it may rarely occur after caesarean section (Shariat et al., 1992). *C. trachomatis* infection of the mother has been associated with prematurity, but the association is confounded by the frequent co-infection of such mothers with *Mycoplasma hominis* and *Ureaplasma urealyticum.* The transmission rate of *C. trachomatis* infection from mother to infant is 50–70% if the rate is measured by the persistence of chlamydia-specific IgG or IgM antibody in early infancy or infant colonization with chlamydia. The rate decreases if the criterion used is infant's conjunctival infection (15–44%) or infant's pneumonia (1–22%) (World Health Organization, 1986).

   C. trachomatis infection in infants may result in two main pathologic conditions, inclusion conjunctivitis and interstitial pneumonia (World Health Organization, 1986). Inclusion conjunctivitis is often secondary to nasopharyngeal chlamydia infection, the nasopharynx being the commonest site of infection. In female infants, conjunctivitis can be accompanied by vulvovaginitis.

Inclusion conjunctivitis

This is the most frequent clinical manifestation of *C. trachomatis* infection and occurs in about 15–44% of infants born to mothers infected with *C. trachomatis* (Schachter et al., 1986; Frommell et al., 1979; Hammerschlag et al., 1979, 1989; Datta et al., 1988; Mardh et al., 1980; Chandler et al., 1977). Half the infants with chlamydial conjunctivitis also have nasopharyngeal infection. Inclusion conjunctivitis typically appears after an incubation period of 1 to 3 weeks after delivery, possibly sooner in case of premature rupture of membranes. Infection is bilateral in 70% of cases and both upper and lower conjunctivae are affected. Conjunctivitis can be mild, with some mucoid discharge or can be severe, with purulent discharge, chemosis and presence of pseudomembranes. In most cases eyelids are swollen and conjunctivae are thick and erythematous. Clinically, neonatal *C. trachomatis* conjunctivitis resembles gonococcal ophthalmia, although the latter condition is now rare in many countries, thanks to widespread use of ocular prophylaxis at birth.

Interstitial pneumonia

The incidence of pneumonia in infants born to chlamydia-infected mothers has been estimated at 1–22% (Schachter et al., 1986; Frommell et al., 1979; Hammerschlag et al., 1979, 1989; Datta et al., 1988). Symptoms usually appear in infected infants before two months of age. Approximately one-third of infants with chlamydial pneumonia also have nasopharyngeal infection. Aspiration of chlamydia-infected cervical secretions, rather than descending infection from the conjunctivae, is the most likely pathogenetic mechanism for pneumonia, since pneumonia may occur without preceding conjunctivitis (Harrison et al., 1983; Hammerschlag et al., 1997).

Diagnosis

Infection in the mother

As in the case of gonococcal infection, the syndrome management approach has been recommended to diagnose and treat symptomatic women with gonococcal and cervical chlamydial infection in developing countries (World Health Organization, 1994). The frequent occurrence of asymptomatic infections is the main limitation of this approach. Laboratory diagnosis with culture or non-culture (antigen detection and DNA amplification) tests is limited, especially in the developing world, to tertiary care centers.

Infection in the neonate

Infant conjunctivitis

Diagnosis is made by clinical examination, cytology, culture or antigen identification. Cytological examination shows characteristic inclusions in conjunctival epithelial cells, stained by Giemsa or by fluorescent antibody stain. Diagnosis by culture, which relies on identification by immunofluorescence of a specific stain in a conjunctival sample, is considered the accepted standard. Non-culture tests include chlamydial antigen detection by direct fluorescence or ELISA in a conjunctival swab, and DNA amplification techniques, such as polymerase chain reaction (PCR). The Amplicor assay is a PCR-based assay manufactured by Roche, which in some countries has only been approved for detection of *C. trachomatis* in genital samples in adults. However, when used in infants with suspected chlamydial conjunctivitis, the assay was found 100% sensitive and 97% specific for the detection of *C. trachomatis* in ocular and nasopharyngeal specimens (Schachter & Dawson, 1978).

Interstitial pneumonia

Infant pneumonia usually has a slow onset, appearing between 1 and 3 months of age with staccato cough and cyanosis, while breath sounds are good and no wheezing is present. Radiographic signs of bilateral interstitial infiltrates with hyperinflation are non-specific. Due to the lack of a specific clinical and radiological picture, laboratory tests are necessary for the diagnosis. Characteristic laboratory findings are peripheral eosinophilia, elevated serum immunoglobulins and anti-chlamydial IgM. Tissue culture using *C. trachomatis*-specific fluorescent antibody is 100% specific in detecting chlamydia in nasopharyngeal swabs, as well as in the genitourinary tract and rectum.

Treatment and management
Infection in the mother

Many antibiotics have proven efficacious against *C. trachomatis* infection (Centers for Disease Control, 1997). Single dose oral azithromycin, 1 g daily is a very practical and cost-effective regimen, but its safety to the fetus is still being evaluated. Erythromycin 2 gm daily can be used, but its efficacy must be confirmed with a test of cure 2 weeks after the end of the course.

Infection in the neonate
Inclusion conjunctivitis

Chlamydial conjunctivitis is often self-limiting, with spontaneous resolution in a few months. However, untreated infection may result in prolonged morbidity, with subclinical infections sometimes persisting for years and occasionally leaving corneal scars. The recommended antibiotic regimen of erythromycin 50 mg/kg per day for 10–14 days is efficacious in most cases, but sometimes a second course is required. Conjunctivitis tends to last for 2–3 weeks even in the presence of treatment.

Interstitial pneumonia

Therapy is the same as for conjunctivitis (oral erythromycin 50 mg/kg per day for 10–14 days) and achieves a similar (about 80%) cure rate.

Prevention and control

Strategies for prevention and control of *C. trachomatis* that have been considered are similar to those for gonorrhoea. For both mothers and infants, these strategies include prevention or antibiotic treatment after screening of at-risk populations. Possible preventive approaches include ocular prophylaxis of the infant or screening and antibiotic treatment of pregnant women. Many studies have illustrated the limited effectiveness of ocular prophylaxis with silver nitrate or antibiotic ointments, such as erythromycin or tetracycline, for the prevention of chlamydial neonatal conjunctivitis (Laga et al., 1988; Isenberg et al., 1995; Hammerschlag et al., 1989). Moreover, ocular prophylaxis does not affect the incidence of nasopharyngeal colonization or pneumonia. Screening and treatment of pregnant women may be a more cost-effective primary prevention measure which would benefit women, by preventing the infection's severe health outcomes, and infants, by preventing the clinical conditions related to vertical transmission of *C. trachomatis*.

Genital mycoplasma infection in pregnancy

Epidemiology

Mycoplasmas are organisms that primarily colonize the genitourinary tract. They are particularly frequent in the lower genital tract of asymptomatic women, where the most commonly found mycoplasmas are *Mycoplasma (Ureaplasma) urealyticum,* present in as many as 80% of healthy women (Cassell et al., 1993; Grattard et al., 1995), *Mycoplasma hominis,* and *Mycoplasma genitalium.* Other colonization sites include the oropharyngeal areas. To date, 14 serotypes of *U. urealyticum* have been detected in humans and have been divided in the parvo biovar (including serotype 1, 3, 6, and 14) and the T960 biovar (including the remaining ten serotypes). Some mycoplasmas (*M. genitalium*) have only been detected by polymerase chain reaction, due to the inability to grow in culture. Others (*M. urealyticum*) require special isolation techniques, which have hindered studies of their biologic and epidemiologic characteristics. In adults, sexual contact is the main mechanism of transmission, particularly for women, who are more prone to colonization than men (Shafer et al., 1985). Genital mycoplasmas have been more commonly found in black than in white populations, after controlling for sexual activity.

Due to their fairly recent recognition and the difficulty of detecting these organisms by culture, studies of prevalence and risk factors for mycoplasma infection in different populations have been limited, unlike similar studies of other causative agents of perinatal infections. Neonatal colonization with mycoplasmas is not only more common in girls than in boys (up to 35% of infant girls have genital colonization and 15% non-genital colonization), but persists longer, with up to 20% of pre-pubertal girls being colonized with *U. urealyticum* and 6% with *M. hominis* (Klein et al., 1969).

Only a few of the genitourinary and reproductive tract conditions associated in published reports with *Ureaplasma urealyticum* and *Mycoplasma hominis* have been conclusively related to these agents. *Mycoplasma hominis,* for example, may be a major cause of post-partum fever. Studies of mother-to-infant transmission of ureaplasmas have often involved patients in sexually transmitted disease clinics and women of low socio-economic status. Cassell et al. (1983, 1986, 1988) have reported extensively on the presumptive role of *U. urealyticum* and adverse pregnancy outcomes such as infertility, spontaneous abortion, prematurity and neonatal infections, including respiratory tract infections and meningitis.

The rate of vertical transmission of *U. urealyticum* from colonized mothers to their offspring can be more than 50% (Sánchez & Regan, 1990). Vertical transmission of *U. urealyticum* can occur *in utero* (Cassell et al., 1983; Waites et al., 1993) or intrapartum (Cassell et al., 1983; Sánchez & Regan, 1980, 1987) and the role of mode of delivery on the transmission rate is still undefined (Sánchez & Regan, 1987). Intrapartum transmission by passage through a mycoplasma-colonized birth canal seems the predominant mechanism of infant colonization and the infant's colonization rate is related to the mother's. Despite previous conflicting results (Sanchez & Regan, 1987), recent studies (Grattard et al., 1995) have documented an association between high maternal colonization and premature rupture of membranes.

Consequences of infection on maternal and child health

Every organ system can be colonized in utero or in the neonatal period (Cassell et al., 1986; Pease et al., 1967; Brus et al., 1991; Waites et al., 1988). Mycoplasma isolation from multiple organs in the presence of an inflammatory response is probably the result of active fetal hematogenous dissemination. In view of the increasing importance of bronchopulmonary dysplasia (BPD) in newborn babies, there is increasing interest in the role of infections in the development of BPD in the high-risk neonate. Studies have examined the association between maternal colonization with mycoplasmas, particularly ureaplasmas, colonization of the newborn's respiratory tract and infant respiratory disease. A recent meta-analysis of four cohorts by Wang et al. (1993) showed that infants with birthweight less than 1250 g in whom *U. urealyticum* was isolated in the respiratory tract within 24 to 72 hours of birth had a 2–3 times higher risk of BPD. A subsequent study by Alfa et al. (1995) also established that very low birthweight children had increased risk of acquiring *U. urealyticum* compared to term infants. In this study, placental rather than vaginal samples were used to assess genital colonization, as it was considered more clinically relevant when assessing the potential of ureaplasmas to cause disseminated infection. *U. urealyticum* is the most common organism isolated from inflamed placentas (Cassell et al., 1986). Possible ways for the fetus to acquire mycoplasmas infection include hematogenous dissemination from infected umbilical vessels, dissemination from infected amnionitic fluid to the fetal lung, meninges and systemic circulation, and intrapartum contact with a colonized birth canal with subsequent spread to skin, mucosa and respiratory tract.

U. urealyticum has been isolated from blood culture of newborn infants and from cord blood. In preterm infants with birthweight < 2500 g, this organism was isolated in 26% of blood cultures from infants with an endotracheal aspirate (Cassell et al., 1988). The actual proportion of subclinical vs. clinical bacteraemia has not been determined and it seems likely that only premature newborns may be at considerable risk of invasive disease due to bloodstream infection with *U. urealyticum.*

As in systemic infection, prevalence, risk factors and clinical picture of central nervous system infections due to *U. urealyticum* have not been resolved. However, the respective frequency of subclinical and clinical central nervous system infections may be substantial, due to the high *U. urealyticum* isolation rate from placenta, amniotic fluid and maternal blood. The culture of cerebrospinal fluid for mycoplasmas has been recommended in ill infants with clinical, laboratory, and radiological evidence of central nervous system infections, but negative bacterial cultures (Waites et al., 1995).

The mycoplasmas have been considered by many as emerging neonatal pathogens that can result in respiratory disease and pneumonitis in low-birth weight infants. Earlier cross-sectional (Cassell et al., 1986, 1988) and prospective (Wang et al., 1988; Sánchez & Regan, 1988) studies showed this association, but subsequent studies have reported contradictory results (Da Silva et al., 1997; Perzigian et al., 1998) about the relationship between recovery of *U. urealyticum* in the lower respiratory tract and later chronic lung disease in very low birthweight (< 1500 g) infants. The association of ureaplasma infection and chronic lung disease was found to be much lower in studies performed after the advent of surfactant to treat respiratory distress syndrome.

Diagnosis

The cultural requirements of mycoplasmas or their inability to grow in culture are currently limiting the widespread diagnosis of mycoplasma colonization and infection. Their detection may increase dramatically with the development and more widespread application of polymerase chain reaction techniques.

Treatment/management

The combined weight of evidence suggests that *U. urealyticum* has the potential to be a true pathogen that may lead to severe pulmonary and systemic disease in very premature infants. However, to establish the role of ureaplasmas in the development of pulmonary lung disease, clinical trials are needed that evaluate soon after birth the effect of anti-ureaplasma antibiotic treatment in low birth-weight infants.

Trichomonas vaginalis infection in pregnancy

Epidemiology

Trichomoniasis is an extremely common infection worldwide and with reported prevalence rates in pregnant women ranging from 2 to 49% (Table 14.1). WHO estimated that in 1995 there were 170 million new cases of trichomoniasis (Gerbase et al., 1998). Studies from the USA indicate that socio-demographic and behavioural risk factors for trichomonal infection in pregnant women are similar to those for non-pregnant women and include minority status, cigarette use, unmarried, lower level of education, previous history of gonorrhoea, and high number of lifetime sexual partners (Cotch et al., 1991).

Consequences of infection on maternal and child health

Several reports have shown an association between maternal trichomonal infection and prematurity, premature rupture of membranes and low birthweight, although not consistently (Table 14.2) (Hardy et al., 1984; Meis et al., 1995; McGregor et al., 1995; Cotch et al., 1997; Read & Klebanoff, 1993; Minkoff et al., 1984; Riduan et al., 1993). In vitro studies suggest that *T. vaginalis* isolates and cell-free filtrates affect the chorioamniotic membranes adversely by decreasing their elastic response, decrease the force necessary to rupture and decrease their bursting tension (Draper et al., 1995). The exact mechanism of action however has not been determined (e.g. direct effect of *T. vaginalis*, proteases produced by *T. vaginalis*, host inflammatory response, or a combination of the above).

An early report in the literature indicated that 48% of antenatal women with untreated trichomonas infection had postpartum fever compared with 25% of women without trichomoniasis (Bland, 1931). This report, however, did not control for other significant confounding factors such as other STDs, bacterial vaginosis or behavioural risk factors. A recent report of a cohort of over 13,000 women found that 6.9% of women with *T. vaginalis* at mid-gestation had postpartum endometritis compared to 4.7% who did not (Cotch et al., 1997). Whether *T. vaginalis* itself or the associated increase in vaginal anaerobic bacteria account for these postpartum infections remains unclear.

Neonatal infection/colonization with *T. vaginalis* is uncommon and colonization appears to be about 5% among exposed female infants (Al Salihi et al., 1980; Bramley 1976). The infection is rarely detected and causes little morbidity. The vaginal mucosa of female infants is susceptible to colonization immediately after birth due to the oestrogenic influence during pregnancy. This susceptibility reverses about 3 to 4 weeks after delivery. There are case reports in the literature of trichomonal vaginitis, urinary tract infection, and possible causes of respiratory tract infection (Postlethwhaite, 1975; McLaren et al., 1983).

Diagnosis

Reported symptoms and clinical signs are poor predictors of trichomonal vaginal infection in pregnant women (Cotch et al., 1991; Pastoreck et al., 1996). All pregnant women with complaints of vaginal discharge should have a direct microscopic examination for trichomonads. Routine screening with direct microscopy is warranted in high prevalence areas. In resource-constrained settings, syndrome management of vaginal discharge, whereby all women with complaints of discharge are treated with metronidazole, has been recommended (World Health Organization, 1994). The diagnosis of *T. vaginalis* is made either microscopically or with culture. Direct microscopy of secretions is the least sensitive method of diagnosis. Compared to culture the sensitivity of direct microscopy for trichomonal vaginitis is 39 to 92%. Direct fluorescent antibody has a sensitivity of 83 to 86% compared to culture (Krieger et al., 1988). Culture capabilities for *T. vaginalis* have been facilitated by the development of a portable culture system (Draper et al., 1993). The diagnosis of *T. vaginalis* indicates the need for further evaluation for other STDs (Pastoreck et al., 1996).

Treatment and management

Metronidazole is the treatment of choice for trichomoniasis (World Health Organization, 1994; Centers for Disease Control, 1997). Systemic therapy is superior to topical therapy as *T. vaginalis* often infects the urethra and periurethal gland in addition to the vagina. A 2 g dose as a single oral dose is highly effective and concomitant treatment of the male sexual partner increases cure rates to over 95% (Lossick, 1990). Nitroimidazoles are mutagenic for bacteria and carcinogenic in some animals after prolonged use. Meta-analyses of studies examining the use of metronidazole in pregnancy have not shown any increased teratogenic risk (Burtin et al., 1995; Caro-Patón et al., 1997). It is therefore recommended that metronidazole can be used in pregnant women after the first trimester of gestation in women with documented trichomonal infection (World Health Organization, 1994; Centers for Disease Control, 1997).

Most cases of neonatal trichomoniasis are self-limited. For those infants with severe symptoms or infections that persist beyond 6 weeks, treatment should be given with 10 to 30 mg of metronidazole per kilogram daily for 5 to 8 days (Lossick, 1990).

Prevention and control

Prevention of trichomonal infection could be accomplished through behaviour change in the mother or the couple to reduce high-risk sexual encounters or to utilize barrier methods. Screening and treatment of trichomonal infection in the women coupled with partner treatment is an approach that would reduce both maternal and infant complications of the disease. Screening with direct microscopy, while it has low sensitivity, is a relatively simple diagnostic that could be implemented in a wide spectrum of clinical sites. Presumptive mass therapy of pregnant women in the setting of population presumptive therapy with metronidazole significantly reduced the prevalence of *T. vaginalis* in women in Uganda (Wawer et al., 1999).

Bacterial vaginosis in pregnancy

Epidemiology

Bacterial vaginosis (BV), a polymicrobial anaerobic overgrowth syndrome, is the most common cause of complaints of vaginal discharge in women of childbearing age in the United States and Europe. It is also a common disorder globally (Table 14.1). BV is more common in women in STD clinics and in women with symptoms of vaginal discharge than women in family planning clinics or antenatal care clinics and the prevalence in the US varies by ethnicity (Sánchez et al., 1998; Meis et al., 1995; Goldenberg et al., 1996; Cohen et al., 1995). The prevalence and natural history of BV in pregnant women does not appear to differ from non-pregnant women (Hillier et al., 1992; Hay et al., 1994).

Risk factors for BV are not well understood. Evidence in the medical literature on the role of sexual transmission is conflicting. BV is significantly less common among college-age women who report no sexual activity compared with those having sexual experience (Amsel et al., 1983). Reports have been contradictory about the association between age of first sexual intercourse and BV and numbers of partners and BV (Amsel et al., 1983; Larsson et al., 1991; Hillier et al., 1995a,b; Evans et al., 1993; Barbone et al., 1990; Hawes et al., 1996; Avonts et al., 1990). Moreover, the treatment of male partners of women with BV does not reduce recurrence or improve the clinical outcome of treatment (Colli et al., 1997; Vejtorp et al., 1988). Other risk factors associated with BV include the lack of hydrogen peroxide producing lactobacilli, douching and IUD use (Amsel et al., 1983; Hawes et al., 1996; Avonts et al., 1990).

Consequences of infection on maternal and child health

BV during pregnancy has been associated with significant increases in adverse pregnancy outcomes including pre-term and low birth weight infants, intra-amniotic infection, chorioamnionitis and premature rupture of membranes (Table 14.2) (Meis et al., 1995; Hillier et al., 1995a, b; Kurki et al., 1992; Newton et al., 1997; Gravett et al., 1986; Joesoef et al., 1993). There are six published studies that evaluate the effect of treating BV in pregnancy as a means to prevent premature births. Two of these studies report on intravaginal clindamycin treatment and neither showed an effect in reducing prematurity (Joesoef et al., 1995; McGregor et al., 1994). Treatment with oral clindamycin resulted in a 50% reduction of BV associated preterm deliveries (McGregor et al., 1995). Three randomized placebo-controlled trials have evaluated metronidazole, either alone or in combination with erythromycin, for the prevention of preterm birth (McDonald et al., 1997; Morales et al., 1994; Hauth et al., 1995). These trials indicated that metronidazole might reduce the incidence of preterm delivery in women with BV who have a history of a previous preterm delivery. The benefit of screening and treating low risk pregnant women for BV is currently the topic of ongoing investigations.

BV is also associated with postpartum endometritis in women undergoing either vaginal deliveries or C-section and in postabortion pelvic inflammatory disease (Newton et al., 1990; Watts et al., 1990; Larsson et al., 1992).The association between BV and infection in the neonate is less well studied. Anaerobic sepsis has been described in 26% of all cases of neonatal bacteraemia at one institution (Chow et al., 1974). The predominant isolates in these cases were *Bacteroides*, *Peptococcus* and *Peptostreptococcus*. The association of anaerobic sepsis in the neonate with material BV, however, has not been evaluated.

Diagnosis
Infection in the mother

The benefit of routine screening and treatment for BV of low risk pregnant women remains unproven. Based on the results of three randomized clinical trials, women with high-risk pregnancies or with a history of premature birth should be screened and treated. The two most common methods of diagnosis are a diagnosis based on clinical and bedside laboratory test criteria or vaginal fluid gram stain. Amsel and colleagues (1983) recommend basing the diagnosis of BV on three of the four criteria: (i) characteristic homogenous white adherent discharge; (ii) vaginal fluid pH over 4.5; (iii) release of a fishy amine odour from the vaginal fluid when mixed with 10% KOH solution (whiff test); and (iv) 20% or more of the vaginal epithelial cells as clue cells. Gram stain has a standardized 0 to 10 point scoring system for vaginal fluid based on three morphotypes (Nugent et al., 1991). Cultures for *G. vaginalis* are not useful in diagnosing BV, since the organism can be isolated from a high proportion of women without BV.

Treatment and management
Infection in the mother

BV diagnosed during pregnancy should be treated with an oral preparation, either oral clindamycin, 300 mg twice daily for 7 days or oral metronidazole, 250 mg three times daily for 7 days. While topical therapy with clindamycin cream or metronidazole gel is effective in eliminating BV, the clinical trial data suggest that oral preparations do not reduce the risk of preterm birth (Centers for Disease Control, 1997). Routine treatment of sexual partners is not suggested for BV.

Prevention

Since the cause and risk factors for the acquisition of BV are poorly understood there are no clear recommendations on preventing it. However, systemic treatment of BV during pregnancy in women with prior preterm births clearly reduces the risk of preterm delivery. Whether universal screening and treatment of pregnant women will be recommended awaits large-scale studies. A presumptive population-based treatment trial of pregnant women in Uganda with a single 2 g dose of metronidazole reduced the prevalence of BV significantly (Wawer et al., 1999).

REFERENCES

Addiss, D. G., Vaughn, M. L., Ludka, D., Pfister, J. & David, J. P. (1993). Decreased prevalence of *Chlamydia trachomatis* infection associated with a selective screening programme in family planning clinics in Wisconsin. *Sex. Transm. Dis.*, **20**, 28–35.

Alfa, M. J., Embree, J. E., Degagne, R. T., Olson, N., Lertsman, J., MacDonald, K. D., MacDonald, N. T. & Hall, P. F. (1995). Transmission of *Ureaplasma urealyticum* from mothers to full and preterm infants. *Pediatr. Infect. Dis. J.*, **14**, 431–5.

Al Salihi, F. L., Curran, J. P. & Wang, J-S. (1980). Neonatal *Trichomonas vaginalis*, report of three cases and review of the literature. *Pediatrics*, **53**, 196–200.

Amsel, R., Totten, P. A., Speigel, C. A., Chen, K. C. S., Eschenbach, D. & Holmes, K. K. (1983). Nonspecific vaginitis, diagnostic criteria and microbial and epidemiologic associations. *Am. J. Med.*, **74**, 14–22.

Amstey, M. S. & Steadman, K. T. (1976). Asymptomatic gonorrhea and pregnancy. *J. Am. Vener. Dis. Assoc.*, **3**, 14–16.

Avonts, D., Sercu, M., Heyerick, P., Vandermeeren, I., Meheus, A. & Piot, P. (1990). Incidence of uncomplicated genital infections in women using oral contraception or an intrauterine device, a prospective study. *Sex. Transm. Dis.*, **17**, 23–9.

Barbone, F., Austin, H., Louv, W. C. & Alexander, W. J. (1990). A follow-up study of methods of contraception, sexual activity and rates of trichomoniasis, candidiasis, and bacterial vaginosis. *Am. J. Obstet. Gynecol.*, **163**, 510–14.

Barnes, R. C. & Holmes, K. K. (1984). Epidemiology of gonorrhea, current perspectives. *Epidemiol. Rev.*, **6**, 1–20.

Barton, L. L. & Shuja, M. (1981). Neonatal gonococcal vaginitis. *J. Pediatr.*, **98**, 171.

Behets, E. M-T., Desormeaux, J., Joseph, D., Adrien, M., Coicou, G., Dallabetta, G., Hamilton, A. H. Moeng, S., Davis, H., Cohen, M. S. & Boulos, R. (1995). Control of sexually transmitted disease in Haiti: results and implications of a baseline study among pregnant women living in Cité Soleil shantytowns. *J. Infect. Dis.*, **172**, 764–71.

Behets, F. M.-T., Ward, E., Fox, L., Reed, R., Spruyt, A., Bennett, L., Johnson, L., Hoffman, I. & Figueroa, J. P. (1998). Sexually transmitted diseases are common in women attending Jamaican family planning clinics and appropriate detection tools are lacking. *Sex. Trans. Infect.*, **74**, S123–7.

Bland, P. B. (1931). Vaginal trichomoniasis in the pregnant woman. *J.A.M.A.*, **96**, 157.

Bourgeois, A., Henzel, D., Malonga-Mouelet, G., Dibanga, G., Tsobou, C., Peeters, M. &

Delaporte, E. (1998). Clinical algorithms for the screening of pregnant women for STDs in Libreville, Gabon, which alternatives? *Sex. Transm. Infect.*, **74**, 35–9.

Braddick, M. R., Ndinya-Achola, J. O., Mirza, N. B., Plummer, F. A., Irungu, G., Sinei, S. K. A. & Piot, P. (1990). Towards developing a diagnostic algorithm for *Chlamydia trachomatis* and *Neisseria gonorrhoeae* cervicitis in pregnancy. *Genitourin. Med.*, **66**, 62–5.

Bramley, M. (1976). Study of female babies of women entering confinement with vaginal trichomonasis. *Br. J. Vener. Dis.*, **52**, 58–62.

Brus, F., Van de Waarde, W. M., Schoots, C. & Oetomo, S. B. (1991). Fatal *Ureaplasma pneumonia* and sepsis in a newborn infant. *Eur. J. Pediatr.*, **150**, 782–3.

Burtin, P., Taddio, A., Ariburnu, O., Einarson, T. R. & Koren, G. (1995). Safety of metronidazole in pregnancy, a meta-analysis. *Am. J. Obstet. Gynecol.*, **172**, 525–9.

Caro-Patón, T., Carvajal, A., de Diego, I. M., Martín-Arias, L. H., Requejo, A. A. & Pinilla, E. R. (1997). Is metronidazole teratogenic? A meta-analysis. *Br. J. Clin. Pharmacol.*, **44**, 179–82.

Cassell, G. H., Davis, R. O., Waites, K. B., Brown, M. B., Marriott, P. A., Stagno, S., Davis, J. K. (1983). Isolation of *Mycoplasma hominis* and *Ureaplasma urealyticum* from amniotic fluid at 16–20 weeks' gestation, potential effect on outcome of pregnancy. *Sex. Transm. Dis.*, **10**, 294–302.

Cassell, G. H., Waites, K. B., Gibbs, R. S. & Davis, J. K. (1986). Role of *Ureaplasma urealyticum* in amniotics. *Pediatr. Infect. Dis.*, **5**, S247–52.

Cassell, G. H., Waites, K. B., Crouse, D. T., Rudd, P. T., Canupp, K. C., Stagno, S., Cutter, G. R. (1988). Association of *Ureaplasma urealyticum* infection of the lower respiratory tract with chronic lung disease and death in very low-birth-weight infants. *Lancet*, **ii**, 240–5.

Cassell, G. H., Waites, K. B., Watson, H. L., Crouse, D. T. & Harasawa, R. (1993). *Ureaplasma urealyticum* intrauterine infection, role in prematurity and disease in newborns. *Clin. Infect. Dis.*, **6**, 69–87.

Cates, W. & Wasserheit, J. M. (1991). Genital chlamydial infections, epidemiology and reproductive sequeleae. *Am. J. Obstet. Gynecol.*, **164**, 1771–81.

Centers for Disease Control (1997). 1998 Guidelines for treatment of sexually transmitted diseases. *M.M.W.R.*, **47**, RR–1.

Chandler, J. W., Alexander, E. R., Pheiffer, T. A., Wang, S. P., Holmes, K. K. & English, M. (1977). Ophthalmia neonatorum associated with maternal chlamydia infections. *Trans. Acad. Ophthalmol. Otolaryngol.*, **83**, 302–8.

Charles, A. G., Cohen, S., Kass, M. B. & Richman, R. (1970). Asymptomatic gonorrhea in prenatal patients. *Am. J. Obstet. Gynecol.*, **108**, 595–9.

Chen, J-Y. (1992). Prophylaxis of ophthalmia neonatorum, comparison of silver nitrate, tetracycline, erythromycin and no prophylaxis. *Pediatr. Infect. Dis. J.*, **11**, 1026–30.

Ching, S., Lee, H., Hook, E. W. 3rd, Jacobs, M. R. & Zenilman, J. (1995). Ligase chain reaction for the detection of *Neisseria gonorrhoeae* in urogenital swabs. *J. Clin. Microbiol.*, **33**, 3111–14.

Chow, A. W., Leake, R. D., Yamauchi, T., Anthony, B. F. & Guze, L. B. (1974). The significance of anaerobes in neonatal bacteremia, analysis of 23 cases and review of the literature. *Pediatrics*, **54**, 736–45.

Cohen, C. R., Duerr, A. N., Pruithithada, N. , Rugpao, S. , Hillier, S., Garcia, P. & Nelson, K. (1995). Bacterial vaginosis and HIV seroprevalence among female commercial sex workers in

Chiang Mai, Thailand. *AIDS*, **9**, 1093–7.

Colli, E., Landoni, M. & Parazzini, F. (1997). Treatment of male partners and recurrence of bacterial vaginosis, a randomised trial. *Genitourin. Med.*, **73**, 267–70.

Costello-Daly, C., Wanger, A-M., Hoffman, I. F., Canner, J. K., Lule, G. S., Lema, V. M., Liomba, N. G. & Dallabetta, G. A. (1998). Validation of the WHO diagnostic algorithm and development of an alternative scoring system for the management of women presenting with vaginal discharge in Malawi. *Sex. Transm. Infect.*, **74**, S50–8.

Cotch, M. F., Pastorek, J. G., Nugent, R. P., Yerg, D. E., Martin, D. H. & Eschenbach, D. A. (1991). Demographic and behavioural predictors of *Trichomonas vaginalis* infections among pregnant women. *Obstet. Gynecol.*, **78**, 1087–92.

Cotch, M. F., Pastorek, J. G. 2nd, Nugent, R. P., Hillier, S. L., Gibbs, R. S., Martin, D. H., Eschenbach, D. A., Edelman, R., Carey, J. C., Regan, J. A., Krohn, M. A., Klebanoff, M. A., Rao, A. V. & Rhoads, G. G. (1997). *Trichomonas vaginalis* associated with low birth weight and preterm delivery. *Sex. Transm. Dis.*, **24**, 353–60.

Curran, J. W., Rendtorff, R. C., Chandler, R. W., Wiser, W. L. & Robinson, H. (1975). Female gonorrhea, its relation to abnormal uterine bleeding, urinary tract symptoms, and cervicitis. *Obstet. Gynecol.*, **45**, 195–8.

Dallabetta, G. A., Gerbase, A. C. & Holmes, K. K. (1998). Problems, solutions and challenges in syndromic management of sexually transmitted diseases. *Sex. Transm. Inf.*, **74** (suppl. 1), S1–11.

Dallabetta, G. A., Miotti, P. G., Chiphangwi, J. D., Saah, A. J., Liomba, G., Odaka, N. Sungami, F. & Hoover, D. R. (1993). High socioeconomics status is a risk factor for human immunodeficiency virus type 1 (HIV-1) infection but not for sexually transmitted diseases in women in Malawi: implications for HIV-1 control. *J. Infect. Dis.*, **167**, 36–42.

Da Silva, O., Gregson, D. & Hammerberg, O. (1997). Role of *Ureaplasma urealyticum* and *Chlamydia trachomatis* in development of bronchopulmonary dysplasia in very low birth weight infants. *Pediatr. Infect. Dis. J.*, **16**, 364–9.

Datta, P., Laga, M. & Plummer, F. A. (1988). Infection and disease after perinatal exposure to *Chlamydia trachomatis* in Nairobi, Kenya. *J. Infect. Dis.*, **158**, 524–8.

D'Auria, A. (1978). Gonococcal scalp wound infection *Am. J. Med. Technol.*, **44**, 471.

Draper, D., Parker, R., Patterson, E., Jones, W., Beutz, M., French, J., Borchardt, K. & McGregor, J. (1993). Detection of *Trichomonas vaginalis* in pregnant women with the InPouch TV culture system. *J. Clin. Microbiol.*, **31**, 1016–18.

Draper, D., Jones, W., Heine, R. P., Beutz, M., French, J. I. & McGregor, J. A. (1995). *Trichomonas vaginalis* weakens human amnio chorion in an in vitro model of premature membrane rupture. *Infect. Dis. Obstet. Gynecol.*, **2**, 267–74.

Edwards, L. E., Barrada, M. I., Hamann, A. A. & Hakanson, E. Y. (1978). Gonorrhea in pregnancy. *Am. J. Obstet. Gynecol.*, **132**, 627–41.

Elliot, B., Brunham, R. C., Laga, M., Piot, P., Ndinya-Achola, J. O., Maitha, G., Cheang, M. & Plummer, F. A. (1990). Maternal gonorrhea as a preventable risk factor for premature birth. *J. Infect. Dis.*, **161**, 531–3.

Erwin, J. O. (1993). Reproductive tract infections among women in Ado-Ekiti, Nigeria: symptoms recognition, perceived causes and treatment choices. *Health Transition*

Rev., **3** (Suppl.), 135–49.

Evans, B. A., Tasker, T. & MacRae, K. D. (1993). Risk profiles for genital infection in women. *Genitourin. Med.*, **69**, 256–61.

Fivush, B., Woodward, C. L. & Wald, E. R. (1980). Gonococcal conjunctivitis in a four-month-old infant. *Sex. Transm. Dis.*, **7**, 24–5.

Fransen, L., Nsanze, H., Klauss, V., Van der Stuyft, P., D'Costa, L., Brunham, R. C. & Piot, P. (1986). *Ophthalmia noenatorum* in Nairobi, Kenya. The roles of *Neisseria gonorrhoeae* and *Chlamydia trachomatis*. *J. Infect. Dis.*, **153**, 862–9.

Frommell, G. T., Rothenberg, R., Wang, S. & McIntosh, K. (1979). Chlamydial infection of mothers and their infants. *J. Pediatr.*, **95**, 28–32.

Galega, F. P., Heymann, D. L. & Nasah, B. T. (1984). Gonococcal ophthalmia neonatorum, the case for prophylaxis in tropical Africa. *Bull. World Health Organ.*, **62**, 95–8.

Gerbase, A. C., Rowley, J. T., Heymann, D. H. L., Berkley, S. & Piot, P. (1998). Global prevalence and incidence estimates of selected curable STDs. *Sex. Transm. Inf.*, **74** (Suppl. 1), S12–16.

Gertig, D. M., Kapiga, S. H., Shao, J. F. & Hunter, D. J. (1997). Risk factors for sexually transmitted disease among women attending family planning clinics in Dar-es-Salaam, Tanzania. *Genitourin. Med.*, **73**, 39–43.

Goldenberg, R. L., Klebanoff, M. A., Nugent, R., Krohn, M. A., Hillier, S. & Andrews, A. A. (1996). Bacterial colonization of the vagina during pregnancy in four ethnic groups. *Am. J. Obstet. Gynecol.*, **174**, 1618–21.

Grattard, F., Soleihac, B., Barbeyrac, B., Bebear, C., Sefert, P. & Pozzetto, B. (1995). Epidemiologic and molecular investigations of genital mycoplasmas from women and neonates at delivery. *Pediatr. Infect. Dis. J.*, **14**, 853–8.

Gravett, M. G., Nelson, P., DeRouen, T., Critchlow, C., Eschenbach, D. A. & Holmes, K. K. (1986). Independent associations of bacterial vaginosis and *Chlamydia trachomatis* infection with adverse pregnancy outcome. *J.A.M.A.*, **256**, 1899–903.

Hale, Y. M., Melton, M. E., Lewis, J. S. & Willis, D. E. (1993). Evaluation of PACE 2 *Neisseria gonorrhoeae* assay by three public health laboratories. *J. Clin. Microbiol.*, **31**, 451–3.

Hammerschlag, M. R., Anderka, M., Semine, D. Z., McComb, D. & McCormack, W. M. (1979). Prospective study of maternal and infantile infection with *Chlamydia trachomatis*. *Pediatrics*, **64**, 142–8.

Hammerschlag, M. R., Cummings, C., Roblin, P. M., Williams, T. H. & Delke, I. (1989). Efficacy of neonatal ocular prophylaxis for the prevention of chlamydia and gonococcal conjunctivitis. *N. Engl. J. Med.*, **320**, 769–72.

Hammerschlag, M. R., Roblin, P. M., Gelling, M., Tsumura, N., Jule, J. E. & Kutlin, A. (1997). Use of polymerase chain reaction for the detection of *Chlamydia trachomatis* in ocular and naso-pharyngeal specimens from infants with conjunctivitis. *Pediatr. Infect. Dis. J.*, **16**, 293–7.

Handsfield, H. H., Hodson, W. A. & Holmes, K. K. (1973). Neonatal gonococcal infection. 1. Orogastric contamination with *Neisseria gonorrhoeae*. *J.A.M.A.*, **225**, 697–701.

Hannenberg, R. S., Rojanapithayakorn, W., Kunasol, P. & Sokal, D. C. (1994). Impact of Thailand's HIV-control programme as indicated by the decline of sexually transmitted diseases. *Lancet*, **224**, 243–5.

Hardy, P. H., Hardy, J. B., Nell, E. E., Grahman, D. A., Spence, M. R. & Rosenbaum, R. C.

(1984). Prevalence of six sexually transmitted disease agents among pregnant inner-city adolescents and pregnancy outcome. *Lancet*, **ii**, 333–7.

Harrison, H. R., Alexander, E. R., Weinstein, L., Lewis, M., Nash, M. & Sim, D. A. (1983). Cervical *Chlamydia trachomatis* and mycoplasmal infections in pregnancy. *J.A.M.A.*, **250**, 1721–7.

Hauth, J. C., Goldenberg, R. L., Andrews, W. W., DuBard, M. B. & Copper, R. L. (1995). Reduced incidence of preterm delivery with metronidazole and erythromycin in women with bacterial vaginosis. *N. Engl. J. Med.*, **333**, 1732–6.

Hay, P. E., Morgan, K. J., Ison, C. A., Bhide, S. A., Romney, M., McKenzie, P., Pearson, J., Lamont, R. F. & Taylor-Robinson, D. (1994). A longitudinal study of bacterial vaginosis during pregnancy. *Br. J. Obstet. Gynaecol.*, **101**, 1048–53.

Hawes, S. E., Hillier, S. L., Benedetti, J., Stevens, C. E., Koutsky, L. A., Wolner-Hanssen, P. & Holmes, K. K. (1996). Hydrogen peroxide-producing lactobacilli and acquisition of vaginal infections. *J. Infect. Dis.*, **174**, 1058–63.

Hawkes, J. S., Alam, N., Gausia, K. de Francisco, A., Chakraborty, J., Williams, L. & Mabey, D. (1997). Using syndromic management in women in areas of low STI prevalance. *12th meeting of the International Society of Sexually Transmitted Diseases Research. Seville, Spain, 19–22 October 1997*, **Abstract 0100**, 78.

Hillier, S. L., Krohn, M., Nugent, R. P. & Gibbs, R. S. (1992). Characteristics of three vaginal flora patterns assessed by Gram stain among pregnant women. *Am. J. Obstet. Gynecol.*, **166**, 938–44.

Hillier, S. L., Nugent, R. P., Eschenbach, D. A., Krohn, M. A., Gibbs, R. S., Martin, D. H., Cotch, M. F., Edelman, R., Pastorek, J. G. 2nd, Rao, A. V. et al. (1995a). Association between bacterial vaginosis and preterm delivery of a low-birth-weight infant. *N. Engl. J. Med.*, **333**, 1737–42.

Hillier, S. L., Krohn, M. A., Cassen, E., Easterling, T. R., Rabe, L. A. & Eschenbach, D. A. (1995b). The role of bacterial vaginosis and vaginal bacteria in amniotic fluid infection in women in preterm labour with intact foetal membranes. *Clin. Infect. Dis.*, **20** (Suppl. 2), S276–8.

Holmes, K. K., Counts, G. W. & Beaty, H. N. (1971). Disseminated gonococcal infection. *Ann. Intern. Med.*, **74**, 979–93.

Hunter, G. W. (1939). Specific urethritis (gonorrhea) in a male newborn. *Am. J. Obstet. Gynecol.*, **38**, 520–1.

Isenberg, S. J., Apt, L. & Wood, M. (1995). A controlled trial of povidone-iodine as prophylaxis against ophthalmia neonatorum. *N. Engl. J. Med.*, **332**, 562–6.

Ison, C. A., Dillon, J. R. & Tapsall, J. W. (1998). The epidemiology of global antibiotic resistance among *Neisseria gonorhoeae* and *Haemophilus ducreyi*. *Lancet*, **351** (suppl. III), 8-11.

Israel, K. S., Rissing, K. B. & Brooks, G. F. (1975). Neonatal and childhood gonococcal infections. *Clin. Obstet. Gynecol.*, **18**, 143–5.

Joesoef, M. R., Hillier, S. L., Utomo, B., Wiknjosastro, G., Linnan, M. & Kandun, N. (1993). Bacterial vaginosis and prematurity in Indonesia, association in early and late pregnancy. *Am. J. Obstet. Gynecol.*, **169**, 175–8.

Joesoef, M. R., Hillier, S. L., Wiknjosastro, G., Sumampouw, H., Linnan, M., Norojono, W., Idajadi, A. & Utomo, B. (1995). Intravaginal clindamycin treatment for bacterial vaginosis, effects on preterm delivery and low birthweight. *Am. J. Obstet. Gynecol.*, **173**, 1527–31.

Kapiga, S. H., Vuylsteke, B., Lyamuya, E. F., Dallabetta, G. & Laga, M. (1998). Evaluation of sexually transmitted diseases diagnostic algorithms among family planning clients in Dar es Salaam, Tanzania. *Sex. Transm. Infect.*, **74**, S132–8.

Kilmarx, P. H., Black, C. M. Limpakarnjanarat, K., Shaffer, N., Yanpaisarn, S., Chaisilwattana, P., Siriwasin, W., Young, W. L., Farshy, C. E., Mastro, T. D. & St Louis, M. E. (1998). Rapid assessment of sexually transmitted diseases in a sentinel population in Thailand; prevalence of chlamydial infection, gonorrhoea, and syphilis among pregnant women – 1996. *Sex. Transm. Infect.*, **74**, 189–93.

Kirkland, H. & Storer, R. V. (1931). Gonococcal rhinitis in an infant. *Br. Med. J.*, **1**, 171.

Kleiman, M. B. & Lamb, G. A. (1973). Gonococcal arthritis in a newborn infant. *Pediatrics*, **52**, 285–7.

Klein, J. O., Buckland, D. & Finland, M. (1969). Colonization of newborn infants by mycoplasmas. *N. Engl. J. Med.*, **280**, 1025–30.

Kohen, D. P. (1974). Neonatal gonococcal arthritis, three cases and review of the literature. *Pediatrics*, **53**, 436–40.

Krieger, J. N., Tam, M. R., Stevens, C. E., Nielsen, I. O., Hale, J., Kiviat, N. B. & Holmes, K. K. (1988). Diagnosis of trichomoniasis. Comparison of conventional wet mount examination with cytologic studies, cultures, and monoclonal antibody staining of direct specimens. *J.A.M.A.*, **259**, 1223–7.

Kurki, T., Sivonen, A., Renkonen, O., Savia, E. & Ylikorkala, O. (1992). Bacterial vaginosis in early pregnancy and pregnancy outcome. *Obstet. Gynecol.*, **80**, 173–7.

Laga, M., Naamara, W., Brunham, R. C., D'Costa, L. J., Nsanze, H., Piot, P., Kunimoto, D., Ndinya-Achola, J. O., Slaney, L., Ronald, A. R., et al. (1986a). Single-dose therapy of gonococcal ophthalmia neonatorum with ceftriaxone. *N Engl J Med*, **315**, 1382–5.

Laga, M., Plummer, F. A., Nzanze, H., Namaara, W., Brunham, R. C., Ndinya-Achola, J. O., Maitha, G., Ronald, A. R., D'Costa, L. J., Bhullar, V. B. et al. (1986b). Epidemiology of ophthalmia neonatorum in Kenya. *Lancet*, **ii**, 1145–9.

Laga, M., Plummer, F. A., Piot, P., Datta, P., Namaara, W., Ndinya-Achola, J. O., Nzanze, H., Maitha, G., Ronald, A. R., Pamba, H. O., et al. (1988). Prophylaxis of gonococcal and chlamydial ophthalmia neonatorum. A comparison of silver nitrate and tetracycline. *N. Engl. J. Med.*, **318**, 653–7.

Laga, M., Meheus, A. & Piot, P. (1989). Epidemiology and control of gonococcal ophthalmia neonatorum. *Bull. World Health Org.*, **67**, 471–7.

Larsson, P. G., Platz-Christensen, J. J. & Sundstrom, E. (1991). Is bacterial vaginosis a sexually transmitted disease? *Intern. J. STD AIDS*, **2**, 362–4.

Larsson, P. G., Platz-Christensen, J. J., Thejls, H., Forsum, U. & Pahlson, C. (1992). Incidence of pelvic inflammatory disease after first-trimester legal abortion in women with bacterial vaginosis after treatment with metronidazole, a double-blind, randomised study. *Am. J. Obstet. Gynecol.*, **166**, 100–3.

Leroy, V., De Clercq, A., Ladner, J., Bogaerts, J., Van, P. & Dabis, F. (1995). Should screening of genital infections be part of antenatal care in areas of high HIV prevalence? A prospective cohort study from Kigali, Rwanda, 1992–1993. *Genitourin. Med.*, **71**, 207–11.

Lossick, J. G. (1990). Treatment of sexually transmitted vaginosis/vaginitis. *Rev. Infect. Dis.*, **6** (suppl.), S665–81.

Linnan, M. (January 1995). Summary report of the STD studies in Surabaya, East Java. The Surabaya STD Study Group, Centers for Disease Control and Prevention.

McCormick, W. M., Stumacher, R. J., Johnson, K. & Donner, A. (1977). Clinical spectrum of gonococcal infections in women. *Lancet*, **ii**, 1182–5.

McDonald, H. M., O'Loughlin, J. A., Vigneswaran, R., Jolley, P. T., Harvey, J. A., Bof, A. & McDonald, P. J. (1997). Impact of metronidazole therapy on preterm birth in women with bacterial vaginosis flora (*Gardnerella vaginalis*), a randomised, placebo controlled trial. *Br. J. Obstet. Gynaecol.*, **104**, 1391–7.

McGregor, J. A., French, J. I., Jones, W., Milligan, K., McKinney, P. J., Patterson, E. & Parker, R. (1994). Bacterial vaginosis is associated with prematurity and vaginal fluid mucinase and sialidase, results of a controlled trial of topical clindamycin cream. *Am. J. Obstet. Gynecol.*, **170**, 1048–60.

McGregor, J. A., French, J. I., Parker, R., Draper, D., Patterson, E., Jones, W., Thorsgard, K. & McFee, J. (1995). Prevention of premature birth by screening and treatment for common genital tract infections, results of a prospective controlled evaluation. *Am. J. Obstet. Gynecol.*, **173**, 157–67.

McLaren, L. C., Davis, L. E., Healy, G. R. & James, C. G. (1983). Isolation of *Trichomonas vaginalis* from the respiratory tract of infants with respiratory disease. *Pediatrics*, **71**, 888–990.

Mardh, P. A., Helin, I., Bobeck, S., Laurin, J. & Nilsson, T. (1980). Colonisation of pregnant and puerperal women and neonates with *Chlamydia trachomatis*. *Br. J. Vener. Dis.*, **56**, 96–100.

Mathai, E., Mathai, M., Baravilala, W. & Schramm, M. (1998). Prevalence of sexually transmitted disease in pregnant women in Suva, Fiji. *Sex. Transm. Infect.*, **74**, 305.

Mayaud, P., Grosskurth, H., Changalucha, J., Todd, J., West, B., Gabone, R., Senkoro, K., Rusizoka, M., Laga, M., Hayes, R. & Mabey, D. (1995). Risk assessment and other screening options for gonorrhoea and chlamydial infections in women attending rural Tanzanian antenatal clinics. *Bull. World Health Organ.*, **73**, 621–30.

Mayaud, P., Uledi, E., Cornelissen, J., Ka-Gina, G., Tood, J., Rwakatare, M. West, B., Kopwe, L., Manoko, D., Grosskurth, H., Hayes, R. & Mabey, D. (1998). Risk scores to detect cervical infections in urban antenatal clinic attenders in Mwanza, Tanzania. *Sex. Transm. Infect.*, **74**, S139–40.

Meda, N., Sangaré, L., Lankoandé, S., Sanou, P. T., Compaoré, P. I., Catraye, J., Cartoux, M. & Soudré (1997). Pattern of sexually transmitted diseases among pregnant women in Burkina Faso, West Africa; potential for a clinical management based on simple approaches. *Genitourin. Med.*, **73**, 188–93.

Meis, P. H., Goldenberg, R. L., Mercer, B., Iams, J. D., Moawad, A. H., Miodovnik, M., Menard, M. K., Caritis, S. N., Thurnau, G. R., Bottoms, S. F., Das, A., Roberts, J. M. & McNellis, D. (1995). The preterm prediction study, significance of vaginal infections. *Am. J. Obstet. Gynecol.*, **173**, 1231–5.

Mertz, K. J., Levine, W. C., Mosure, D. J., Berman, S. M., Dorian, K. J. & Hadgu, A. (1997). Screening women for gonorrhea, demographic screening criteria for general clinical use. *Am. J. Public Health*, **87**, 1535–8.

Minkoff, H., Brunebaum, A. N., Schwarz, R. H., Feldman, J., Cummings, M., Crombleholme, W., Clark, L., Pringle, G. & McCormack, W. M. (1984). Risk factors for prematurity and premature rupture of membranes. A prospective study of the vaginal flora in pregnancy. *Am. J. Gynecol.*, **150**, 965–72.

Morales, W. J., Schorr, S. & Albritton, J. (1994). Effect of metronidazole in patients with preterm birth in preceding pregnancy and bacterial vaginosis. A placebo-controlled, double-blind study. *Am. J. Obstet. Gynecol.*, **171**, 345–9.

Newton, E. R., Prihoda, T. J. & Gibbs, R. S. (1990). A clinical and microbiological analysis of risk factors for puerperal endometritis. *Obstet. Gynecol.*, **298**, 402–6.

Newton, E. R., Piper, J. & Peairs, W. (1997). Bacterial vaginosis and intraaminiotic infection. *Am. J. Obstet. Gynecol.*, **176**, 672–7

Nugent, R. P., Krohn, M. A. & Hillier, S. L. (1991). Reliability of diagnosing bacterial vaginosis is improved by a standardized method of Gram stain interpretation. *J. Clin. Microbiol.*, **29**, 297–301.

O'Farrell, N., Hoosen, A. A., Kharsany, A. B. M. & Van Den Ende, J. (1989). Sexually transmitted pathogens in pregnant women in a rural South African community. *Genitourin. Med.*, **65**, 276–80.

Panke, E. S., Yang, L. I., Leist, P. A., Magevney, P., Fry, J. R. & Lee, R. F. (1991). Comparison of Gen-Probe DNA probe test and culture for the detection of *N. gonorrhoeae* in endocervical specimens. *J. Clin. Microbiol.*, **29**, 883–8.

Passey, M., Mgone, C. S., Lupiwa, S., Suve, N., Tiwara, S., Lupiwa, T., Clegg, A. & Alpers, M. P. (1998). Community based study of sexually transmitted diseases in rural women in the highlands of Papua New Guinea; prevalence and risk factors. *Sex. Transm. Infect.* **74**, 120–7.

Pastoreck, J. G., Cotch, M. F., Martin, D. H. & Eschenbach, D. A. (1996). Clinical and microbiological correlates of vaginal trichomoniasis during pregnancy. *Clin. Infect Dis.*, **23**, 1075–80.

Pease, P., Rogers, K. B. & Cole, B. C. (1967). A cytopathogenic strain of *Mycoplasma hominis* type 1 isolated from the lung of a stillborn infant. *J. Pathol. Bacteriol.*, **84**, 460–2.

Perine, P. L., Duncan, M. E., Krause, D. W. & Awoke, S. (1980). Pelvic inflammatory disease and puerperal sepsis in Ethiopia. *Am. J. Obstet. Gynecol.*, **138**, 969–73.

Perzigian, R., Adams, J., Weiner, G., Dipietro, M., Blythe, L., Pierson, C. & Faix, R. (1998). *Ureaplasma urealyticum* and chronic lung disease in very low birth weight infants during the exogenous surfactant era. *Pediatr. Infect. Dis. J.*, **17**, 620–5.

Plummer, F. A., Laga, M., Brunham, R. C., Piot, P., Ronald, A. R., Bhullar, V., Mati, J. Y., Ndinya-Achola, J. O., Cheang, M. & Nsanze, H. (1987). Postpartum upper genital tract infection in Nairobi, Kenya. Epidemiology, etiology and risk factors. *J. Infect. Dis.*, **156**, 92–8.

Postlethwaite, R. J. (1975). *Trichomonas vaginitis* and *Escherichiae coli* urinary infection in a newborn infant. *Clin. Pediatr. (Phila)*, **14**, 866–7.

Quinn, P. A., Gillian, J. E., Markestad, T., St John, M. A., Daneman, A., Lie, K. I., Li, H. C., Czegledy-Nagy, E. & Klein, A. (1985). Intrautrine infection with *Ureaplasma urealyticum* as a cause of fetal neonatal pneumonia. *Pediatr. Infect. Dis. J.*, **4**, 538–43.

Read, J. S. & Klebanoff, M. A. (1993). Sexual intercourse during pregnancy and preterm delivery, effects of vaginal microorganism. *Am. J. Obstet. Gynecol.*, **168**, 514–19.

Riduan, J. M., Hillier, S. L., Utomo, B., Wiknjosastro, G., Linnan, M. & Kandun, N. (1993). Bacterial vaginosis and prematurity in Indonesia, association in early and late pregnancy. *Am. J. Obstet. Gynecol.*, **169**, 175–8.

Ryan, C. A. & Gorbach, P. M. (1997). HIV and sexually transmitted diseases in Cambodia: prevalence of infections, evaluation of treatment flowcharts and assessments of risk and health seeking behaviours. *Final Report*, Family Health International.

Ryan, C. A., Courtois, B. N., Hawes, S. E., Stevens, C. E., Eschenbach, D. A. & Holmes, K. K. (1998a). Risk assessment, symptoms, and sign as predictors of vulvovaginal and cervical infections in an urban US STD clinic, implications for use of STD algorithms. *Sex. Transm. Infect.*, **74**, S59–76.

Ryan, C. A., Zidouh, A., Manhart, L. E., Selka, R., Xia, M., Moloney-Kitts, M., Mahjour, J., Krone, M., Courtois, B. N., Dallabetta, G. & Holmes, K. K. (1998b). Reproductive tract infections in primary health care, family planning, dermatovenereology clinics, evaluation of syndromic management in Morocco. *Sex. Transm. Infect.*, **74** (Suppl. 1), S95–S105.

Sánchez, P. J. & Regan, J. A. (1987). Vertical transmission of *Ureaplasma urealyticum* in full-term infants. *Pediatr. Infect. Dis. J.*, **6**, 825–8.

Sánchez, P. J. & Regan, J. A. (1988). *Ureaplasma urealyticum* colonization and other chronic lung disease in low-birth-weight infants. *Pediatr. Infect. Dis. J.*, **7**, 542–6.

Sánchez, P. J. & Regan, J. A. (1990). Vertical transmission of *Ureaplasma urealyticum* from mothers to pre-term infants. *Pediatr. Infect. Dis. J.*, **9**, 398–401.

Sánchez, S. E., Koutsky, L. A., Sánchez, J., Fernandez, A., Casquero, J., Kreiss, J., Catlin, M., Xia, M. & Holmes, K. K. (1998). Rapid and inexpensive approaches to managing abnormal vaginal discharge or lower abdominal pain, an evaluation in women attending gynaecology and family planning clinics in Peru. *Sex. Transm. Infect.*, **74**, S85–S94.

Sarrel, P. M. & Pruett, K. A. (1968). Symptomatic gonorrhea during pregnancy. *Obstet. Gynecol.*, **32**, 670–3.

Schachter, J. & Dawson, C. R. (1978). *Human Chlamydial Infections*, pp. 111–20. Littleton, MA: PSG Publishing.

Schachter, J., Grossman, M., Sweet, R. L. Holt, J., Jordan, C. & Bishop, E. (1986). Prospective study of perinatal transmission of *Chlamydia trachomatis*. *J.A.M.A.*, **255**, 3374–7.

Schmale, J. D., Martin, J. E. Jr. & Domescik, G. (1969). Observation on the culture diagnosis of gonorrhea in women. *J.A.M.A.*, **210**, 312–14.

Schneider, H., Coetzee, D. J., Fehler, H. G., Bellingan, A., Dangor, Y. Radebe, F. & Ballard, R. C. (1998). Screening for sexually transmitted disease in rural South African women. *Sex. Transm. Infect.* **74**, S147–52.

Shafer, M. A., Sweet, R. L., Ohm-Smith, M. J., Shalwitz, J., Beck, A. & Schachter, J. (1985). Microbiology of the lower genital tract in post-menarchal adolescent girls, difference by sexual activity, contraception and presence of non-specific vaginitis. *J. Pediatr.*, **107**, 974–81.

Shariat, H., Young, M. & Abedin, M. (1992). An interesting case presentation, a possible new route for perinatal acquisition of *Chlamydia*. *J. Perinatol.*, **12**, 300–2.

Sheller, J. P., Johannessen, G., Olsen, T. & Maruping, S. (1990). *Neisseria gonorrhoeae, Trichomonas vaginalis*, and yeast reported from attendees at an antenatal clinic in a rural area in Botswana. *Genitourin. Med.*, **66**, 460.

Smith, K. R., Ching, S., Lee, H., Ohhashi, Y., Hu, H. Y., Fisher, H. C. 3rd, & Hook, E. W. 3rd (1995). Evaluation of ligase chain reaction for use with urine for identification of *Neisseria gonorrhoeae* in females attending a sexually transmitted disease clinic. *J. Clin. Microbiol.*, **33**, 455–7.

Spiegel, C. A. (1991). Vaginitis. In *Laboratory Methods for the Diagnosis of Sexually Transmitted Diseases*, ed. B. B. Wentworth, F. M. Judson, M. J. Gilchrist, pp. 181–202. Washington, DC: American Public Health Association.

Teles, E., Hardy, E., Oliverira, U. M., Elias, C. J. & Faúndes, A. (1997). Reassessing risk assessment: limits to predicting reproductive tract infection in new contraceptive users. *International Family Planning Perspectives*, **23**, 179–82.

Temmerman, M., Kidula, K., Tyndall, M., Rukaria-Kaumbutho, R., Muchiri, L. & Ndinya-Achola, J. O. (1998a). The supermarket for women's reproductive health: the burden of genital infections in a family planning clinic in Nairobi, Kenya. *Sex. Transm. Infect.*, **74**, 202–4.

Temmerman, M., Laga, M., Ndinya-Achola, J. O., Paraskevas, M., Brunham, R. C., Plummer, F. A. & Piot, P. (1988b). Microbial aetiology and diagnostic criteria of postpartum endometritis in Nairobi, Kenya. *Genitourin. Med.*, **64**, 172–5.

Temmerman, M., Plummer, F. A., Farah, A., Wamola, I. A., Brunham, R. C. & Piot, P. (1992). Gonorrhea in pregnancy. *J. Obstet. Gynecol.*, **12**, 162–6.

Temmerman, M., Njagi, E., Nagelkerke, N., Ndinya-Achola, J., Plummer, F. A. & Meheus, A. (1995). Mass antimicrobial treatment in pregnancy, a randomised placebo-controlled trial in a population with high rates of sexually transmitted diseases. *J. Reprod. Med.*, **40**, 176–80.

Thomas, T., Choudhri, S., Kariuki, C. & Moses, S. (1996). Identifying cervical infection among pregnant women in Nairobi, Kenya; limitations of risk assessment and symptoms-based approaches. *Genitourin. Med.*, **72**, 334–8.

Vejtorp, M., Bollerup, A. C. & Vejtorp, L. (1988). Bacterial vaginosis, a double-blind randomised trial of the effect of treatment of the sexual partner. *Br. J. Obstet. Gynecol.*, **95**, 920–6.

Vuylsteke, B., Laga, M., Alary, M., Geniers, M.-M., Lebughe J.-P., Nzila, N., Behets, F., Van Dyck, E. & Piot, P. (1993). Clinical algorithms to screen women for gonococcal and chlamydial infection: evaluation for pregnant women and prostitutes in Zaire. *Clin. Infect. Dis.*, **17**, 82–8.

Waites, K. B., Rudd, P. T., Crouse, D. T., Canupp, K. C., Nelson, K. G., Ramsey, C. & Cassell, G. H. (1988). Chronic *Ureaplasma urealyticum* and *Mycoplasma hominis* infections of central nervous system in pre-term infants. *Lancet*, **i**, 17–21.

Waites, K. B., Duffy, L. B., Crouse, D. T., Dworsky, M. E., Strange, M. J., Nelson, K. G. & Cassell, G. H. (1990). Mycoplasmal Infections of cerebrospinal fluid in newborn infants from a community hospital population. *Pediatr. Infect. Dis. J.*, **9**, 241–5.

Waites, K. B., Crouse, D. T. & Cassell, G. H. (1993). Systemic neonatal infection due *to Ureaplasma urealyticum. Clin. Infect. Dis.*, **17**, S131–5.

Waites, K. B., Casell, G. H., Duffy, L. B., Searcey, K. B., Crouse, D. T., Reese, J. M., Heggie, A. D., Jacobs, M. R., Butler, V. T., Baley, J. E. & Boxerbaum, B. (1995). Isolation of *Ureaplasma urealyticum* from low birth weight infants. *J. Paediatr.*, **126**, 502–4.

Wang, E. E., Frayha, H., Watts, J., Hammerberg, O., Chernesky, M. A., Mahony, J. B. & Cassell, G. H. (1988). Role of *Ureaplasma urealyticum* and other pathogens in the development of chronic lung disease of prematurity. *Pediatr. Infect. Dis. J.*, **7**, 547–51.

Wang, E. E., Cassell, G. H., Sanchez, P. J., Regan, J. A., Payne, N. R. & Liu, P. P. (1993). *Ureaplasma urealyticum* and chronic lung disease of prematurity, critical appraisal of the literature on causation. *Clin. Infect. Dis.*, **17**, S112–16.

Watts, D. H., Krohn, M. S., Hillier, S. L. & Eschenbach, D. A. (1990). Bacterial vaginosis as a risk factor for post caesarean endometritis. *Obstet. Gynecol.*, **75**, 52–8.

Wawer, M., Sewankambo, N. K., Serwadda, D., Quinn, T. C., Paxton, L. A., Kiwanuka, N., Wabwire-Mangen, F., Li, C., Lutalo, T., Nalugoda, F., Gaydos, C. A., Moulton, L. H., Meehan, M. O., Ahmed, S. & Gray, R. H. (1999). Control of sexually transmitted diseases for AIDS prevention in Uganda, a randomised community trial. *Lancet*, **353**, 525–35.

Winceslaus, J., Goh, B. T., Dunlop, E. M. C., Mantell, J., Woodland, R. M., Forsey, T. & Treharne, J. D. (1987). Diagnosis of ophthalmia neonatorum. *Br. Med. J.*, **295**, 1377–9.

World Health Organization. (1986). *Conjunctivitis of the Newborn, Prevention and Treatment at the Primary Health Care Level.* Geneva: World Health Organization.

World Health Organization. (1988). *Maternal and Perinatal Infections – Report of a WHO Consultation (22/11–2/12, 1988).* Geneva: Division of Family Health, World Health Organization.

World Health Organization. (1991). *Maternal and Perinatal Infections, a Practical Guide. WHO/MCH/91.10.* Geneva: World Health Organization.

World Health Organization. (1994). Global Programme on AIDS. *Management of Sexually Transmitted Diseases. WHO/GPA/TEM/94.1.* Geneva: World Health Organization.

15

Toxoplasmosis

Ruth Gilbert

Introduction

Toxoplasma gondii occurs throughout the world and is one of the most common parasitic infections of humans. Infection is acquired by ingestion of viable tissue cysts in undercooked meat, or of oocysts excreted by cats and contaminating soil or water (Remington et al., 1995). Acquisition of toxoplasma infection for the first time (primary infection) is usually asymptomatic although a significant minority of people suffer fever, malaise and lymphadenopathy (Ho-Yen, 1992a). As the primary infection resolves, the parasite forms latent cysts throughout the body. In approximately 1% or less of people infected with *T. gondii*, latent cysts in the retina and choroid can reactivate, often years after infection, and give rise to inflammatory lesions, which may affect vision (Gilbert & Stanford, 2000). Toxoplasma infection is a major cause of morbidity and mortality in immunodeficient patients (Ho-Yen, 1992b).

When primary infection occurs during pregnancy, *T.gondi* may be transmitted from the mother to the fetus. Fetal infection can result in inflammatory lesions in the brain, retina and choroid that may lead to permanent neurological damage and visual impairment. Rarely, disseminated fetal infection causes fetal or postnatal death. Approximately 1–10 per 10 000 babies are born with congenital toxoplasmosis (Ancelle et al., 1996; Conyn-van-Spaedonck, 1991; Guerina et al., 1994; Lebech et al., 1999).

How best to prevent symptoms and disability due to congenital toxoplasmosis is a question that has caused controversy among clinicians for the last three decades. At the core of the debate is uncertainty about the effectiveness of prenatal treatment on the risk of congenital toxoplasmosis, and of prenatal and postnatal treatment on the risk of clinical signs and symptoms in the long term.

In this chapter, options available for the prevention of congenital toxoplasmosis and its sequelae will be outlined for the most reliable evidence based on the potential benefits and harms of alternative strategies.

Prenatal screening

The main aim of prenatal screening is to offer early treatment to the mother in order to reduce the risks of neurological or visual impairment in the child due to congenital toxoplasmosis. These serious outcomes occur in a small minority of babies born to women who acquire toxoplasma infection during pregnancy. The potential benefits of screening depend on three factors: first, accurate identification of women who acquired infection during pregnancy; secondly, the effect of prenatal treatment on the risk of transmission of infection to the fetus; and thirdly, the effect of prenatal treatment on the risk of an infected child developing symptoms.

Identification of infected women

As primary toxoplasma infection is usually asymptomatic (Ho-Yen, 1992a), infected women can only be detected reliably by serological testing. Of the two strategies involved (Raeber et al., 1995), both start by testing all women at their first prenatal visit. In the first strategy, women who have no detectable antibodies to *T. gondii* are re-tested at intervals throughout pregnancy and once after delivery. Seroconversion (a change from undetectable to detectable toxoplasma-specific IgG and/or IgM) indicates acquisition of infection during pregnancy. In France, the prevalence of past infection is high (54%) (Ancelle et al., 1996), and less than half the women require repeated testing during pregnancy. In contrast, in the UK (Allain et al., 1998) and Norway (Jenum et al., 1998a), only 10% have been infected in the past and 90% require repeated testing. The costs of re-testing clearly depend on the prevalence of toxoplasma infection. This varies according to country and ethnic group (see Table 15.1) and decreases with altitude and latitude (Ancelle et al., 1996; Gilbert et al., 1993; Guimaraes et al., 1993; Jeannel et al., 1988; Ljungstrom et al., 1995; Remington et al., 1995; Zuber et al., 1995). The prevalence has fallen in many European countries over the last three decades (Ades & Nokes, 1993; Bornand & Piguet, 1991; Horion et al., 1990; Nokes et al., 1993).

Susceptible pregnant women are re-tested monthly in France (Thulliez, 1992) and Switzerland (Raeber et al., 1995), and three-monthly in Austria, Germany (Raeber et al., 1995), and Italy (Buffolano et al., 1994). Monthly testing has the advantage of earlier treatment, which is thought to reduce the risk of infection and of damage in the fetus. However, frequent testing has the disadvantage of lowering the detection rate with each additional test, thereby increasing the number of women falsely identified as positive, the number of prenatal visits, and costs (Anon, 1990). For example in France, the incidence of confirmed infection is 8/1000 susceptible pregnancies (Ancelle et al., 1996). In any 1-month period, the incidence will therefore be 0.83/1000. If susceptible women are re-tested monthly

Table 15.1. Prevalence of toxoplasma IgG antibodies in pregnant women

Study	Country and year of survey	Number of pregnant women	% IgG positive
Ancelle et al. (1996)	France (all) 1995	13 459	54%
Berger et al. (1995)	Switzerland, Basel 1986–1994	30 000	29%
Jacquier et al. (1995)	Switzerland (most) 1990–1991	9059	46%
Buffolano et al. (1993)	Italy, Naples 1993	3518	40%
Valcavi et al. (1995)	Italy, Parma 1987–1991	19 432	49%
Roos et al. (1993)	Germany, Wurzburg 1989–1990	2104	42%
Aspock & Pollak (1992)	Austria, Vienna 1981–1991	167 041	43%
Conyn van Spaendonck (1991)	Netherlands 1987	28 049	45%
Ljungstrom et al. (1995)	Sweden 1987–1988: north	3654	12%
	south		26%
Foulon et al. (1988)	Belgium 1979–1990	11 286	56%
Allain et al. (1988)	UK, Eastern 1992	13 000	8%
Zadik et al. (1995)	UK, Sheffield 1989–1992	1621	10%
Lappalainem et al. (1995)	Finland, south 1988–189	16 733	20%
Jenum et al. (1997)	Norway 1992 north	35 940	7%
	south		13%
Lebech et al. (1993)	Denmark 1992	5 402	27%
Decavalas et al. (1990)	Greece	217	52%
Remington et al. (1995)	USA, seven different regions 1986–1993		10–30%
Walpole et al. (1991)	Australia, Western 1986–1989	10 207	35%
Guimares et al. (1993)	Brazil, Sao Paulo 1989	1286	59–78%
Altintas et al. (1997)	Turkey, Aegean region 1991–1995	2287	55%
Sun et al. (1995)	China, Chengdu 1987	1211	39%
Ashrafunnessa et al. (1998)	Bangladesh 1995	286	38%

with one test of 98% specificity, 20/1000 women will be false-positives and 0.8/1000 true-positives. The relative proportion of false-positive test results is higher in areas with a lower incidence rate. Performing several tests at the same time and repeating tests reduces the rate of false-positive results but at a cost. Less frequent re-testing balances the costs of investigating falsely positive results and the possible harms of delayed treatment.

The second strategy is based on the interpretation of tests of recent infection in women who are IgG positive at their first prenatal test, to assess the risk of postconceptional infection. Many centres test simultaneously for IgG and IgM *T.gondii* specific antibodies (Aspock & Pollak, 1992; Hengst, 1992; Thulliez, 1992). Specific IgM in the absence of IgG indicates infection in the previous 2 weeks, but

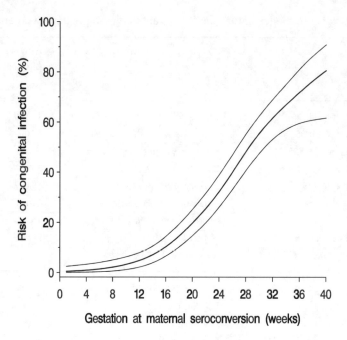

Figure 15.1 Risk of congenital infection according to gestation at maternal seroconversion. Thin lines represent 90% confidence interval.

requires confirmation, as false positives are common. If both IgM and IgG are positive, further tests for high or rising IgG titre, low IgG avidity, IgA antibodies or a combination of these are undertaken, although none reliably distinguishes between infection acquired before and after conception. One of the most promising single sample tests for recent infection is IgG avidity (Jenum et al., 1997; Lappalainen et al., 1993), which appears to have moderate specificity for infection within the past year. Reliance on tests for recent infection in the first trimester inevitably results in unnecessary treatment or pregnancy termination (Buffolano et al., 1994) in a large number of women who acquired infection preconception. In such women, the risk of fetal infection is negligible and limited to a few case reports in the world literature (Desmonts et al., 1990; Marty et al., 1991; Pons et al., 1995).

Mother to child transmission of infection and prenatal treatment

The risk of congenital toxoplasmosis increases with gestation at acquisition of maternal infection (Desmond & Couvreur, 1984). A recent study of women in France, where seronegative women are tested monthly, Dunn et al. (1999) provides precise and reliable estimates of the risk of congenital toxoplasmosis according to gestation at first detection of seroconversion that can be used for counselling women. Overall, the risk of congenital toxoplasmosis is 29%, but this masks a steep increase with gestation (see Fig. 15.1). The risk is low in early pregnancy and only 6% (3–9%) at 13 weeks' gestation. Thereafter, the risk rises sharply reaching 40% (34–46%) at 26 weeks, 72% (61–80%) at 36 weeks and 81% just before delivery.

Congenital infection can be diagnosed by the persistence of toxoplasma specific IgG antibodies in serum beyond 12 months of age or by identifying the parasite in amniotic fluid or fetal products by detection of *T. gondii* DNA by PCR analysis or isolation of the parasite by mouse inoculation (Lebech et al., 1996). False-positive PCR results are a concern and depend on the rigour of the technique (Guy et al., 1996). The reported sensitivity of PCR is approximately 90–97% (Hohlfeld et al., 1994; Jenum et al., 1998b). In France, amniocentesis is delayed until 4 weeks after estimated maternal infection (Dunn et al., 1999). The rationale is to allow time for mother-to-child transmission to occur, but the evidence to support this reasoning is lacking.

Once the child is born, congenital infection can be excluded if IgG becomes negative during infancy but only after discontinuation of treatment. This is because antitoxoplasma treatment depresses antibody production, often to un-detectable levels. In infected children, antibody production increases to detectable levels soon after treatment is stopped (Fortier et al., 1997).

Treatment to prevent mother-to-child transmission of infection usually consists of spiramycin (9×10^6 units/day), which is prescribed immediately after confirmation of maternal infection. In some French centres, women infected after 32 weeks are started on a more potent regimen of pyrimethamine (50 mg/day) and sulphadiazine (3 g/day) plus folinic acid alternating 3 weekly with spiramycin (Dunn et al., 1999). The rationale for the latter regimen is to reduce the risk of fetal damage in view of the high risk of fetal infection (over 50%). Pyrimethamine and sulphadiazine are transmitted to the fetus in higher concentrations than spi-ramycin and, unlike spiramycin, penetrate the fetal brain and cerebrospinal fluid (Schoondermark van de Ven et al., 1994, 1995). Adverse effects of spiramycin include nausea, vomiting, abdominal pain, dry mouth and, rarely, skin rash. Pyrimethamine and sulphadiazine are associated with bone marrow depression, rash, vomiting, respiratory distress, tachycardia or convulsions. Pyrimethamine is teratogenic in rats in doses similar to those used in humans but this effect is attenuated if folinic acid is given. This drug is therefore only given in the second half of pregnancy (Remington et al., 1995).

Evidence for the effectiveness of any prenatal treatment regimen in reducing mother-to-child transmission is lacking. Two systematic reviews found no con-trolled trials (Eskild et al., 1996; Wallon et al., 1999) and none of the observational studies has taken account of the steep rise in the risk of transmission with gestation at maternal infection (Dunn et al., 1999). However, a recent study (Foulon et al.,

1999) found no effect of any prenatal treatment on transmission after adjustment for gestation at maternal infection. One explanation may be that treatment is given after mother-to-child transmission has occurred. In animal models, transmission mostly occurs during the parasitaemic phase, which lasts for 2–3 weeks after infection (Remington et al., 1995). In most women, parasitaemia is thought to have ceased by the time seroconversion occurs (Remington et al., 1995), usually within 2 weeks of infection (Sulzer et al., 1986). Consequently, if mother-to-child transmission coincides with parasitaemia, the treatment of women identified by serological testing will always be given too late to prevent fetal infection.

In many centres, treatment is continued throughout pregnancy, due to a theoretical risk of delayed transmission. This is controversial. The evidence for delayed transmission is based on a small number of reports of false-negative PCR analyses of amniotic fluid samples in fetuses who later proved to be infected (Hohlfeld et al., 1994; Jenum et al., 1998b). However, such results may be due to insensitivity of the test or the possibility that amniocentesis may cause mother-to-child transmission, as reported for HIV infection (Tess et al., 1998).

Risk of signs and symptoms due to congenital toxoplasmosis

For children with congenital toxoplasmosis, the risk of clinical signs, such as hydrocephalus, intracranial calcification and retinochoroiditis, is inversely related to gestation at maternal infection (Desmonts & Couvreur, 1984; Dunn et al., 1999). Dunn et al. found that 41 of the 153 (27%) congenitally infected children had at least one of the following clinical signs by 3 years of age: intracranial calcification (14 children), retinochoroiditis (33) or hydrocephalus (2). Development of clinical signs was strongly related to gestation at maternal seroconversion, declining from an estimated 61% (37–83%) at 13 weeks, to 25% (19–31%) at 26 weeks, and 9% (4–16%) at 36 weeks (see Fig. 15.2). However, for pregnant women with a diagnosis of primary toxoplasma infection, knowledge of the risks of clinical sequelae is not relevant as they first need to decide whether to undergo prenatal diagnosis or not. The risk of clinical signs in a fetus born to an infected woman is obtained by multiplying the risk of congenital infection by the risk of signs among congenitally infected children. For example, at 26 weeks' gestation the risk of maternal–fetal transmission is 40% and the risk of clinical signs in an infected fetus is 25%. The overall risk is therefore 10% (0.4×0.25). If this calculation is repeated for all gestational ages, an 'n' shaped distribution is produced which reaches a maximum of 10% at 24–30 weeks' gestation (see Fig. 15.3). In the second and third trimesters, the risk never falls below 5% and is 6% just before delivery.

Knowledge of these risks allows women to balance the risks of harm and benefit when deciding about treatment, amniocentesis or termination. For example, a

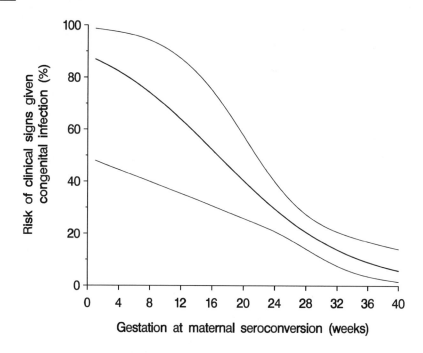

Figure 15.2   Risk of developing clinical signs (not necessarily symptomatic) before 3 years given congenital infection, according to gestation at maternal seroconversion. Thin lines represent 90% confidence interval.

woman with a positive test at 12 weeks' gestation would have a risk of giving birth to a child with clinical signs of 3% or less depending on how well the test predicts postconceptional infection. The possible reduction in this risk which might be achieved by prenatal treatment must be balanced against the risk of fetal loss of 0.9% associated with amniocentesis (Tabor et al., 1986). However, women really need to know the risk of ocular lesions in the long term, not just at 3 years. Most importantly, they need to know the risk of disability due to neurological damage or visual impairment. Unfortunately, information on these latter outcomes is less reliable and the effect of gestation is not known.

Ocular lesions can appear at any age. However, the limited available data suggest a decline in the risk of lesions appearing for the first time in children with normal ophthalmologic examinations during the first 2 years of life. Of 91 children with congenital toxoplasmosis followed for 1 to 6 years in four cohort studies (Conyn-van-Spaedonck, 1991; Guerina et al., 1994; Lappalainen et al., 1995; Lebech et al., 1999), 20 developed retinochoroidal lesions, and only one was first found to be affected after 2 years of age. At a 20-year follow-up of 11 infected children (Koppe et al., 1986), nine had retinochoroidal lesions and five of them

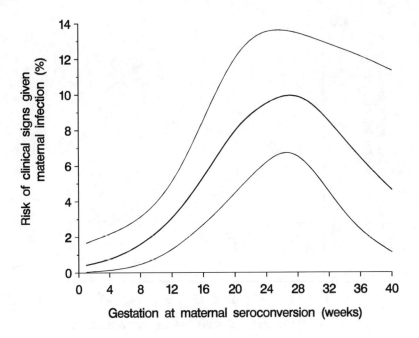

Figure 15.3 Risk of developing clinical signs (not necessarily symptomatic) before age 3 years given maternal infection, according to gestation at maternal seroconversion. Thin lines represent 90% confidence interval.

had lesions first noted during infancy. Approximately half the children with retinochoroidal lesions followed in five cohort studies (Conyn-van-Spaedonck, 1991; Guerina et al., 1994; Koppe et al., 1986; Lappalainen et al., 1995; Lebech et al., 1999) had macula lesions (likely to cause some degree of permanent visual impairment) or some degree of unilateral visual impairment. In the study by Dunn et al., eight of 33 children with retinochoroiditis had unilateral visual impairment of less than 1/10 (Dunn et al., 1999). Symptoms of transient visual impairment, due to reactivation of retinochoroidal lesions, are common in adults with ocular toxoplasmosis. Such episodes usually resolve spontaneously, after 6–8 weeks but the duration of symptoms and size of lesions may be attenuated by treatment (Mets et al., 1996; Rothova et al., 1993).

Few studies have adequately assessed neurological impairment in children with congenital toxoplasmosis. However, reports of severe impairment are rare: of 3/102 children followed in five cohort studies (Conyn-van-Spaedonck, 1991; Guerina et al., 1994; Koppe et al., 1986; Lappalainen et al., 1995; Lebech et al., 1999), 1 had severe neurological impairment. Other studies report that children with intracranial calcification or hydrocephalus detected prenatally (usually after 22 to 24 weeks' gestation) appear to be asymptomatic (Berrebi et al., 1994; Patel et al., 1996).

Once fetal infection has been diagnosed, pyrimethamine and sulphadiazine is prescribed alternating 3 weekly with spiramycin in order to reduce the risk of clinical signs and symptoms in the infected child. The evidence for benefit is inconclusive. Foulon et al. (1999) reported an odds ratio of 0.3 (95% confidence interval 0.1 to 0.9) for clinical signs at 1 year in children whose mothers were treated prenatally compared with those not treated. However, the study included referral centres for prenatal diagnosis, and there was no attempt to exclude women referred due to suspicion of signs in the fetus or infant. Selection bias may therefore account for the apparent effect of treatment: untreated women with fetuses or children with clinical signs may have been more likely to be included in the study than untreated women with unaffected fetuses/children. In an earlier study, Desmonts and Couvreur compared the risk of clinical sequelae in children whose mothers received prenatal treatment with pyrimethamine and sulfadiazine and those born to mothers infected at a similar gestation but treated only with spiramycin (Couvreur et al., 1993). They reported no significant difference in clinical sequelae.

Neonatal screening

Neonatal screening aims to identify neonates with congenital toxoplasmosis in order to offer treatment and clinical follow-up. The vast majority of congenitally infected infants are asymptomatic in early infancy and would be missed by routine paediatric examinations. Neonatal screening is based on the detection of toxoplasma specific IgM on Guthrie card blood spots and has been found to detect 85% of infected infants (Lebech et al., 1999). However the proportion may be lower if the mothers have been treated prenatally due to depression of antibody levels (Pinon et al., 1996).

In France, infected infants are treated with pyrimethamine (3 mg/kg/3 days) and sulphadiazine (75 mg/kg/day for 3 weeks), followed by spiramycin (0.375×10^6 units/kg/day) for 5 weeks, followed by pyrimethamine (6 mg/kg/10 days) and sulfadoxine (125 mg/kg/10 days) with folinic acid to at least one year of age (Dunn et al., 1999). Duration of treatment varies. Some centres treat for up to 2 years (Fortier et al., 1997), while in Denmark treatment is for 6 months (Lebech et al., 1999). Pyrimethamine and sulphadiazine (or sulphadoxine) has been shown to be effective against the tachyzoite form of the parasite in patients with AIDS (Porter & Sande, 1992) but adverse effects are common. Although treatment of infants with disseminated infection or with lesions causing acute inflammation is justified, these drugs do not penetrate toxoplasma cysts which harbour the latent form of the parasite (bradyzoite). The benefits for infants without signs of infection or who have quiescent lesions is therefore uncertain. There are no published studies which have determined the effect of postnatal treatment compared with no treatment, or treatment of short duration vs. 1 year or more on the long-term risk of clinical signs or impairment in children with congenital toxoplasmosis (Remington et al., 1995). Information from the treatment of ocular toxoplasmosis in adults is also limited. One trial, by Rothova et al. (1993) compared treated and untreated adults with active retinochoroiditis. Treatment reduced the size of the lesion but had no effect on the risk of recurrence of ocular lesions (Rothova et al., 1993). Despite the lack of evidence of benefit, most centres treat infected children, even if they have no signs of congenital toxoplasmosis. However, 12 infected children in a recent Dutch study were not treated (Conyn-van-Spaedonck, 1991). The results of their long-term follow-up are awaited.

Treatment of infants is not without clinical costs. Blood tests are required every 3–6 weeks to monitor leucocyte counts as pyrimethamine and sulphadiazine cause bone marrow suppression. Anecdotal reports suggest that clinicians frequently have to lower drug dosages due to falling leukocyte counts, and permanent or temporary discontinuation of therapy due to adverse side effects has been reported in 10–35% of children (Guerina et al., 1994; Mombro et al., 1995). Pyrimethamine and sulphadiazine, or sulphadoxine (fansidar) have a non-specific and profound depressive effect on IgG production and whether this has any effects on childhood response to infective agents is not known. Toxic shock syndrome (Lyell's disease) is a rare, potential adverse effect of fansidar (Joss, 1992).

Harms of screening

Bader et al. (1997) estimated that, assuming a 60% reduction in the risk of congenital infection with prenatal treatment, 18 fetuses would be lost due to amniocentesis for every infected child prevented. Other costs include the unnecessary treatment or termination of uninfected or unaffected fetuses and the distress and discomfort of repeated examinations and investigations, both prenatal and postnatal. A further problem is that, even when prenatal diagnostic tests are negative, absence of congenital toxoplasmosis cannot be confirmed until the child is 12 months old (Lebech et al., 1996). Finally, children with confirmed congenital toxoplasmosis, most of whom are asymptomatic, are labelled as at risk of sudden blindness, or even mental impairment, throughout childhood and adolescence.

Crude estimates of the cost of monthly serological testing in France for 780 000 pregnant women were approximately £32 million in France at 1992 prices (Veron & Petithory, 1993). This compares with a cost of £3 million to screen a similar number according to the Danish programme, which involves testing of neonatal blood spot samples for toxoplasma IgM (E. Petersen, personal communication).

The benefits, in terms of costs due to disability that may be prevented by early treatment, are uncertain.

Primary prevention

There is general consensus that women should be provided with information about how to avoid toxoplasma infection before or early in pregnancy. However, the quality of information given is variable and it is not known whether giving health information to pregnant women has any effect on the risk of toxoplasma infection (Newton & Hall, 1995). In a French study, only 17% of women who knew they were susceptible and had received health information reported taking any action to avoid infection (Wallon et al., 1994). One study showed a small change in the incidence of infection over time, when health information was given, but this effect cannot be separated from random chance or secular trends (Foulon et al., 1988).

Typically women are advised to cook meat thoroughly, avoid contact with cat faeces, wash their hands after touching soil, wash vegetables thoroughly and avoid cured meat products (Buffolano et al., 1996; Ho-Yen et al., 1995). A recent study in six European centres identified undercooked meat and cured meat products as the principal factor contributing to toxoplasma infection in pregnant women. Contact with soil contributed to a substantial minority of infections (Cook et al., 2000).

Future research

Reliable information is needed on the effect of prenatal treatment on the risks of mother-to-child transmission of toxoplasma infection and clinical signs. Clinical trials to address these questions would require the enrolment of whole countries and considerable resources. In the meantime, a longitudinal cohort study – EMSCOT (European Multicentre Study on Congenital Toxoplasmosis) – was established in 1997 to address questions of prenatal treatment effectiveness and provide reliable data on the risks of clinical sequelae in the long term. The study has recruited over 1300 mother–child pairs in 14 centres in seven European countries. Analyses will compare the effect of the varying delay between maternal seroconversion and prenatal treatment inherent in different screening schedules on the risk of mother to child transmission, clinical signs and neurodevelopmental outcomes in the long term. Unfortunately, EMSCOT will not be able to address the important question of the effect of postnatal treatment on long-term symptoms and signs, particularly in infants without signs at birth. This question can only be adequately addressed by a large multicentre trial of postnatal treatment.

REFERENCES

Ades, A. E. & Nokes, D. J. (1993). Modeling age- and time-specific incidence from sero-prevalence: toxoplasmosis, *Am. J. Epidemiol.*, **137**, 1022–34.

Allain, J. P., Palmer, C. R. & Pearson, G. (1998). Epidemiological study of latent and recent infection by *Toxoplasma gondii* in pregnant women from a regional population in the UK *J. Infect.*, **36**, 189–96.

Altintas, N., Kuman, H. A., Akisu, C., Aksoy, U. & Atambay, M. (1997). Toxoplasmosis in last four years in Aegean region, Turkey. *J. Egypt. Soc. Parasitol,* **27**, 439–43.

Ancelle, T., Goulet, V., Tirard-Fleury, V., Baril, L., Mazaubrun, C. du, Thulliez, P., Wcislo, M. & Carme, B. (1996). La Toxoplasmose chez la femme enceinte en France en 1995. Resultats d'une enquete nationale perinatale. *Bull. Epidemiol. Hebdomadiare,* **51**, 227–9.

Anonymous (1990). Antenatal screening for toxoplasmosis in the UK. *Lancet,* **336**, 346–8.

Ashrafunnessa, Khatun, S., Islam, M. N. & Huq, T. (1998). Seroprevalence of toxoplasma antibodies among the antenatal population in Bangladesh. *J. Obstet. Gynaecol. Res.,* **24**, 115–9.

Aspock, H. & Pollak, A. (1992). Prevention of prenatal toxoplasmosis by serological screening of pregnant women in Austria. *Scand. J. Infect. Dis. Suppl.,* **84**, 32–7.

Bader, T. J., Macones, G. A. & Asch, D. A. (1997). Prenatal screening for toxoplasmosis. *Obstet. Gynecol.,* **90**, 457–64.

Berger, R., Merkel, S. & Rudin, C. (1995). [Toxoplasmosis and pregnancy – findings from umbilical cord blood screening in 30,000 newborn infants]. *Schweiz. Med. Wochenschr.,* **125**, 1168–73.

Berrebi, A., Kobuch, W. E., Bessieres, M. H., Bloom, M. C., Rolland, M., Sarramon, M. F., Roques, C. & Fournie, A. (1994). Termination of pregnancy for maternal toxoplasmosis. *Lancet,* **344**, 36–9.

Bornand, J. E. & Piguet, J. D. (1991). [Toxoplasma infestation: prevalence, risk of congenital infection and development in Geneva from 1973 to 1987]. *Schweiz. Med. Wochenschr.,* **121**, 21–9.

Buffolano, W., Del, Pezzo. M., Avagliano, G. & Di, Costanzo, P. (1993). Prevalenza degli anticorpi anti-Toxoplasma nelle donne campane in eta fertile. *Microbiol. Med.* **8**, 189–91.

Buffolano, W., Sagliocca, L., Fratta, D., Tozzi, A., Cardone, A. & Binki, N. (1994). Prenatal toxoplasmosis screening in Campania region, Italy. *Ital. J. Gynaecol. Obstet.,* **6**, 70–4.

Buffolano, W., Gilbert, R. E., Holland, F. J., Fratta, D., Palumbo, F. & Ades, A. E. (1996). Risk factors for recent toxoplasma infection in pregnant women in Naples. *Epidemiol. Infect.,* **116**, 347–51.

Conyn-van-Spaedonck, M. A. E. (1991). Prevention of congenital toxoplasmosis in the Netherlands. (Thesis). National Institute of Public Health and Environmental Protection [Netherlands].

Cook, A. J. C., Gilbert, R. E., Buffolano, W., Zufferey, J., Petersen, E., Jenum, P. A., Foulon, W., Semprini, A. E. & Dunn, D. T. on behalf of the European Rsearch Network on Congenital Toxoplasmosis (2000). Sources of toxoplasma infection in pregnant women: a European multicentre case-control study. *Br. Med. J.* (in press).

Couvreur, J., Thulliez, P., Daffos, F., Aufrant, C., Bompard, Y., Gesquiere, A. & Desmonts, G. (1993). In utero treatment of toxoplasmic fetopathy with the combination pyrimethamine-sulfadiazine. *Fetal Diagn. Ther.*, **8**, 45–50.

Decavalas, G., Papapetropoulou, M., Giannoulaki, E., Tzigounis, V. & Kondakis, X. G. (1990). Prevalence of *Toxoplasma gondii* antibodies in gravidas and recently aborted women and study of risk factors, *Eur. J. Epidemiol.*, **6**, 223–6.

Desmonts, G. & Couvreur, J. (1984). [Congenital toxoplasmosis. Prospective study of the outcome of pregnancy in 542 women with toxoplasmosis acquired during pregnancy]. *Ann. Pediatr. Paris*, **31**, 805–9.

Desmonts, G., Couvreur. J. & Thulliez, P. (1990). [Congenital toxoplasmosis. Five cases of mother-to-child transmission of pre-pregnancy infection]. *Presse Med.*, **19**, 1445–9.

Dunn, D., Wallon, M., Peyron, F., Petersen, E., Peckham, C. S. & Gilbert, R. E. (1999). Mother to child transmission of toxoplasmosis: risk estimates for clinical counselling. *Lancet*, **353**, 1829–33.

Eskild, A., Oxman, A., Magnus, P., Bjorndal, A. & Bakketeig, L. S. (1996). Screening for toxoplasmosis in pregnancy: what is the evidence of reducing a health problem? *J. Med. Screen.*, **3**, 188–94.

Fortier, B., Coignard Chatain, C., Dao, A., Rouland, V., Valat, A. S., Vinatier, D. & Lebrun, T. (1997). [Study of developing clinical outbreak and serological rebounds in children with congenital toxoplasmosis and follow-up during the first 2 years of life]. *Arch. Pediatr.*, **4**, 940–6.

Foulon, W., Naessens, A., Lauwers, S., de Meuter, F. & Amy, J. J. (1988). Impact of primary prevention on the incidence of toxoplasmosis during pregnancy. *Obstet. Gynecol.*, **72**, 363–6.

Foulon, W., Naessens, A. & Derde, M. P. (1994). Evaluation of the possibilities for preventing congenital toxoplasmosis. *Am. J. Perinatol.*, **11**, 57–62.

Foulon, W., Villena, I., Stray-Pedersen, B., Decoster, A., Lappalainen, M., Pinon, J-M., Jenum, P. A., Hedman, K. & Naessens, A. (1999). Treatment of toxoplasmosis during pregnancy: a multicentre study of impact on fetal transmission and children's sequelae at age 1 year. *Am. J. Obstet. Gynecol.*, **180**, 410–15.

Gilbert, R. E., & Stanford, M. R. (2000). Is ocular toxoplasmosis caused by prenatal or postnatal infection? *Br. J. Ophthalmol.*, **84**, 224–6.

Gilbert, R. E., Tookey, P. A., Cubitt, W. D., Ades, A. E., Masters, J. & Peckham, C. S. (1993). Prevalence of toxoplasma IgG among pregnant women in west London according to country of birth and ethnic group, *Br. Med. J.*, **306**, 185.

Gilbert, R. E., Dunn, D., Lightman, S., Murray, P. I., Pavesio, C., Gormley, P., Masters, J., Parker, S. P. & Stanford, M. R. (1999). Incidence of symptomatic toxoplasma eye disease: aetiology and public health implications. *Epidemiol. Infect.*, **123**, 283–9.

Guerina, N. G., Hsu, H. W., Meissner, H. C., Maguire, J. H., Lynfield, R., Stechenberg, B., Abroms, I., Pasternack, M. S., Hoff, R., Eaton, R. B. et al. (1994). Neonatal serologic screening and early treatment for congenital *Toxoplasma gondii* infection. The New England Regional Toxoplasma Working Group. *N. Engl. J. Med.*, **330**, 1858–63.

Guimaraes, A. C., Kawarabayashi, M., Borges, M. M., Tolezano, J. E. & Andrade, H. F. Junior. (1993). Regional variation in toxoplasmosis seronegativity in the São Paulo metropolitan region. *Rev. Inst. Med. Trop. Sao. Paulo*, **35**, 479–83.

Guy, E. C., Pelloux, H., Lappalainen, M., Aspock, H., Hassl, A., Melby, K. K., Holberg Petersen, M., Petersen, E., Simon, J. & Ambroise Thomas, P. (1996). Interlaboratory comparison of polymerase chain reaction for the detection of *Toxoplasma gondii* DNA added to samples of amniotic fluid, *Eur. J. Clin. Microbiol. Infect. Dis.*, **15**, 836–9.

Hengst, P. (1992). Screening for toxoplasmosis in pregnant women: presentation of a screening programme in the former East Germany, and the present status in Germany, *Scand. J. Infect. Dis. Suppl.*, **84**, 38–42.

Ho-Yen, D. O. (1992a). Clinical features. In *Human Toxoplasmosis*, 1st edn, ed. D. O. Ho-Yen & A. W. L. Joss, pp. 56–78, Oxford: Oxford University Press.

Ho-Yen, D. O. (1992b). Immunocompromised patients. In *Human Toxoplasmosis*, 1st edn, ed. D. O. Ho-Yen & A. W. L. Joss, pp. 184–203, Oxford: Oxford University Press.

Ho-Yen, D. O., Dargie, L., Chatterton, J. M. W. & Petersen, E. (1995). Toxoplasma health education in Europe. *Health Educ. J.*, **54**, 415–20.

Hohlfeld, P., Daffos, F., Costa, J-M., Thulliez, P., Forestier, F. & Vidaud, M. (1994). Prenatal diagnosis of congenital toxoplasmosis with a polymerase- chain reaction test on amniotic fluid. *N. Engl. J. Med.,* **331**, 695–9.

Horion, M., Thoumsin, H., Senterre, J. & Lambotte, R. (1990). [20 years of screening for toxoplasmosis in pregnant women. The Liege experience in 20,000 pregnancies]. *Rev. Med. Liege,* **45**, 492–7.

Jacquier, P., Hohlfeld, P., Vorkauf, H. & Zuber, P. (1995). [Epidemiology of toxoplasmosis in Switzerland: national study of seroprevalence monitored in pregnant women 1990–1991]. *Schweiz. Med. Wochenschr. Suppl.,* **65**, 29S-38S.

Jeannel, D., Niel, G., Costagliola, D., Danis, M., Traore, B. M. & Gentilini, M. (1988). Epidemiology of toxoplasmosis among pregnant women in the Paris area, *Int. J. Epidemiol.,* **17**, 595–602.

Jenum, P. A., Stray Pedersen, B. & Gundersen, A. G. (1997). Improved diagnosis of primary *Toxoplasma gondii* infection in early pregnancy by determination of antitoxoplasma immunoglobulin G avidity. *J. Clin. Microbiol.,* **35**, 1972–7.

Jenum, P. A., Kapperud, G., Stray Pedersen, B., Melby, K. K., Eskild, A. & Eng, J. (1998a). Prevalence of *Toxoplasma gondii* specific immunoglobulin G antibodies among pregnant women in Norway. *Epidemiol. Infect.,* **120**, 87–92.

Jenum, P. A., Holberg Petersen, M., Melby, K. K. & Stray Pedersen, B. (1998b). Diagnosis of congenital *Toxoplasma gondii* infection by polymerase chain reaction (PCR) on amniotic fluid samples. The Norwegian experience. *APMIS,* **106**, 680–6.

Joss, A. W. L. (1992). Treatment. In *Human Toxoplasmosis*, 1st edn, ed. D. O. Ho-Yen & A. W. L. Joss, pp. 119–43. Oxford: Oxford University Press.

Koppe, J. G., Loewer Sieger, D. H. & de Roever Bonnet, H. (1986). Results of 20-year follow-up of congenital toxoplasmosis. *Lancet,* **i**, 254–6.

Lappalainen, M., Koskela, P., Koskiniemi, M., Ammala, P., Hiilesmaa, V., Teramo, K., Raivio, K. O., Remington, J. S. & Hedman, K. (1993). Toxoplasmosis acquired during pregnancy: improved serodiagnosis based on avidity of IgG. *J. Infect. Dis.,* **167**, 691–7.

Lappalainen, M., Koskiniemi, M., Hiilesmaa, V., Ammala, P., Teramo, K., Koskela, P., Lebech, M., Raivio, K. O. & Hedman, K. (1995). Outcome of children after maternal primary Toxoplasma infection during pregnancy with emphasis on avidity of specific IgG. The Study Group. *Pediatr. Infect. Dis. J.,* **14**, 354–61.

Lebech, M., Larsen, S. O. & Petersen, E. (1993). Prevalence, incidence and geographical distribution of *Toxoplasma gondii* antibodies in pregnant women in Denmark, *Scand. J.*

Infect. Dis., **25**, 751–6.

Lebech, M., Joynson, D. H., Seitz, H. M., Thulliez, P., Gilbert, R. E., Dutton, G. N., Ovlisen, B. & Petersen, E. (1996). Classification system and case definitions of *Toxoplasma gondii* infection in immunocompetent pregnant women and their congenitally infected offspring. *Eur. J. Clin. Microbiol. Infect. Dis.,* **15**, 799–805.

Lebech, M., Andersen, O., Christensen, C. N., Hertel, J., Neilsen, H. E., Peitersen, B., Rechnitzer, C., Larsen, S. O., Norgaard-Pedersen, B., Petersen, E. & Danish Congenital Toxoplasmosis Study Group. (1999). Feasibility of neonatal screening for toxoplasma infection in the absence of prenatal treatment. *Lancet,* **353**, 1834–7.

Ljungstrom, I., Gille, E., Nokes, J., Linder, E. & Forsgren, M. (1995). Seroepidemiology of *Toxoplasma gondii* among pregnant women in different parts of Sweden. *Eur. J. Epidemiol.,* **11**, 149–56.

Marty, P., Le-Fichoux, Y., Deville, A. & Forest, H. (1991). [Congenital toxoplasmosis and preconceptional maternal ganglionic toxoplasmosis (letter)]. *Presse Med.,* **20**, 387.

Mets, M. B., Holfels, E., Boyer, K. M., Swisher, C. N., Roizen, N., Stein, L., Stein, M., Hopkins, J., Withers, S., Mack, D., Luciano, R., Patel, D., Remington, J. S, Meier, P. & McLeod, R. (1996). Eye manifestations of congenital toxoplasmosis. *Am. J. Ophthalmol.,* **122**, 309–24.

Mombro, M., Perathoner, C., Leone, A., Nicocia, M., Moiraghi Ruggenini, A., Zotti, C., Lievre, M. A. & Fabris, C. (1995). Congenital toxoplasmosis: 10-year follow up. *Eur. J. Pediatr.,* **154**, 635–9.

Newton, L. H. & Hall, S. M. (1995). A survey of health education material for the primary prevention of congenital toxoplasmosis. *Commun. Dis. Rep. CDR. Rev.,* **5**, R21–7.

Nokes, D. J., Forsgren, M., Gille, E. & Ljungstrom, I. (1993). Modelling toxoplasma incidence from longitudinal seroprevalence in Stockholm, Sweden. *Parasitology,* **107**, 33–40.

Patel, D. V., Holfels, E. M., Vogel, N. P., Boyer, K. M., Mets, M. B., Swisher, C. N., Roizen, N. J., Stein, L. K., Stein, M. A., Hopkins, J., Withers, S. E., Mack, D. G., Luciano, R. A., Meier, P., Remington, J. S. & McLeod, R. L. (1996). Resolution of intracranial calcifications in infants with treated congenital toxoplasmosis. *Radiology,* **199**, 433–40.

Pinon, J. M., Chemla, C., Villena, I., Foudrinier, F., Aubert, D., Puygauthier Toubas, D., Leroux, B., Dupouy, D., Quereux, C., Talmud, M., Trenque, T., Potron, G., Pluot, M., Remy, G. & Bonhomme, A. (1996). Early neonatal diagnosis of congenital toxoplasmosis: value of comparative enzyme-linked immunofiltration assay immunological profiles and anti-*Toxoplasma gondii* immunoglobulin M (IgM) or IgA immunocapture and implications for postnatal therapeutic strategies, *J. Clin. Microbiol.,* **34**, 579–83.

Pons, J. C., Sigrand, C., Grangeot Keros, L., Frydman, R. & Thulliez, P. (1995). [Congenital toxoplasmosis: transmission to the fetus of a pre-pregnancy maternal infection]. *Presse Med.,* **24**, 179–82.

Porter, S. B. & Sande, M. A. (1992). Toxoplasmosis of the central nervous system in the acquired immunodeficiency syndrome. *N. Engl. J. Med,* **327**, 1643–8.

Pratlong, F., Boulot, P., Villena, I., Issert, E., Tamby, I., Cazenave, J. & Dedet, J. P. (1996). Antenatal diagnosis of congenital toxoplasmosis: evaluation of the biological parameters in a cohort of 286 patients. *Br. J. Obstet. Gynaecol,* **103**, 552–7.

Raeber, P. A., Biedermann, K., Just, M. & Zuber, P. (1995). [Prevention of congenital toxoplasmosis in Europe], *Schweiz. Med. Wochenschr. Suppl.,* **65**, 96S–102S.

Remington, J. S., McLeod, R. & Desmonts, G. (1995). Toxoplasma In *Infectious Disease of the Fetus and Newborn Infant*, 4th edn, ed. J. S. Remington & J. O. Klein, pp. 140–267. Philadelphia: W. B. Saunders.

Roos, T., Martius, J., Gross, U. & Schrod, L. (1993). Systematic serologic screening for toxoplasmosis in pregnancy. *Obstet. Gynecol.*, **8**, 243–50.

Rothova, A., Meenken, C., Buitenhuis, H. J., Brinkman, C. J., Baarsma, G. S., Boen Tan, T. N., de Jong, P. T., Klaassen Broekema, N., Schweitzer, C. M., Timmerman, Z. et al. (1993). Therapy for ocular toxoplasmosis. *Am. J. Ophthalmol.*, **115**, 517–23.

Schoondermark van de Ven, E., Galama, J., Camps, W., Vree, T., Russel, F., Meuwissen, J. & Melchers, W. (1994). Pharmacokinetics of spiramycin in the rhesus monkey: transplacental passage and distribution in tissue in the fetus. *Antimicrob. Agents Chemother.*, **38**, 1922–9.

Schoondermark van de Ven, E., Galama, J., Vree, T., Camps, W., Baars, I., Eskes, T., Meuwissen, J. & Melchers, W. (1995). Study of treatment of congenital *Toxoplasma gondii* infection in rhesus monkeys with pyrimethamine and sulfadiazine. *Antimicrob. Agents Chemother.*, **39**, 137–44.

Sulzer, A. J., Franco, E. L., Takafuji, E., Benenson, M., Walls, K. W. & Greenup, R. L. (1986). An oocyst-transmitted outbreak of toxoplasmosis: patterns of immunoglobulin G and M over one year. *Am. J. Trop. Med. Hyg.*, **35**, 290–6.

Sun, R. G., Liu, Z. L. & Wang, D. C. (1995). [The prevalence of Toxoplasma infection among pregnant women and their newborn infants in Chengdu]. *Chung. Hua. Liu. Hsing. Ping. Hsueh. Tsa. Chih*, **16**, 98–100.

Tabor, A., Madsen, M., Obel, E., Philip, J., Bank, J. & Norgaard-Pedersen, B. (1986). Randomised controlled trial of genetic amniocentesis in 4606 low risk women. *Lancet*, **i**, 1287–93.

Tess, B. H., Rodrigues, L. C., Newell, M. L., Dunn, D. T. & Lago, T. D. (1998). Breastfeeding, genetic, obstetric and other risk factors associated with mother-to-child transmission of HIV-1 in Sao Paulo State, Brazil. *AIDS*, **12**, 513–20.

Thulliez, P. (1992). Screening programme for congenital toxoplasmosis in France. *Scand. J. Infect. Dis. Suppl.*, **84**, 43–5.

Valcavi, P. P., Natali, A., Soliani, L., Montali, S., Dettori, G. & Cheezi, C. (1995). Prevalence of anti-*Toxoplasma gondii* antibodies in the population of the area of Parma (Italy). *Eur. J. Epidemiol.*, **11**, 333–7.

Veron, M. & Petithory, J-C. (1993). *Formation Continue Conventionelle des Directeurs de Laboratoires Prives d'Analyses de Biologie Medicale 1992*. Paris: Bioforma.

Wallon, M., Mallaret, M. R., Mojon, M. & Peyron, F (1994). Congenital toxoplasmosis, assessment of prevention policy. *Presse Med.*, **23**, 1467–70.

Wallon, M., Liou, C., Garner, P. & Peyron, F. (1999). Congenital toxoplasmosis: what is the evidence that treatment in pregnancy prevents congenital disease? *Br. Med. J.*, **318**, 1511–14.

Walpole, I. R., Hodgen, N. & Bower, C. (1991). Congenital toxoplasmosis: a large survey in western Australia. *Med. J. Aust.*, **154**, 720–4.

Zadik, P. M., Kudesia, G. & Siddons, A. D. (1995). Low incidence of primary infection with toxoplasma among women in Sheffield: a seroconversion study. *Br. J. Obstet. Gynaecol.*, **102**, 608–10.

Zuber, P. L., Jacquier, P., Hohlfeld, P. & Walker, A. M. (1995). Toxoplasma infection among pregnant women in Switzerland: a cross-sectional evaluation of regional and age-specific lifetime average annual incidence. *Am. J. Epidemiol.*, **141**, 659–66.

16

Neonatal sepsis

Daynia E. Ballot

Introduction

The issue of neonatal sepsis remains a vexing problem, despite great advances in neonatal care, as it is a potentially fatal condition that is difficult to diagnose. Clinical signs are vague and non-specific and there is no easily available, reliable marker of infection. If left untreated, a baby with sepsis can deteriorate rapidly and may die. As a consequence, many neonates are evaluated and treated for 'suspected sepsis' unnecessarily, with associated costs in terms of drugs, prolonged hospitalisation and parental anxiety. It is estimated that between 11 and 23 neonates are treated for each documented case of sepsis (Gerdes, 1991). In a recent study, less than 20% of neonates evaluated for suspected sepsis were subsequently confirmed to have definite or probable sepsis (Magudumana et al., 1999). Neonatal sepsis classically occurs in two distinct time periods – early (<7 days) or late (>7 days). The most typical example of this infection is group B streptococcus, with early onset infection affecting 0.1 to 0.4% of neonates and a mortality rate of 15 to 45%. Late onset, or nosocomial, infection occurs in as many as 25% of hospitalised neonates and mortality rates are between 10 and 20% (Harris, 1993). It should be noted, however, that the incidence and mortality rates of neonatal sepsis vary greatly between different geographical areas. Neonatal sepsis will be discussed in this chapter, with special emphasis on the more recent advances that have taken place in the diagnosis and management of these neonates.

Risk factors

General

Neonates presenting with infection during the first week of life were almost certainly exposed to microorganisms colonizing the maternal genital tract during the intrapartum period (Harris, 1993). The fetus is either exposed to the bacterial pathogen by ascending infection or during the passage through the birth canal. Risk factors include evidence of chorioamnionitis (e.g. maternal fever, uterine tenderness, foul smelling liquor, fetal tachycardia), premature and/or prolonged (>24 hours) rupture of membranes (ROM), maternal urinary tract infection, interference in the pregnancy and heavy colonization of the mother with virulent organisms (Harris, 1993). A recent retrospective review of 1657 women found a significant association between epidural analgaesia in labour and maternal fever, neonatal sepsis evaluation and treatment of the neonate with antibiotics. It was not clear whether the epidural caused maternal fever or was an associated risk factor (Lieberman et al., 1997). Antenatal corticosteroids significantly improve outcome in preterm infants but concern has been expressed that their use could increase the incidence of neonatal sepsis. The use of antenatal steroids is recommended, however, even in pregnancies complicated by preterm ROM (Gardner et al., 1997). The risks of nosocomial infection are related to prolonged hospital stay, interruption of normal defence mechanisms such as the integrity of the skin and mucous membranes, in-dwelling catheters and many invasive procedures.

The neonatal immune system

Neonates are particularly susceptible to infection due to the immature structure and function of most components of the immune system and should be regarded as immunocompromised patients. The newborn infant has low levels of specific antibodies, low levels of complement, and deficient T-lymphocyte activity. There are abnormalities in the number and function of neutrophils with a decreased bone marrow neutrophil storage pool (NSP) reserve and an inability to increase neutrophil production (Hill, 1991; Bracho et al., 1998). Neonatal mononuclear cells are deficient in their production of granulocyte colony stimulating factor (G–CSF) and granulocyte macrophage stimulating factor (GM–CSF), which may explain the tendency for neonates to respond to sepsis with depletion of the NSP and the development of peripheral neutropenia (Goldman et al., 1998; Bracho et al., 1998). Neonatal polymorphonuclear (PMN) function is depressed in comparison to adults, while the PMN function of preterm infants as measured by chemiluminescence and chemotactic motility is depressed in comparison to full-term infants (Usmani et al., 1991). Transplacental passage of IgG antibodies confers some degree of passive immunity on the newborn infant. Preterm infants are at increased risk of infection due to low levels of passive immunity as most of the antibody transfer occurs in the last 10 weeks of gestation (Harris, 1993). The neonate is prone to developing Gram-negative sepsis as immunologic defences against these organisms are mediated by IgM antibodies which are too large to cross the placenta (Harris, 1993).

Bacterial infection activates monocytes and macrophages that produce and secrete proinflammatory cytokines including tumour necrosis factor alpha (TNFa) and interleukin 6 (IL6). TNFa is believed to be responsible for the lethal injury and organ failure in septic shock, including that in group B streptococcal sepsis (Williams et al., 1993). IL6 acts as a hepatocyte stimulating factor and gives rise to leukocytosis, increased immature neutrophilia and the acute phase response, including the production of C reactive protein (CRP) (de Bont et al., 1994).

Likely organisms

Neonates behave as immunocompromised individuals and hence are prone to infection from organisms in the immediate environment which may be relatively non-virulent (Harris, 1993). The majority of early onset neonatal sepsis in the developed world is due to Group B streptococcus and *Escherichia coli* (Harris, 1993). A recent survey at Chris Hani Baragwanath Hospital in Soweto (H. Saloojee, 1999, personal communication) showed an incidence of neonatal sepsis (both early and late) of 37/1000 live births. Early infection (<3 days) occurred in 48% of which 21.6% were due to Group B streptococcus, 6% to *E. coli* and 23% *Staphylococcus epidermidis* (although the majority of the early *S. epidermidis* isolated was considered to be due to contamination). The remaining 52% presented after 3 days and the most common pathogens isolated were *Klebsiella* (36%,), *S. epidermidis* (26%) and *Pseudomonas aerugenosa* (23%). The *Klebsiella* was a multiresistant organism with an extended spectrum beta lactamase activity and has recently been the most common cause of nosocomial sepsis in the Johannesburg hospital neonatal unit as well.

Evaluation of a neonate with suspected sepsis

The approach to a neonate with suspected sepsis should begin with a history of risk factors as mentioned above. The clinical presentation should then be evaluated. The signs of sepsis are vague and non-specific (See Table 16.1) (Gerdes, 1991; Harris, 1993). Neonatal jaundice in an otherwise well child is not regarded as a sign of sepsis and does not warrant a sepsis evaluation (Maisels & Kring, 1992). Septic neonates with neutropenia, metabolic acidosis, increased prothrombin time and refractory septic shock have a high risk of mortality (Mathur et al., 1996).

A neonate with suspected sepsis should then be subjected to special investigations, referred to as a 'septic work up' (SWU), which generally includes a full blood count (FBC), with differential white cell count (WBC) and platelets, blood cultures and detection of C-reactive protein (CRP). Lumbar punctures should only be performed if there is strong suspicion of meningitis or if a blood culture is positive. Similarly, urine cultures (suprapubic specimens) are only carried out if there is clinical evidence to suggest underlying renal abnormalities or if the urine

Table 16.1. Signs of neonatal sepsis

Lethargy	Poor feeding
Vomiting	Abdominal distension
Respiratory distress	Hypo- or hyperthermia
Hypotonia	Apnoea
Poor perfusion	Shock
Seizures	Skin rashes – petechiae, sclerema
Jaundice	Hypotension
Tachycardia	Cyanotic spells

dipstick screening is abnormal. These special investigations are done in some neonates who, although asymptomatic, have maternal risk factors such as premature rupture of membranes. Investigations are indicated in suspected neonatal sepsis whether or not the mother received antibiotics (Heimler et al., 1995).

Cultures

The gold standard for the diagnosis of neonatal sepsis is culture of normally sterile body fluids, especially blood. However, the gold standard itself is unreliable, as only 81 to 82% of antemortem cultures were found to be positive in neonates who died of infection proven by immediate post mortem cultures and autopsy (Squire et al., 1979). In addition, a positive blood culture alone does not mean the neonate definitely had sepsis, as certain blood cultures may be contaminated.

The volume of blood sent for culture is important as microsampling is usually practised in neonates. Sending a single larger volume of blood for culture will achieve a better yield than sending several smaller volumes (Isaacman et al., 1996). A blood specimen of at least 1 ml is required to detect a low level of bacteraemia (<1 colony forming unit [cfu] per ml) (Schelonka et al., 1996). However, clinical sepsis usually occurs with >100 cfu per ml and a blood sample of 0.5 ml should yield positive results in >97% of cases (Brown et al., 1995). The final blood culture results are normally available after 72 hours of incubation by which time 98% of positive cultures will have been identified (Pichichero & Todd, 1979).

The use of surface cultures for the diagnosis of neonatal sepsis has largely disappeared because of the poor correlation between colonisation and infection. The routine use of surface cultures does not influence the incidence of infection or the duration of antibiotic therapy (Dobson et al., 1992). Urine cultures are difficult to obtain in the first 72 hours of life and have a low yield (Visser & Hall, 1979).

Lumbar puncture

The value of lumbar punctures as part of routine sepsis evaluation in the early newborn period has been questioned. The procedure itself carries certain risks including trauma, infection, clinical deterioration, hypoxaemia and epidermoid tumours; while up to 50% of samples are inadequate for evaluation (Schwerenski et al., 1991). The incidence of meningitis in the early neonatal period is low (0.25 per 1000 live births) (Wiswell et al., 1995). Furthermore, the occurrence of meningitis in asymptomatic babies with risk factors alone is almost zero (Fielkow et al., 1991) and although meningitis can occur in infants with uncomplicated respiratory distress or negative blood cultures, this is most unusual (Schwerenski et al., 1991; Weiss et al., 1991). Thus the risks of the procedure, frequent inadequate specimens and low yield do not justify the inclusion of routine lumbar punctures in the sepsis evaluation of neonates during the first week of life. It is recommended that lumbar puncture in the first week of life be limited to those neonates with suggestive symptoms or who have positive blood cultures (Fielkow et al., 1991; Weiss et al., 1991). Using this approach the diagnosis of meningitis may be delayed in a small number of infants presenting in the early neonatal period (Wiswell et al., 1995).

Markers of infection

A single rapid reliable marker of sepsis in the neonate would greatly assist in the management of babies with suspected infection. As mentioned above, blood cultures, the current gold standard, provide definitive results after 72 hours. Most babies with suspected infection are hospitalized and treated with intravenous antibiotics while awaiting blood culture results. While it is very important to commence antibiotic therapy early in a neonate with sepsis, unnecessary treatment in babies shown to be without infection on culture should be stopped as soon as possible. There are many reports of other markers of infection including the white blood cell count (WBC), increased immature to total neutrophil ratio (I/T ratio), platelet count, CRP, IL6, IL1beta, CD11b, TNFa, procalcitonin and CD14. The use of serial and multiple markers of infection (as discussed below) increases the accuracy of predicting the presence of sepsis (Ng et al., 1997).

Full blood count, including WBC, differential count and platelets

The WBC is routinely performed as part of the investigation of suspected neonatal sepsis. Leukopenia, rather than leukocytosis, is considered to be a significant sign of sepsis in the neonate. The lower limit of normal for the WBC is 1800/mm³, rising to 7200/ mm³ and then declining to 1800/ mm³ at 72 hours and beyond (Manroe et al., 1979). An increased number of immature white cells in the peripheral blood is a sensitive but not very specific marker of infection (see

Table 16.2. Predictive value of white cell parameters

Test	Sensitivity (%)	Specificity (%)	Positive predictive value (%)	Negative predictive value (%)
Neutropenia	38–96	61–92	20–77	96–99
Raised I/T ratio	90–100	50–78	11–51	99–100
Leukopenia (WBC <5000)	29	91	27	91
Platelet count < 150 000	22–38	82–99	20–60	92–93

Modified from Gerdes (1991).

Table 16.2). The immature to total white cell ratio (I/T ratio) is ≥ 0.16 at birth declining to ≤ 0.12 at 72 hours (Manroe et al., 1979). Total immature neutrophils peak at 1400 cells/mm3 at 12 hours of age. Normal white cell indices may be useful in ruling out infection. Manroe et al., (1979) found a 100% negative predictive value if the total WBC, I/T ratio and total immature neutrophil count were all normal. These results vary between different units, however, and these criteria may need to be modified according to local experience (Philip & Hewitt, 1980).

There are several problems regarding the WBC as a marker of infection. An ideal test is both sensitive (will detect all affected cases) and specific (a positive result is confined to that condition). As can be seen in Table 16.2, WBC markers are specific but not very sensitive, which means that a patient with sepsis may have normal WBC results. The WBC varies considerably even in infants without infection (Gerdes, 1991). There is interobserver variability in doing the differential white cell count. Neutropenia can occur in conditions other than infection e.g. maternal pre-eclampsia, perinatal asphyxia or intraventricular haemorrhage. There are differences in the WBC between arterial and venous specimens and the timing of venesection in the course of the disease can determine whether the WBC is normal or not (Gerdes, 1991). Thrombocytopenia may be associated with neonatal sepsis, but is not a very reliable marker of infection, with a low sensitivity and positive predictive value (See Table 16.2).

C-reactive protein

The detection of C-reactive protein (CRP) is widely used in the assessment of neonates with suspected sepsis. It is a good discriminatory marker of bacterial infection and is unaffected by perinatal conditions, such as asphyxia, prolonged ROM, jaundice and respiratory distress syndrome (Schouten van Meeteren et al., 1992). The predictability of CRP improves with time; it is most predictive if measured between 24 and 48 hours after presentation with signs of infection. Serial measurements, rather than a single estimation, are therefore recommended (Benitz et al., 1998; Messer et al., 1996; Ng et al., 1997; Pourcyrous et al., 1993). Serial CRP assessments that remain negative after 24 hours have a very good negative predictive value and may allow early discontinuation of antibiotic therapy (Ehl et al., 1997). The negative predictive value of serial CRP assessments was 99% in a recent study in Johannesburg (H. N. Bomela & D. E. Ballot, 1999, unpublished data).

Interleukin 6

IL6 obtained from cord blood has been shown to predict poor outcome in preterm infants, including sepsis, pneumonia, necrotizing enterocolitis and intraventricular haemorrhage (Weeks et al., 1997). Unfortunately, raised IL6 is not specific for sepsis, as perinatal asphyxia and periventricular leukomalacia are also associated with increased IL6 levels (Martin-Ancel et al., 1997; Yoon et al., 1996). IL6 rises rapidly after exposure to a pathogen and peaks earlier than CRP; it can therefore provide an earlier indication of the presence of infection than CRP. Serum IL6 obtained in the first 12 hours of life is both sensitive and specific for the presence of early neonatal infection (Buck et al., 1994; Messer et al., 1996). IL6 levels return to normal within 24 hours in the vast majority of neonates with sepsis (Buck et al., 1994), and serial measurements of IL6 are not warranted. The combined use of IL6 and CRP provides a more reliable indication of infection than the use of either alone (Doellner et al., 1998; Messer et al., 1996; Ng et al., 1997). Performing IL6 and CRP at the initial presentation and repeating CRP after 24 to 48 hours may allow antibiotics to be stopped before final cultures results are available (Magudumana et al., 1999; Ng et al., 1997). One limitation to the widespread use of IL6 is cost (±US $20) as compared to that of CRP (±US $2).

Other markers of infection

There are a number of other markers of infection that are discussed below. The majority of these investigations are not readily available to most laboratories and should still be regarded as experimental. Tumour necrosis factor (TNF) alpha may be useful in the early diagnosis of neonatal sepsis, especially if used in combination with IL6 or CRP (de Bont et al., 1994; Ng et al., 1997). CD11b is a beta integrin involved in neutrophil adhesion, diapedesis and phagocytosis. It is stored in primary and secondary intracellular granules in unstimulated neutrophils and levels rise rapidly after exposure to pathogens. A recent report shows that surface neutrophil CD11b is an excellent marker of early infection that correlates well with CRP, but peaks earlier (Weirich et al., 1998). CD14 levels are raised in newborns with sepsis and this increase is significantly higher in babies with Gram-negative sepsis, while TNF, CRP and IL6 levels were similar for Gram-positive and Gram-negative organisms. Thus CD14 may allow Gram-positive and Gram-negative infection to be distinguished (Blanco et al., 1996) with practical application to guiding antibiotic therapy. IL1beta levels are decreased in neonates with sepsis (Atici et al., 1996). The serum levels of IgG and its subclasses, IgM, C3 and C4, have no value in the diagnosis of neonatal sepsis (Kalayci et al., 1997). Serum procalcitonin was found to be increased in neonates with bacterial sepsis (Gendrel et al., 1996).

Management

General measures

The neonate with suspected sepsis must be given symptomatic and supportive treatment according to the basic principles of neonatal care. The baby's general condition must be stabilized. Metabolic derangement must be corrected. Anaemia, poor perfusion, and hypothermia must be treated as required with blood transfusions, intravenous fluids, inotropes and warming. Feeding intolerance is common in sepsis so the baby may need to be placed nil per os and on intravenous fluids. Exchange transfusion may be of benefit in neonates with sepsis and sclerema. A small study in India showed a reduction in mortality and significant increases in IgM, IgA and IgG in neonates treated with exchange compared to controls (Sadana et al., 1997).

Antibiotic treatment

Neonatal sepsis carries a grave prognosis, so empirical antibiotic therapy is generally started in a baby with suspected sepsis and only stopped once sepsis has been ruled out. Antibiotics are chosen according to the organisms thought to be most likely to cause the sepsis. In most instances, early infection is due to Group B streptococcus, Gram-negative organisms (especially *E. coli*) or *Listeria monocytogenes*. A combination of penicillin or ampicillin together with an aminoglycoside, will cover these organisms (Yurdakök, 1998). This antibiotic combination is beneficial as the drugs act synergistically. Ampicillin would be the antibiotic of choice rather than penicillin if listeria were prevalent. Where congenital syphilis is a significant problem and listeria is extremely uncommon (as in Southern Africa), penicillin should be the first-line antibiotic. Gentamycin may be used as the aminoglycoside in initial antibiotic therapy, netilmicin or amikacin are generally preferred in cases of nosocomial sepsis (Yurdakök, 1998). If there is a strong suspicion of meningitis, the antibiotic combination should be penicillin together with a third generation cephalosporin, as aminoglycosides do not cross the blood–brain barrier readily. The combination of two beta-lactam antibiotics is not ideal as antagonistic interactions have been demonstrated (Yurdakök, 1998). One of the drugs should be discontinued as soon as an organism has been identified.

Nosocomial sepsis should be treated with empirical antibiotic therapy appropriate to the organisms present in the neonatal unit. It is thus very important to review cultures for both the type of organisms and patterns of sensitivity in order to guide empirical antibiotic treatment. Generally these organisms would be *S. epidermidis*, *S. aureus* and Gram-negative organisms, including *Pseudomonas* and *Klebsiella*. A combination of a third-generation cephalosporin, together with an aminoglycoside or vancomycin, would be an appropriate combination. There is, however, rapid emergence of resistance to third-generation cephalosporins. For example, approximately half the Gram-negative organisms isolated in significant nosocomial infections in the Johannesburg Hospital neonatal unit during the last 3 years were resistant to cefotaxime. Of particular concern is the high rate of resistance exhibited by *Klebsiella* – 73% at Johannesburg and 85% at Chris Hani Baragwanath (H. Saloojee, 1999, personal communication). In this setting, the empirical antibiotic therapy for nosocomial sepsis is therefore piperacillin/ tazobactam together with an aminoglycoside or vancomycin. In a recent outbreak of nosocomial sepsis with the multiresistant *Klebsiella*, neonates presenting with symptoms of sepsis were commenced on a carbapenam. Teicoplanin has been shown to be safe and efficacious in preterm infants with staphylococcal sepsis. The dose used is a loading dose of 15 mg /kg intravenously followed by 8 mg/kg every 24 hours (Degraeuwe et al., 1998). Doses of the other antibiotics mentioned above are shown in Table 16.3 (adapted from NEOFAX, 1998). Note that the aminoglycosides and vancomycin require monitoring of blood levels.

Adjunctive treatment

Intravenous immune globulin (IVIG)

IVIG has been proposed as a means of both preventing and treating nosocomial infection and early onset sepsis in neonates. This proposal is attractive in theory as neonates lack adequate levels of specific antibody and are thus prone to infection. Passive immunity by means of administering IVIG would simulate that provided by transplacental passage of maternal antibodies. The prophylactic use of IVIG has been extensively evaluated. IVIG is well tolerated by neonates and has few adverse effects (Christensen et al., 1991; Kinney et al., 1991; Magny et al., 1991). However, there appears to be no overall benefit in reducing rates of neonatal sepsis (Adhikari et al., 1996; Fanaroff et al., 1994; Kinney et al., 1991; Magny et al., 1991; Weisman et al., 1994). At best, there may be marginal benefit (Lacy & Ohlson, 1995; Jenson & Pollock, 1997, 1998). In view of the expense of IVIG and lack of obvious benefit, the routine use of IVIG to prevent neonatal sepsis is not recommended (Jenson & Pollock, 1997, 1998). The lack of efficacy of IVIG appears to be related to the fact

Table 16.3. Doses of intravenous antibiotics commonly used in neonates

(a) Aminoglycosides

Postmenstrual age (weeks)	Amikacin (mg/kg/dose)	Gentamycin (mg/kg/dose)	Dosing interval (hours)
≥29	15	5	48
30 to 33	14	4.5	48
34 to 37	12	4	36
≤38	12	4	24
>1 week	12	4	12 to 24

(b) Vancomycin

Postmenstrual age (weeks)	Dose mg/kg/ dose	Dosing interval (hours)
≥29	20	24
30 to 33	20	18
34 to 37	20	12
≤38	15	8
>1 week	10	6

(c) Penicillins and cephalosporins

Postmenstrual age (weeks)	Chronological age (days)	Dosing interval (hours)
≤29	0 to 28	12
	>28	8
30 to 36	0 to 14	12
	>14	8
37 to 44	0 to 7	12
	>7	8
≥45	All	6

Source: NEOFAX (1998).

Note: higher doses recommended for meningitis and Group B streptococcal infection.

Ampicillin: 25 to 100 mg/kg/dose; cefotaxime: 50 mg/kg/dose; penicillin G: 50 000 to 100 000 IU/kg/dose; piperacillin/tazobactam 50 to 100 mg/kg/dose; carbapenems–imipenem/cilastatin: 20 to 25 mg/kg/dose, 12 hourly; meropenem: 20 mg/kg/dose, 12 hourly; meningitis: 40 mg/kg/dose, 8 hourly.

that polyvalent serum from adult donors lacks adequate antibody levels to Gram-negative and other organisms causing neonatal sepsis and hyperimmune globulin may be more effective (Magny et al., 1991).

The use of IVIG for the treatment of neonatal sepsis has been less well evaluated. IVIG stimulates release of PMN from the bone marrow NSP resulting in increased neutrophil count and ratio of immature to total neutrophil count. IVIG also stimulates complement and enhances opsonic activity (Christensen et al., 1991; Weisman et al., 1994). In a recent meta-analysis of three studies evaluating IVIG used as an adjunct to standard treatment in neonates with early onset sepsis, Jenson and Pollock (1997, 1998) found a sixfold reduction in mortality. They therefore recommend considering the use of IVIG in the treatment of neonates with sepsis in addition to standard therapies.

Myelopoetic cytokines: G–CSF, GM–CSF

Neonates respond to overwhelming sepsis with depletion of the bone marrow NSP and the development of peripheral neutropenia (Bracho et al., 1998). Theoretically, improved PMN numbers and function should enhance the outcome of neonates with sepsis. Granulocyte transfusions have been shown to improve survival in preterm infants with sepsis and neutropenia (Cairo et al., 1992). More recently, G–CSF and GM–CSF have been shown to be safe and well tolerated, to increase the absolute neutrophil count by expansion of the marrow NSP and to enhance neutrophil function (Bracho et al., 1998; Goldman et al., 1998). The use of G–CSF and GM–CSF in the prevention and treatment of neonatal sepsis is still under investigation. There are two recent reports of the use of therapeutic G–CSF which give conflicting results. The first suggests benefit in reducing the incidence of neonatal sepsis in a group of critically ill, ventilated neonates with prolonged neutropenia associated with maternal pre-eclampsia (Kocherlakota & La Gamma, 1998). The second study showed no benefit in a group of newborns with neutropenia and early-onset sepsis (Schibler et al., 1998). Sample numbers are small and larger studies are under way. A recently published large randomized controlled trial failed to show any reduction in the incidence of nosocomial infections in very low birthweight infants with the use of prophylactic GM–CSF (Cairo et al., 1999).

Prevention

The maxim that prevention is better than cure applies to neonatal sepsis. Early onset neonatal sepsis due to Group B streptococcus can be prevented by the use of intrapartum chemoprophylaxis (Committee on Infectious Disease, 1997). The use of IVIG and myelopoetic factors to prevent neonatal sepsis has been ineffective (see pp. 329–331). In a study from Malawi, cleansing the birth canal with chlorhexidine reduced early neonatal sepsis and postpartum infectious problems in the mothers (Taha et al., 1997). This is a safe, simple and cheap means to improve neonatal outcome (Hofmeyr & McIntyre, 1997). The simple measure of meticulous observation of hand-washing is the single most effective means of preventing nosocomial sepsis (Nenstiel et al., 1997). Feeding preterm neonates human milk has been shown to decrease the incidence of necrotizing enterocolitis and late onset sepsis (Schanler et al., 1999). The extensive use of prophylactic antibiotics results in increased resistance of microorganisms. In well babies born to mothers with risk factors, our approach is to do a SWU and observe the baby. If the clinical condition deteriorates, or if there is suggestion of infection on the blood results, then the baby is treated as for suspected sepsis. This approach applies whether or not the mother received antibiotics.

Conclusion

Neonatal sepsis remains a significant problem, despite many technological advances. Some new tests may aid the more rapid diagnosis of sepsis, or at least allow the duration of antibiotic therapy and hospitalization to be reduced. Many promising adjunctive therapies such as IVIG and GCSF infusions have been very disappointing. Simple measures such as cleansing the birth canal, providing intrapartum chemoprophylaxis to at-risk mothers and observing hand-washing would go a long way to reducing the incidence of infection and improving neonatal outcome.

REFERENCES

Adhikari, M., Wesley, A. G. & Fourie, P. B. (1996). Intravenous immunoglobulin prophylaxis in neonates on artificial ventilation. *S. Afr. Med. J.*, **86**, 542–5.

Atici, A., Satar, M. & Alparslan, N. (1996). Serum interleukin-1 beta in neonatal sepsis. *Acta Paediatr.*, **85**, 371–4.

Benitz, W. E., Han, M. Y., Madan, A. & Ramchandra, P. (1998). Serial serum C reactive protein levels in the diagnosis of neonatal infection. *Pediatrics*, **102**, E4.

Blanco, A., Solis, G., Arranz, E., Coto, G. D., Ramos, A. & Telleria, J. (1996). Serum levels of CD14 in neonatal sepsis by gram positive and gram negative bacteria. *Acta Paediatr.*, **85**, 728–32.

Bracho, F., Goldman, S. & Cairo, M. S. (1998). Potential uses of granulocyte colony-stimulating factor and granulocyte–macrophage colony stimulating factor in neonates. *Curr. Opin. Hematol.*, **5**, 215–20.

Buck, C., Bundschu, J., Gallati, H., Bartmann, P. & Pohlandt, F. (1994). Interleukin 6, a sensitive parameter for the early diagnosis of neonatal bacterial infection. *Pediatrics*, **93**, 54–8.

Cairo, M. S., Worcester, C. C., Rucker, R. W., Hanten, S., Amlie, R. N., Sender, L. & Hicks, D. A. (1992). Randomised trial of granulocyte transfusions versus intravenous immune globulin therapy for neonatal neutropenia and sepsis. *J. Pediatr.*, **120**, 281–5.

Cairo, M. S., Agosti, J., Ellis, R., Laver, J. J., Puppala, B., deLemos, R., Givner, L., Nesin, M., Wheeler, G., Seth, T., van de Ven, C., Fanaroff, A. & the Very Low Birthweight GM–CSF consortium (1999). A randomised double blind, placebo-controlled trial of prophylactic recombinant granulocyte–macrophage colony-stimulating factor to reduce nosocomial infections in very low birth weight neonates. *J. Pediatr.*, **134**, 64–70.

Christensen, R. D., Brown, M. S., Hall, D. C., Lassiter, H. A. & Hill, H. R. (1991). Effect on neutrophil kinetics and serum opsonic capacity of intravenous administration of immune globulin to neonates with clinical signs of early onset sepsis. *J. Pediatr.*, **118**, 606–14.

Committee on Infectious Disease and Committee on Fetus And Newborns (1997). Revised guidelines for prevention of early onset group B streptococcal infection. *Pediatrics*, **99**, 489–96.

de Bont, E. S., Martens, A., van Raan, J., Samson, G., Fetter, W. P., Okken, A., de Leij, L. H. & Kimpen, J. L. (1994). Diagnostic value of plasma levels of tumour necrosis factor alpha and interleukin 6 in newborns with sepsis. *Acta Paediat.*, **83**, 696–9.

Degraeuwe, P. L., Beuman, G. H., van Tiel, F. H., Maertzdorf, W. J. & Blanco, C. E. (1998). Use of teicoplanin in preterm neonates with staphylococcal late-onset neonatal sepsis. *Bio Neonate*, **73**, 287–94.

Dobson, S. M. R., Isaacs, D., Wilkinson, A. R. & Hope, P. L. (1992). Reduced use of surface cultures for suspected neonatal sepsis and surveillance. *Arch. Dis. Child.*, **67**, 44–7.

Doellner, H., Arntzen, K. J., Haereid, P. E., Aag, S. & Austgulen, R. (1998). Interleukin 6 concentrations in neonates evaluated for sepsis. *J. Pediatr.*, **132**, 295–9.

Ehl, S. (1997). C reactive protein and duration of antibiotic therapy in neonates. *Pediatrics*, **99**, 216–21.

Ehl, S., Gering, B., Bartmann, P., Hogel, J. & Pohlandt, F. (1997). C-reactive protein is a useful marker for guiding duration of antibiotic therapy in suspected neonatal bacterial infection. *Pediatrics*, **99**, 216–21.

Fanaroff, A. A., Korones, S. B., Wright, L. L., Wright, E. C., Poland, R. L., Bauer, C. B., Tyson, J. E., Philips, J. B. 3rd, Edwards, W., Lucey, J. F. et al. (1994). A controlled trial of intravenous immune globulin to reduce nosocomial infections in very low birth weight infants. *N. Engl. J. Med.*, **330**, 1107–13.

Fielkow, S., Reuter, S. & Gotoff, S. P. (1991). Cerebrospinal fluid examinations in symptom free infants with risk factors for infection. *J. Pediatr.*, **119**, 971–3.

Gardner, M. O., Papile, L. A. & Wright, L. L. (1997). Antenatal corticosteroids in pregnancies complicated by preterm premature rupture of membranes. *Obstet. Gynecol.*, **90**, 851–3.

Gendrel, D., Assicot, M., Raymond, J., Moulin, F., Francoual, C., Badoaul, J. & Bohoun, C. (1996). Procalcitonin as a marker for the early diagnosis of neonatal infection. *J. Pediatr.*, **128**, 570–3.

Gerdes, J. S. (1991). Clinicopathological approach to the diagnosis of neonatal sepsis. *Clin.*

Perinatol., 18, 361–81.

Goldman, S., Ellis, R., Dhar, V. & Cairo, M. S. (1998). Rationale and potential use of cytokines in the prevention and treatment of neonatal sepsis. *Clin. Perinatol.*, **25**, 699–710.

Harris, M. C. (1993). Neonatal septicaemia. In *Workbook in Practical Neonatology*, ed. R. A. Polin, M. C. Yoder & F. D. Burg, pp. 227–50. Philadelphia: W. B. Saunders.

Heimler, R., Nelin, L. D., Billman, D. O. & Sasidharan, P. (1995). Identification of sepsis in neonates following maternal antibiotic therapy. *Clin. Pediatr. (Phila.)*, **34**, 133–7.

Hill, H. (1991). Is prophylaxis of neonates with intravenous immunoglobulin beneficial? (Editorial). *Am. J. Dis. Child.*, **145**, 1229–30.

Hofmeyr, G. J. & McIntyre, J. A. (1997). Preventing perinatal infections (Editorial) *Br. Med. J.*, **315**, 199–200.

Isaacman, D. J., Karasic, R. B., Reynolds, E. A. & Kost, S. I. (1996). Effect of number of blood cultures and volume of blood on detection of bacteraemia in children. *J. Pediatr.*, **128**, 190–5.

Jenson, H. B. & Pollock, B. H. (1997). Meta-analyses of the effectiveness of intravenous immune globulin for prevention and treatment of neonatal sepsis. *Pediatrics*, **99**, E2.

Jenson, H. B. & Pollock, B. H. (1998). The role of intravenous immunoglobulin for the prevention and treatment of neonatal sepsis. *Semin. Perinatol.*, **22**, 50–63.

Kalayci, A. G., Adam, B., Yilmazar, F., Uysal, S. & Gurses, N. (1997). The value of immunoglobulin and complement levels in the early diagnosis of neonatal sepsis. *Acta Paediatr.*, **86**, 999–1002.

Kinney, J., Mundorf, L., Gleason, C., Lee, C., Townsend, T., Thibault, R., Nussbaum, A., Abby, H. & Yolken, R. (1991). Efficacy and pharmacokinetics of intravenous immunoglobulin administration to high-risk neonates. *Am. J. Dis. Child.*, **145**, 1233–8.

Kocherlakota, P. & La Gamma, E. F. (1998). Preliminary report, rhGCSF may reduce the incidence of neonatal sepsis in prolonged preeclampsia-associated neutropenia. *Pediatrics*, **102**, 1107–11.

Lacy, J. B. & Ohlsson, A. (1995). Administration of intravenous immunoglobulins for prophylaxis or treatment of infection in preterm infants, meta-analysis. *Arch. Dis. Child.*, **72**, F151–5.

Lieberman, E., Lang, J. M., Frigoletto, F. Jr, Richardson, D. K., Ringer, S. A. & Cohen, A. (1997). Epidural analgesia, intrapartum fever, and neonatal sepsis evaluation. *Pediatrics*, **99**, 415–19.

Magny, J. F., Bremard-Oury, C., Brault, D., Menguy, C., Voyer, M., Landais, P., Dehan, M. & Gabilan, J. C. (1991). Intravenous immunoglobulin therapy for the prevention of infection in high-risk premature infants, Report of a multicentre double blind trial. *Pediatrics*, **88**, 437–43.

Magudumana, M. O., Ballot, D. E., Cooper, P. A., Trusler, J., Cory, B. J., Viljoen, E. & Carter, A. C. (1999). Serial interleukin 6 measurements in the early diagnosis of neonatal sepsis. *J. Trop. Paediat.* (in press)

Maisels, J. & Kring, E. (1992). Risk of sepsis in newborns with severe hyperbilirubinaemia. *Pediatrics*, **90**, 741–3.

Manroe, B. L., Weinberg, A. G., Rosenfeld, C. R. & Browne, R.(1979). The neonatal blood count in health and disease. I: Reference values for neutrophilic cells. *J. Pediatr.*, **95**, 89.

Martin-Ancel, A., Garcia-Alix, A., Pascual-Saleedo, D., Cabanas, F., Valcarce, M. & Quero, J. (1997) Interleukin 6 in the cerebrospinal fluid after perinatal asphyxia is related to early and late neurological manifestations. *Pediatrics*, **100**, 789–94.

Mathur, N. B., Singh, A., Sharma, V. K. & Satanarayana, L. (1996). Evaluation of risk factors for fatal neonatal sepsis. *Indian Pediatr.*, **33**, 817–22.

Messer, J., Eyer, D., Donato, L., Gallati, H., Matis, J. & Simeoni, U. (1996) Evaluation of interleukin 6 and soluble receptors of tumour necrosis factor for early diagnosis of neonatal infection. *J. Pediatr.*, **129**, 574–80.

Nenstiel, R. O., White, G. L. & Aikens, T. (1997). Handwashing – a century of evidence ignored. *Clin. Rev.*, **7**, 55–8, 61–2.

NEOFAX (1998). *A Manual of Drugs Used in Neonatal Care.* 11th edn, ed. T. E. Young & O. B. Mangum. Raleigh NC: Acorn Publishing.

Ng, P. C., Cheng, S. H., Chui, K. M., Fok, T. F., Wong, M. Y., Wong, W., Wong, R. P. & Cheung, K. L. (1997). Diagnosis of late onset neonatal sepsis with cytokines, adhesion molecule and C-reactive protein in preterm very low birth weight infants. *Arch. Dis. Child. Fetal Neonatal Ed.*, **77**, F221–7.

Philip, A. G. S. & Hewitt, J. R. (1980). Early diagnosis of neonatal sepsis. *Pediatrics*, **65**, 1036–42.

Pichichero, M. E. & Todd, J. K. (1979). Detection of neonatal bacteremia. *J. Paediatr.*, **94**, 958–60.

Pourcyrous, M., Bada, H. S., Karones, S. B., Baselski, V. & Wong, S. P. (1993). Significance of serial C reactive protein responses in neonatal infection and other disorders. *Pediatrics*, **92**, 431–5.

Sadana, S., Mathur, N. B. & Thakur, A. (1997). Exchange transfusion in septic neonates with sclerema, effect on immunoglobulin and complement levels. *Indian Pediatr.*, **34**, 20–5.

Schanler, R. L., Schulman, R. J. & Lau, C. (1999). Feeding strategies for premature infants: beneficial outcomes of feeding fortified human milk versus preterm formula. *Pediatrics*, **103**, 1150–7.

Schelonka, R. L., Chai, M. K., Yoder, B. A., Hensley, D., Brockett, R. M. & Ascher, D. P. (1996). Volume of blood required to detect common neonatal pathogens. *J. Pediatr.*, **129**, 275–8.

Schibler, K. R., Osborne, K. A., Leung, L. Y., Le, T. V., Baker, S. I. & Thompson, D. D. (1998). A randomized placebo-controlled trial of granulocyte colony-stimulating factor administration to newborn infants with neuropenia and clinical signs of early onset sepsis. *Pediatrics*, **102**, 6–13.

Schouten van Meeteren, N. Y., Rietveld, A., Moolenaar, A. J. & Van Bal, F. (1992). Influence of perinatal conditions on C reactive protein production. *J. Pediatr.*, **120**, 621–4.

Schwersenski, J., Mckintyre, L. & Bauer, C. (1991). Lumbar puncture frequency and cerebrospinal fluid analysis in the neonate. *Am. J. Dis. Child.*, **145**, 54–8.

Squire, E., Favara, B. & Todd, J. (1979). Diagnosis of neonatal bacterial infection; hematologic and pathologic findings in fatal and nonfatal cases. *Pediatrics*, **64**, 60–4.

Taha, T. E., Biggar, R. J., Broadhead, R. L., Mtimavalye, L. A., Justesen, A. B., Liomba, G. N., Chiphangwi, J. D. & Miotti, P. G. (1997). Effect of cleansing the birth canal with antiseptic solution on maternal and newborn morbidity and mortality in Malawi. *Br. Med. J.*, **315**, 216–19.

Usmani, S. S., Schlessel, J. S., Sia, C. G., Kamran, S. & Orner, S. D. (1991). Polymorphonuclear leukocyte function in preterm neonates. *Pediatrics*, **87**, 675–9.

Visser, V. E. & Hall, R. T. (1979). Urine culture in the evaluation of suspected neonatal sepsis. *J. Pediatr.*, **94**, 635–8.

Weeks, J. W., Reynolds, L., Taylor, D., Lewis, J., Wan, T. & Gall, S. A. (1997). Umbilical cord blood interleukin 6 levels and neonatal morbidity. *Obstet. Gynecol.*, **90**, 815–18.

Weirich, E., Rabin, R. L., Maldonado, Y., Benitz, W., Modler, S., Herzenberg, L. A. & Herzenberg, L. A. (1998). Neutrophil CD11b expression as a marker for early onset neonatal infection. *J. Pediatr.*, **132**, 445–51.

Weisman, L. E., Stoll, B. J., Kueser, T. J., Rubio, T. T., Frank, C. G., Heiman, H. S., Subramanian, K. N., Hankins, C. T., Cruess, D. F., Hemming, V. G. et al. (1994). Intravenous immune globulin prophylaxis of late onset sepsis in premature neonates. *J. Pediatr.*, **125**, 922–30.

Weiss, M. G., Ionides, S. P. & Anderson, C. L. (1991). Meningitis in premature infants with respiratory distress: role of admission lumbar puncture. *J. Pediatr.*, **119**, 973–5.

Williams, P. A., Bohnsack, J. F., Augustine, N. H., Drummond, W. K., Rubens, C. E. & Hill, H. R. (1993). Production of tumour necrosis factor by human cells in vitro and in vivo by group B streptococci. *J. Pediatr.*, **123**, 292–300.

Wiswell, T. E., Baumgart, S., Gannon, C. M. & Spitzer, A. R. (1995). No lumbar puncture in the evaluation for early neonatal sepsis: will meningitis be missed? *Pediatrics*, **95**, 803–6.

Yurdakök, M. (1998). Antibiotic use in neonatal sepsis. *Turk. J. Pediatr.*, **40**, 17–33.

Yoon, B. H., Romero, R., Yang, S. H, Jun, J. K., Kim, I. O., Choi, J. H. & Syn, H. C. (1996). Interleukin 6 concentrations in umbilical cord plasma are elevated in neonates with white matter lesions associated with periventricular leukomalacia. *Am. J. Obstet. Gynecol.*, **174**, 1433–40.

Index